Medicaid and Devolution

⟨...⟩

Medicaid and Devolution
A View from the States

Frank J. Thompson
and
John J. DiIulio Jr.

Editors

BROOKINGS INSTITUTION PRESS
Washington, D.C.

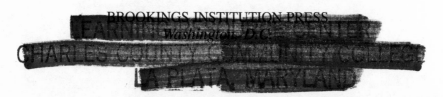

Copyright © 1998
THE BROOKINGS INSTITUTION
1775 Massachusetts Avenue, N.W., Washington, D.C. 20036

Library of Congress Cataloging-in-Publication data

Medicaid and devolution : a view from the states / [edited by] Frank J.
  Thompson and John J. DiIulio Jr.
      p.   cm.
    Includes bibliographical references and index.
    ISBN 0-8157-8450-3 (cloth : alk. paper). — ISBN 0-8157-8451-1
  (pbk. : alk. paper)
    1. Medicaid—Management. I. Thompson, Frank J. II. DiIulio, John J., Jr.
  RA412.4.M425   1998
  368.4'2'00973—dc21   97-45316
                                                                   CIP

9 8 7 6 5 4 3 2 1

The paper used in this publication meets the minimum requirements of the American National Standard for Information Sciences—Permanence of Paper for Printed
Library Materials, ANSI Z39-48-1984.

Typeset in Times Roman

Composition by Cynthia Stock
Silver Spring, Maryland

Printed by R. R. Donnelley and Sons Co.
Harrisonburg, Virginia

For Elizabeth

Foreword

Hard questions of how to provide Americans with access to health care of high quality at a reasonable cost will continue to preoccupy policymakers in the indefinite future. Medicaid, the country's primary program to provide health insurance to the needy, will be at the center of their deliberations.

Federalism, a fundamental feature of American governance, profoundly shapes Medicaid. The joint responsibility of the national and state governments for funding and implementing the program has enmeshed it in perennial debates about the appropriate division of labor, or balance of power, between levels of government in the federal system. As momentum for devolution grew in the 1990s, policymakers sought to augment the already substantial discretion states have over Medicaid. Proposals range from major block grants to more incremental, but nonetheless important, measures. What are the implications for Medicaid policymaking and implementation of shifting more power to the states? The authors in this volume provide some answers.

This book arose from a project launched in 1996 with support from the Robert Wood Johnson Foundation. Working through the Nelson A. Rockefeller Institute of Government, the public policy research arm of the State University of New York at Albany, and the Brookings Center for Public Management, a conference was held in May 1996. This conference brought together top officials from eight states and other experts to ponder the implications of devolution for the Medicaid program. The transcript resulting from this conference provided the base for subsequent research into the topic.

The editors are greatly indebted to those who made this volume possible. The project would not have gone forward without critical, timely support from the Robert Wood Johnson Foundation. They also wish to thank the conference participants (listed at the end of the volume), who gave so generously of their time and insights. Others also provided invaluable assistance. Donald Kettl offered constructive comments on an earlier draft of the book. Todd French, a graduate assistant in Albany, worked diligently and creatively to track down and analyze Medicaid information. Matt Atlas, Fred Dews, Laurel Imig, and Carole Plowfield verified references and other data in the book. Nancy Campbell and Inge Lockwood edited the manuscript; Carlotta Ribar proofread the book; and Deborah Patton constructed the index.

The views expressed in this volume are those of the authors and should not be attributed to the persons or organizations whose assistance is acknowledged or to the trustees, officers, or other staff members of the Brookings Institution.

Michael H. Armacost
President

May 1998
Washington, D.C.

Contents

1

Introduction

John J. DiIulio Jr. and Richard P. Nathan

THE 1990s have become the decade of devolution. Whatever the exact magnitude and pace of this development, few would question that political momentum exists to shift power from the national government to the states. Leaders in both political parties trumpet its importance, with some of them going so far as to call for constitutional revision to bolster the rights of the states. Policy developments also reflect this momentum. In 1995, for example, Congress approved and the president signed the Unfunded Mandates Reform Act, which limited the federal government's authority to adopt future mandates for state and local governments without paying for them. In 1996 the same Congress abolished a welfare program that had been in place since the Great Depression and approved a new block grant that gives the states appreciably greater discretion in this sphere. For its part, the Supreme Court handed down several decisions in the mid-1990s that bolstered the prerogatives of the states—among other things, making it more difficult for the federal government to justify intervention on the basis of a flexible reading of the Constitution's commerce clause. These policymakers did not appear to be out of sync with American public opinion. Survey after survey indicated that large majorities preferred that state governments rather than federal officials take the lead in a spectrum of policy arenas.[1]

Not surprisingly, the trend toward devolution has sparked heated debate about governance and policy in the United States. Just as the Founding

Fathers and subsequent generations have differed about the appropriate division of labor in the federal system, politicians, pundits, experts, and other stakeholders currently advance conflicting views on this matter. This debate is fueled by many forces—normative and empirical. For some proponents of devolution, for instance, the need to shift power to the states springs from core constitutional concerns. In this vein Governor Mike Leavitt of Utah asserts, "Never have those wielding federal power . . . been so imperious in their assertion of federal supremacy." He goes on to argue, "Because nothing less than the constitutionally guaranteed freedom of Americans to govern themselves is at stake, usurpations by federal legislators and bureaucrats of powers not delegated to them under the Constitution must be resisted with whatever tools are at hand and in whatever forums are available."[2] For their part, opponents of devolution often portray it as a distraction from the pursuit of more meaningful reform. In a recent book, for instance, John D. Donahue argues, "On balance, devolution will prove to be a detour, a disappointment, or a misstep toward engaging (the country's) fundamental problems." He calls for "debunking today's prevailing sentiment that devolution offers an easy alternative to national reform."[3]

To a considerable degree—although not completely—the devolution debate revolves around differing assessments of the governing and fiscal capacity of the states—whether they have the resources and general wherewithal to cope with the increased responsibilities that devolution would bring. It also has roots in varying assessments of the kind of policy commitments likely to emanate from state political processes as opposed to those at the federal level—whether, for example, state governments will in the aggregate be less likely to adopt policies sympathetic to the least-advantaged segments of American society. Whatever the validity of their specific assessments, disputants correctly sense that decisions about devolution may well profoundly affect who gets what from government in the years ahead.

The unfolding of this devolutionary trend—this latest chapter in the ongoing history of American federalism—can appropriately be viewed through multiple lenses; it intersects with fundamental questions of governance and public policy in myriad ways. While respecting this diversity, the perspective offered in this book rests on two pillars. First, it posits that the analysis of specific policy arenas can advance knowledge of the appropriate division of labor in the federal system. This approach does not discount the contribution that broader theories and studies of federalism can make toward understanding the implications of devolution.[4] It instead recognizes that detailed assessment, policy by policy, can yield valuable insights for those seeking to fathom and encourage a suitable balance of power between the national government and the states.

Second, this book adheres to the view that the devolution debate will be much less fruitful than it should be if it fails to consider issues of implementation and management. Although considered to be dreary and dull by the citizenry, the media, policymakers, and any number of scholars, the details of administration often make the critical difference in whether government policies succeed or fail. In this regard, devolution raises a host of important questions. Do states have the administrative capacity—highly skilled personnel, information systems, facilities, funds, authority structures, and more—to shoulder increased responsibility for federal programs? In the realm of intergovernmental management, how far exactly should the scale be tipped toward empowering state officials in their day-to-day dealings with their federal counterparts? These and countless other implementation issues must be taken into account in any serious assessment of the potential and limits of devolution.

The conviction that policy-by-policy analysis and implementation are important provides the foundation for this book's assessment of Medicaid and devolution. Medicaid is truly the colossus of intergovernmental programs in the United States. It accounts for roughly 40 percent of all federal grant monies to the states, consumes a major share of federal and state budgets, and plays a critical role in providing access to medical and long-term care for low-income Americans. No general assessment of devolution in the United States can safely proceed without considering this program.

The Medicaid Colossus

Fiscally, politically, and administratively, Medicaid—a joint federal-state program that provides health care insurance to over 35 million low-income, elderly, and disabled Americans—is the single most costly, complicated, and consequential of all intergovernmental programs. Medicaid's legislative politics, fiscal stresses, and administrative complexities are each interesting and important in their own right, and they condition each other in countless ways. But as the contributors to this volume argue, it is the administrative dimension of Medicaid—how the program's major statutory provisions governing eligibility standards are interpreted, how claims are filed and filtered, how payments are processed, how everything from pediatric care to long-term nursing care services is delivered—

that ultimately matters most. In short, how, how well, and by whom is the program implemented?

Severe Fiscal Pressures, Hard Political Limits

Between 1988 and 1995 Medicaid spending grew from about $54 billion to $157 billion, roughly $90 billion of which were federal dollars. It is widely estimated that between 1995 and 2002 total Medicaid spending will continue to grow rapidly—by between 7 and 10 percent a year, leading Medicaid spending to total well over $250 billion annually just five years from now.[5]

Some analysts view Medicaid cost escalation as an untreated symptom of health care system inflation, which for years has exceeded the general inflation rate. Others are more inclined to blame Medicaid's spending increases on its acute and long-term care expenditures on behalf of the elderly and disabled persons, who represent less than one-third of all program beneficiaries but consume about two-thirds of all program dollars. Still others emphasize a different budget-busting Medicaid demographic: about one-half of all program beneficiaries are low-income children, an eligible population that will almost certainly continue to grow over the next decade. Whatever the best explanation, no one denies that Medicaid expenditures have steadily risen and will continue to fuel fiscal stress for federal and state policymakers.

Politically, Medicaid was born alongside Medicare in 1965, but the two programs were hardly legislative twins. The idea of having the government pay the medical and hospital bills of the elderly and the poor had been discussed since the drafting of the Social Security Act in the 1930s. The talk went nowhere until the Johnson landslide in 1964 produced large Democratic majorities in Congress. Suddenly the powerful House Ways and Means Committee, which for years had prevented all manner of national health care plans from reaching the floor, had two Democrats for every one Republican, new Johnson-backed Democrats who were strongly committed to a federal role in financing health care. In short, Johnson had a ready-made majority that favored having Washington pay for part of the cost of hospital care for retired or disabled people covered by Social Security. Unexpectedly, however, the committee broadened the coverage of the plan beyond what Johnson had thought was politically possible. To the federally administered Medicare plan the committee added Medicaid, which provided funds to the states to enhance access to medical and long-term care for those on welfare or who were otherwise needy.

The 1970s and 1980s witnessed a stream of legislation that, as Frank Thompson documents in chapter 2, made significant adjustments in the original Medicaid program—some bolstering state prerogatives and others enhancing federal power. During this period no far-reaching proposals for the devolution of Medicaid received serious attention. This circumstance began to change in the late 1980s, when Medicaid expenditures began to soar. Between 1988 and 1993 Medicaid costs grew at a compound annual rate of nearly 20 percent, resulting in a growth rate of over 140 percent in five years.[6] By 1996 about half of every new dollar of state revenue was being spent on Medicaid, and projected federal spending on the program was being counted in the tens of billions of dollars per year as far as the budgetary eye could see. In the meantime the number of citizens with no health insurance grew.

On taking office, President Clinton responded to the simmering problems of Medicaid by pursuing a mix of centralizing and devolutionary initiatives. His comprehensive health reform plan of 1993 would have radically altered and, in many respects, replaced Medicaid. Although calling on states to play a major role, his plan represented an effort to shift greater responsibility for health insurance to the central government. Simultaneously, however, the Clinton administration proved much more willing than its predecessors to grant states comprehensive waivers to reform their Medicaid programs.

In 1995 sweeping Medicaid reform was part of the "devolution revolution" espoused by many key lawmakers in the Republican-led 104th Congress. During March 1995 total cuts up to $500 billion in Medicaid and Medicare spending were proposed in the House. In February 1996 the National Governors' Association (NGA) adopted a devolution-spirited bipartisan resolution on Medicaid. As summarized by then NGA chairman Governor Tommy Thompson of Wisconsin, the "challenge for the nation, and governors as the stewards of this program, is to redesign Medicaid so that health care costs are more effectively contained and those that truly need health care coverage continue to gain access to that care while giving states the needed flexibility to maximize the use of these limited health care dollars to most effectively meet the needs of low income individuals."[7] Responding to the exhortations of Thompson and many others, Congress took a major step toward devolution by transforming Medicaid into a block grant called Medigrant. President Clinton, however, concluded that the measure went too far and vetoed it. By 1997 more incremental proposals for devolution had displaced discussions of a Medicaid block grant. Several of these proposals to enhance state discretion found their way into the Balanced Budget Act of 1997.

After three decades of incremental program changes, some initiated by the federal government, others catalyzed in the states, Medicaid is today, as James Tallon and Lawrence Brown observe in chapter 7, "replete with paradox. It is a federal 'entitlement' that gives states wide discretion on many substantive matters of policy; a 'poor people's program' that covers little more than half of those whose incomes fall below 100 percent of the federal poverty level; . . . a venture in 'welfare medicine' whose benefit package equals or exceeds that found in many private health insurance plans."

Fifty Administrative Possibilities, and More

Medicaid is an intergovernmental program that varies so much from one state to the next that it makes considerable sense to see it as fifty different programs (more if one includes the District of Columbia and U.S. territories). These programs are tethered in varying degrees to federal funding, rules, and regulations, each struggling with a critical set of political, fiscal, and—above all—administrative challenges. Even the mantra of "fifty states, fifty programs" fails to do justice to Medicaid's diversity. In a sense Medicaid in each state consists of two programs: one that provides access to medical care mostly for mothers and children and another that provides access to long-term care mostly for the elderly and the disabled. In this latter capacity Medicaid serves as a safety net for many middle-class Americans who in their later years become infirm and impoverished (at times, but not frequently, through decisions to transfer their assets to others) or who have children with acute disabilities.

In part because of this, those components of Medicaid focused on long-term care enjoy certain political advantages that other programs for the poor often lack. In addition to support from advocates for the elderly and disabled, health care providers—especially nursing home operators—back the program. As James Fossett and Joshua Wiener point out later in this book, mothers and children on Medicaid cannot usually count on as much political support as those with chronic conditions who need long-term care. This raises the question of whether devolution will unleash political dynamics within the states that tilt Medicaid still further toward meeting the interests of the elderly and disabled at the expense of needy mothers and children. The fact remains, however, that all Medicaid beneficiaries benefit to a degree from their somewhat higher status as compared to the beneficiaries of other welfare programs. Medicaid enrollees can more readily escape being stigmatized as indolent, shiftless, and generally undeserving. While Medicaid officials can count on an array of defenders, this support cannot compare with that engendered by more thoroughly middle-class entitlement programs such as Medicare.

More Medicaid Devolution?

By the late 1990s the increased White House commitment to providing states with waivers had enhanced the substantial discretion over Medicaid that states already possessed. The reelection of President Clinton in 1996 made it unlikely that a block grant proposal would resurface on the policy agenda in this century. But this does not signal an end to Medicaid devolution.

Understanding why this is so requires a clarified definition of devolution—especially since the term conjures up different images for different people. According to Webster's Dictionary, devolution refers to the "transference (as of rights, powers, property, or responsibility) to another, especially the surrender of powers to local authorities by a central government."[8] Of course, this definition begs the question of just how much transference one needs to label a development as devolution. Some might reserve the term exclusively for change of the magnitude involved in converting a categorical program to a block grant. This book, however, argues that devolution can follow a more incremental path. It suggests that ostensibly small technical changes (such as those related to provider payment and more flexible waiver processes) can have great implications for the intergovernmental balance of power—for the ability of states to shape their Medicaid programs. In this regard devolution might constructively be seen as a continuum. At the "big devolution" end would be federal government withdrawal from a policy sphere with the surrender of all responsibilities to the states. Somewhere toward the middle would be a move from categorical to block grants. At the other end of the continuum would be more incremental devolution—relatively small steps to give states more power. Of course, several small steps pursued over time can lead to big change; in this sense incrementalism can be a major force for Medicaid devolution.[9]

Given this definition, devolution seems highly likely to remain on the Medicaid policy agenda for the foreseeable future. The general forces that fuel devolution show no sign of abating. Were the Republicans to win the presidency and retain control of Congress in the year 2000, a block grant proposal similar to the one approved by the 104th Congress could well resurface. But leaving this prospect aside, the facts are that President Clinton, the NGA, and other players in the Medicaid issue network continue to propose changes that could significantly empower the states in the Medicaid arena. In this regard, the agreement on a balanced budget forged between President Clinton and Congress in August 1997 contains provisions that significantly expand state discretion over such matters as provider payment and managed care. Given the persistent pressures for devolution and the substantial leeway states already have, it is more important than ever to fathom the potential and limits of state capacity and commitment. This book seeks to contribute to that effort.

The Approach

In 1994 we edited a volume, *Making Health Reform Work: The View from the States*, that was based on a series of meetings with leading health program administrators from seven states.[10] The group initially met in Albany, New York, at the Nelson A. Rockefeller Institute of Government in 1993, when the consideration of President Clinton's national health reform plan was in high gear. A follow-up seminar in May 1996, jointly sponsored by the Rockefeller Institute and the Brookings Institution and funded by the Robert Wood Johnson Foundation, brought together another group of state officials and policy experts (see Conference Participants). This conference, at which eight states were represented—Alabama, Colorado, Florida, Michigan, Minnesota, New York, Washington, and Wisconsin— focused on the implications of devolution for Medicaid.

The transcript from the second meeting became a primary reference for the authors of this volume. The conference sought to foster a dialogue, to create a two-sided learning experience for both practitioners and policy experts. For scholars the session presented a special opportunity: in effect to conduct comparative field research efficiently. All but one of the authors in this book attended the 1996 conference. More than any other single factor, the conference shaped the topics covered and the arguments developed in this book. Subsequently, the authors supplemented insights gleaned from the session with exhaustive reviews of primary and secondary documents as well as continued conversations with key Medicaid players.

In chapter 2, Frank Thompson places issues of Medicaid devolution in historical perspective. He portrays devolution as a complex process that can occur with respect to five key dimensions of the Medicaid program: eligibility determination, service packages, the selection and payment of providers, program financing, and administrative structure (especially reporting requirements). Thompson's analysis of federal-state relationships with respect to each dimension challenges any notion that the history of Medicaid represents a steady march toward greater centralization. Instead, the image of federalism that emerges is one of ebb and flow—movement toward greater state discretion on some fronts and toward less on others. He also drives home a central theme of this book: that states have always enjoyed considerable leeway under Medicaid. If the program has been a source of fiscal stress for the states, it is less attributable to federal mandates than to choices that states themselves have made.

Donald Boyd's analysis of the fiscal dimensions of Medicaid in chapter 3 reinforces Thompson's point about state discretion. Reviewing a spectrum of indicators, such as Medicaid expenditures per poor person, Boyd concludes that "states have enormous flexibility, and they use it." He raises the most fundamental of questions—"With all this flexibility, who needs devolution?"—and ultimately concludes that fiscal forces will continue to galvanize pressures to devolve more responsibility to the states. Boyd analyzes the factors that have caused Medicaid to be a source of fiscal stress in the past and why these fiscal pressures have recently moderated. He also examines a factor that makes major devolution such a complex political task: crafting the formula that determines federal and state shares of the program's costs and how funds get distributed among the states. Critics have pointed to the limits of the current formula as a device for targeting Medicaid monies to the neediest states. But Boyd shows how proposals to improve this allocation mechanism, in several instances, go well beyond the current information capacity of the federal government. Boyd's analysis also cuts through the incredibly dense thicket of fifty state programs to present a glimpse of the entire Medicaid program. Offering a typology of states based on two critical variables—their Medicaid enrollment as a percentage of citizens in poverty and their expenditures per enrollee—Boyd sheds some light on the degree to which various states are committed to the program and have the fiscal capacity to support it.

The devolution debate is, of course, about more than money. It also involves what states propose to do with their enhanced discretion to bolster the efficiency and effectiveness of Medicaid. In this regard, managed care has been a particularly conspicuous byproduct of devolution. But, as Fossett reveals in chapter 4, the race to managed care is occurring with widely varying degrees of political determination and administrative skill from one state to the next. The safest prediction about how that race will end is that most states will "underinvest in the management capacity required to realize the potential improvements in access and quality that managed care represents." Managed care works best when applied to the least-expensive enrollees in the Medicaid program: women and children seeking preventive and acute medical care. Limits to state administrative capacity and various political obstacles make it much more difficult to apply managed care to the enrollees who consume the lion's share of the Medicaid budget: the disabled and aged institutional populations. If the barriers to placing these recipients in managed care cannot be surmounted, managed care's ability to produce significant savings for the states will be limited. For this and other reasons, Fossett predicts that, contrary to many expectations, significant new strides toward devolution may well reduce momentum toward enrolling greater numbers of Medicaid beneficiaries in managed care.

The movement toward managed care noted by Fossett, as well as the prospect that states will acquire still more flexibility to select providers and determine their payment rates, has significant implications for those safety net providers that have traditionally done so much to deliver services to Medicaid enrollees and other disadvantaged individuals. As Michael Sparer notes in chapter 5, this safety net has primarily consisted of public hospitals, academic medical centers, community health centers, public health clinics, and community-based specialty clinics. Will devolution erode the capacity of these institutions? Will any such decline be offset by the willingness of other providers to offer medical services to Medicaid enrollees? Sparer concludes that in a devolutionary era "Safety net providers are not only likely to receive less reimbursement for each Medicaid beneficiary, but also to have fewer of these publicly insured patients." Unless states adopt aggressive safety net protection plans (and Sparer is skeptical that most will), "the poor and the uninsured will have a harder time obtaining care." Sparer's chapter also highlights a more general issue concerning devolution and governance: since state governments themselves directly provide very few health care services, sustaining and building their capacity in an era of devolution compose only one small piece of the implementation puzzle. Preserving and buttressing the capacity of the third parties that deliver services to Medicaid enrollees may well be more important.

The chapters by Fossett and Sparer focus primarily on issues of getting services delivered to the great majority of Medicaid enrollees: mothers and children. But as Wiener reminds us in chapter 6, the bulk of Medicaid dollars goes to long-term care for the disabled and elderly. Wiener, like Boyd, documents the great variation in state approaches to this segment of the Medicaid population. He credits states with developing many innovative approaches and notes the special flexibility they have in devising ways to provide home- and community-based care to the elderly and disabled (as distinct from services provided in nursing homes). Wiener also considers the potential and limits of a range of alternatives for reforming Medicaid's approach to dealing with this segment of its clientele. Like Fossett, he expresses skepticism that managed care provides ready answers for improving the efficiency and effectiveness of Medicaid in serving the elderly and disabled. He also points to the perennial problem of unanticipated consequences in the pursuit of reform. For instance, expanded home- and community-based services tend to increase Medicaid costs to the states rather than reduce them as many reformers predicted. Wiener also sounds a cautionary note about major steps toward additional devolution. "Current national standards regarding nursing home reimbursement are clearly not working as intended," he writes, "but complete repeal could open the way for inadequate reimbursement and quality problems in an industry that has been plagued by more than its share of substandard providers."

Chapters 7 and 8 place issues of devolution, state capacity, and state commitment in broad perspective. In the former chapter, Tallon and Brown review the implications of radical (major block grants) and restrained (more incremental) devolution. They argue that radical devolution could well bring cuts in eligibility and service packages along with reduced payment to providers—developments that create "justified anxiety" about the wisdom of this approach. They urge consideration of three state-based approaches that they think would be less likely to have deleterious consequences. One such approach, modeled on an initiative attempted in the state of Washington, seeks to dissolve the stark categorical definitions that make Medicaid an all-or-nothing proposition. Instead it seeks to expand insurance coverage to many of the working poor not now eligible through subsidies or premiums linked to a sliding income-based scale. The second approach advanced by Tallon and Brown is the public health model whereby state and local governments would play a more significant role in delivering health care, not just insuring people. A third approach would be to move toward a system of broad coverage like the one in Canada. In this model the states would continue to possess vast discretion, but the central government would impose certain basic mandates (such as universal coverage). Tallon and Brown indicate, however, that political dynamics make major movement toward any of the three approaches unlikely in the foreseeable future. Hence they suggest the appropriateness of a restrained devolution that would lead to the preservation of a grant system "devised precisely to accommodate a measure of purposive national leadership to the centrifugal values of American federalism."

In chapter 8, Thompson returns to the core questions that undergird the debate about devolution: do states have the governing (especially administrative) and fiscal capacity to take on significantly enlarged Medicaid responsibilities? Faced with devolution, will their political systems yield sufficient commitment to dealing with the health care needs of the disadvantaged? Thompson notes that existing knowledge about state government capabilities and proclivities does not permit a definitive answer to either question. But he warns against ready assumptions that states in the aggregate will measure up well to the challenges of Medicaid devolution. He concludes, for example, that while some states have increased their capacity on some fronts, many have lost ground on others. Although questioning the degree to which a race-to-the-bottom dynamic would characterize the response of states to Medicaid devolution, he suggests that, overall, states would lack the commitment to compensate adequately for the reduction in federal dollars that major devolution would probably bring. These conclusions prompt Thompson to urge a more calibrated approach to devolution, one that closely resembles the restrained approach advocated by Tallon and Brown. Whatever the degree of devolution attempted, Thompson believes that policy learning will in no small measure depend on the federal government continuing to play a major role as data collector and scorekeeper. Progress will also depend on paying more attention to issues of implementation and management. In this regard, he notes that federal initiatives to provide uninsured children with more access to health care by channeling additional funds to the states could well founder on the perennial problem of American governance: inadequate attention to implementation details, especially those related to enrolling needy populations.

On balance the detailed analyses embedded in this volume present a cautionary tale about the movement toward devolution in one important policy sphere. There are few, if any, policy elixirs in American political life—and the authors suggest that major Medicaid devolution is certainly not one of them. To be sure, increasing state prerogatives with respect to many aspects of the Medicaid program may well yield better health care outcomes. But the details of the balancing act between federal and state authority matter. Appropriately pursued, greater freedom for the states could very well chart a course to constructive and lasting reform. Inappropriately imposed, it could just as easily lead to a loss of decent and dependable health coverage for millions of vulnerable low-income Americans.

Notes

1. See Roper Center for Public Opinion Research, "Devolution in the Polls," in Michael J. Malbin, ed., *Rockefeller Institute Bulletin* (Albany, N.Y.: Nelson A. Rockefeller Institute of Government, 1996), pp. 14–16; and John D. Donahue, *Disunited States* (Basic Books, 1997).

2. Mike Leavitt, "The Williamsburg Resolves," *Rockefeller Institute Bulletin*, pp. 17–18.

3. Donahue, *Disunited States*, pp. 159, 169.

4. See, for example, Paul E. Peterson, *The Price of Federalism* (Brookings, 1995); Daniel J. Elazar, "From Statism to Federalism: A Paradigm Shift," *Publius*, vol. 25 (Spring 1995), pp. 5-18; John Kincaid, "Values and Value Tradeoffs in Federalism," *Publius*, vol. 25 (Spring 1995), pp. 29–44.

5. See John Holahan and David Liska, "The Slowdown in Medicaid Spending Growth: Will It Continue?" *Health Affairs*, vol. 16 (March/April 1997), pp. 157–63.

6. See Donald Boyd in chapter 3 of this book.

7. Tommy Thompson, "The Governors on Medicaid and Welfare," *Rockefeller Institute Bulletin*, p. 31.

8. *Merriam Webster's Collegiate Dictionary*, 10th ed. (Springfield, Mass.: Merriam-Webster, 1993), p. 317.

9. Obviously some changes can be so marginal as to fall off the entire continuum of devolution.

10. John J. DiIulio Jr. and Richard P. Nathan, eds., *Making Health Reform Work: The View from the States* (Brookings, 1994).

2

The Faces of Devolution

Frank J. Thompson

As the Federal government consolidated its authority, America resumed its rank among the nations, peace returned to its frontiers, and public credit was restored. . . . Delivered from the cares that oppressed them, [Americans] easily returned to their ordinary habits. . . . When a powerful government no longer appeared to be necessary, they once more began to think it irksome.

Alexis de Tocqueville, *Democracy in America*

THE DEMISE of President Clinton's health care proposal in 1994 and the Republican takeover of Congress in 1995 radically altered the debate over health policy in the United States. For decades health care reformers envisioned the two major federal programs, Medicaid and Medicare, as way stations on the road to nationally guaranteed health insurance for all Americans. Greater centralization of policy responsibility in the federal government was assumed. To be sure, these reformers had increasingly acknowledged the possibilities of federalism. In this regard, the approaches of Canada and Germany attracted considerable attention and President Clinton's comprehensive reform package assigned important duties to the states.[1] But neither the Clinton plan nor the other major proposals left any doubt that the national government would be in the driver's seat in steering basic policy.

The triumph of the Republican party in the 1994 election both in Congress and in many statehouses signaled a retreat from the goal of an integrated national health insurance system. It promptly moved the spotlight to devolution—shifting responsibility for social programs to the states. Although a program that already afforded states substantial policy and administrative discretion, Medicaid quickly became a target. The 104th Congress moved to bolster the role of the states in providing health care to the poor by transforming Medicaid into a block grant. Although approved by Congress as part of the Balanced Budget Act of 1996, President Clinton vetoed the measure.

In doing so, however, the president offered his own version of Medicaid devolution—an action that was but the latest manifestation of his interest in providing states with more freedom to mold Medicaid. Soon after taking office, the Clinton administration began to provide states with waivers to redesign their Medicaid programs. Earlier administrations had also used this tool. Throughout the 1980s the Health Care Financing Administration (HCFA) had approved over 170 waiver requests from state Medicaid programs allowing them to launch specific initiatives such as the delivery of home- and community-based care.[2] But the scope of previous waivers paled beside that of many that the Clinton administration approved. Drawing on the demonstration authority embedded in Section 1115 of the Social Security Act, HCFA approved dramatic changes in the Medicaid programs of some states. Officials in Tennessee, for instance, gained approval of a plan that would massively restructure its Medicaid program. The new initiative, TennCare, promised to open the eligibility gates to an anticipated half million new enrollees and to place primary responsibility for service delivery in the hands of managed-care organizations that contracted with the state on a capitated, rather than fee-for-service, basis. Prior to the arrival of the Clinton administration, only Arizona had received permission to operate a Medicaid program under a comprehensive waiver. As of April 1997, fifteen additional states had received these passports to greater discretion; another ten still had their waiver requests under review, and four more had announced their intention to submit these petitions.[3]

The split decision of the 1996 election, with President Clinton in the White House and the Republicans in control of Congress, is unlikely to curtail interest in devolution. To the contrary, persistent pressures to balance the budget and cut taxes will encourage national policymakers to intensify their search for greater economy and efficiency in entitlement programs. Mingled with the widespread view that the time has come to tilt power back to the states—to make the central government smaller and less intrusive—Medicaid devolution in one form or another seems sure to remain on the policy agenda.

The enduring political interest in the devolution of Medicaid makes it important to fathom the policy and management implications of such action. Proponents of devolution typically express confidence that states can meet the challenges it will pose for them. Early in 1996, for instance, the National Governors' Association (NGA) urged federal policymakers to see them "as the stewards of the program" who should be "unburdened" from the "heavy hand of (federal) oversight."[4] But the degree to which states in fact have the capacity and commitment to use enhanced discretion to sustain or improve health care for the poor remains an open question. Even where there is a will, there may not be a way. The propensity of policymakers to neglect issues of capacity, implementation, and management could derail devolution initiatives and lead to disappointment.

This chapter sets the stage for the more specific contributions of the other authors. Two characteristics of the Medicaid backdrop seem particularly important to highlight. First, devolution needs to be understood as a complex process involving multiple program dimensions. Movement to shift more responsibility to the states could therefore assume myriad forms depending on the choices of federal policymakers with respect to each of these dimensions. Second, coming to grips with the devolution debate necessitates that we assess the degree of discretion states currently have in implementing the Medicaid program. Since its birth in 1965, has the program evolved in ways that increasingly shackled states in their dealings with it? To address these issues, we shine the spotlight on five Medicaid dimensions: beneficiaries, the scope and quality of service, provider selection and payment, finance, and general program administration (especially reporting requirements).

The Medicaid Lifeline

Medicaid devolution is a high-stakes proposition. In the most literal sense, the program extends a lifeline to millions of the poor and near-poor. As of 1994 Medicaid provided health insurance to nearly one in ten citizens under the age of sixty-five; it also assisted one in twenty among the group eligible for Medicare, those sixty-five and older. As the private sector slowly retreated from providing health insurance to its workers in the period from 1984 to 1994 (from insuring 77 percent of those under sixty-five to 71 percent), the proportion of the population covered by Medicaid slowly crept upward (from 5.6 percent in 1984). Medicaid expansion has not been sufficient to prevent the proportion of the population without any health insurance from growing to over 18 percent of those under sixty-five by 1994. But without Medicaid, this problem would surely have been much worse.[5]

Medicaid also looms very large in the fiscal life of health care providers and governments at all levels of the federal system. In 1995 government outlays for the program amounted to some $157 billion, roughly 15 percent of all national health expenditures. Barring changes in law, these outlays are projected to grow to over $300 billion by 2005. The role of Medicaid in paying the nation's bills for long-term care (both nursing home and home health care) is especially dramatic. Nearly half of all payments for such care come from the program.[6]

Any effort to adjust fiscal and institutional arrangements under the banner of devolution would therefore unleash dynamics that could conceivably have great effects on very large numbers of people. It could reshape the balance among the three core values that compete so tenaciously in the health care arena: access, quality, and cost. Most important, it could well affect the degree to which different segments of society will suffer from the five "Ds" that health care policy seeks to ameliorate: death, disease, disability, discomfort, and dissatisfaction.[7]

In considering the implications of devolution for the Medicaid lifeline, it is critical to acknowledge the complex, protean qualities of devolution. In the context of federalism, the concept implies the transfer of rights, powers, and responsibilities from the national government to the states. But this general view should not mask the fact that devolution can emerge in countless forms and in greatly varying degrees. Some reserve use of the concept for particularly momentous shifts in responsibilities such as a move from categorical programs to block grants. The position taken in this chapter is, however, that less dramatic, incremental steps toward enhancing state discretion can also qualify as devolution and have a major impact on the division of labor in the federal system.

In the case of Medicaid, devolution would be more fully present to the extent that federal policymakers enlarge states' authority to:

—Define which categories of citizens can receive Medicaid benefits;

—Specify the nature, amount, and quality of the services provided to beneficiaries;

—Determine which providers will deliver care to beneficiaries and how much they will be paid;

—Choose how much they will spend on Medicaid and the sources of funding for the program; and

—Craft an administrative structure to carry out the program—everything from designating the agency that will lead the implementation effort to forging standard operating procedures that will govern program operations to determining the program information that will be collected and transmitted to the federal government.

As this list indicates, proponents of devolution can conceivably choose to enhance state discretion on some fronts while retaining more centralized control on others. Indeed, the proposals for devolution that surfaced in 1995 and 1996, ranging from the Medigrant proposal approved by Congress to the Clinton plan to a compromise proposal offered by the NGA, selected different options from this menu. This will become evident as we review each of the five dimensions.

Beneficiaries: Federal Assertiveness Grows

How much discretion should states have to determine who is eligible for Medicaid services? In general, national policymakers have answered "quite a lot." Nonetheless, in the more than three decades since the birth of the program, the federal government has inched toward greater centralization of eligibility policy. This movement, which was almost imperceptible in the early period from 1966 through 1983, became much more obvious in the late 1980s, as the federal government ordered states to extend Medicaid benefits to new categories of their citizens.

Marginal Centralization in the Early Period (1966–83)

The initial Medicaid legislation approved in 1965 allowed states vast freedom to determine eligibility for the program. During Medicaid's early years, three core groups of beneficiaries stood front and center: (1) those deemed eligible by the states for aid to families with dependent children (AFDC); (2) the blind, disabled, and elderly poor who eventually became categorized as supplemental security income (SSI) recipients; and (3) a group known as the medically needy—individuals who possessed too much income to qualify for welfare programs but who could not afford the health care services they required. States initially possessed enormous discretion to set eligibility standards for all of these groups and varied widely in the stringency of income and asset criteria they applied to determine who made it through Medicaid's gates.

The decade following 1965 featured two developments that constrained states' freedom over eligibility policy. The first came in response to aggressiveness by some states in extending Medicaid benefits to a large percentage of their citizens. Section 1903 of the founding statute had urged states to move "in the direction of liberalizing the eligibility requirements for medical service." Some states took this exhortation quite seriously. New York State, for instance, initially adopted eligibility definitions for the medically needy that entitled about 45 percent of the state's population to Medicaid benefits. Confronted with the fiscal ramifications of these developments, Congress in 1967 passed amendments that more closely tied the family income of a medically needy individual (after deducting health care expenses) to a state's eligibility criteria for its welfare programs. This action slammed the door on states that wanted to use the medically needy category as a means to obtain federal subsidies to insure large segments of their populations. In 1972 federal policymakers sent another signal about constraining the number of recipients when it repealed the original provision that had pushed states toward more liberal eligibility standards.

A second development—the nationalization of the SSI program in 1974—also set in motion pressures that would reduce state discretion to determine Medicaid beneficiaries. In assuming responsibility for SSI, federal policymakers showed substantial deference to less-generous states by permitting them to deny Medicaid coverage to individuals who became eligible for Medicaid only as a result of the federal takeover. As of the early 1990s, twelve states continued to take advantage of this loophole to block certain SSI recipients from becoming eligible for Medicaid. On balance, however, the SSI centralization caused some erosion in state control over this path to Medicaid eligibility.

Mandates, Waivers, and Expansion (1984–94)

The division of labor between the federal government and the states during the early period kept the number of Medicaid recipients quite stable. But beginning in 1984 Congress moved increasingly to require states to cover certain categories of the poor and near-poor. These changes, combined with a major Supreme Court decision in 1990, put states under increasing pressure to provide Medicaid to greater numbers of citizens.

Congress in the 1980s passed a spate of mandates that steadily decoupled Medicaid eligibility from AFDC and SSI status. These measures allowed new categories of the poor and near-poor (including those with jobs) to qualify for Medicaid. The pattern quickly became clear. Congress would initially give states the option of covering new categories of poor women and children. Then in ensuing years it would require such coverage. In 1986, for instance, federal legislation made it easier for states to choose to insure pregnant women and children with incomes below 100 percent of poverty regardless of whether they qualified for AFDC. In 1988 Congress required coverage of pregnant women and infants who were poor. Other mandates quickly followed. Legislation in 1989 ordered state Medicaid programs to insure pregnant women and children under six up to 133 percent of poverty. In 1990 Congress directed states to phase in eligibility for Medicaid for all poor children up to age nineteen, an expansion that was to be achieved by 2002.[8]

The federal government also mandated that states extend Medicaid coverage to new groups of the elderly. These provisions sprang from a concern that out-of-pocket medical costs for low-income Medicare beneficiaries had mushroomed. The Medicare program for the elderly charges beneficiaries a monthly premium as well as various copayments and deductibles. From its inception federal officials allowed state programs to buy into Medicare, thereby covering these out-of-pocket expenses for Medicaid beneficiaries. Although many states had chosen to do so, Congress in 1988 mandated that state Medicaid programs provide buy-ins for all qualified medicare beneficiaries (QMBs) who were poor. And in 1990 Congress insisted that states eventually pay Part B Medicare premiums for elderly people with incomes up to 120 percent of poverty.

As if these pressures were not enough, a 1990 Supreme Court decision also opened the Medicaid door to new recipients. In determining eligibility under SSI, the Social Security Administration had set up a system that provided more opportunity for adults to demonstrate their disability than children. The agency's system tended to emphasize narrower, more restrictive medical criteria in evaluating disability claims by children and provided them with fewer opportunities to make the case that they were functionally impaired—that is, unable to perform gainful activity in the broader society. The approach prompted a class action suit on behalf of Brian Zebley, a child who had been denied SSI disability status. In February 1990 the Supreme Court in a seven-to-two decision sided with Zebley. Writing for the majority, Justice Blackmun emphasized that administrators must apply a "functional analysis" to children just as they did to adults. In his words:

> An inquiry into the impact of an impairment on the normal daily activities of a child of the claimant's age—speaking, walking, washing, dressing, feeding oneself, going to school, playing, etc.—is in our view, no more amorphous or unmanageable than an inquiry into the impact of an adult's impairment on his ability to perform "any other kind of substantial gainful work which exists in the national economy" (the standard applied to adults).[9]

Sullivan v. *Zebley* made it easier for children who had such difficult-to-calibrate mental problems as attention deficit disorders to become eligible for SSI and, hence, Medicaid. The states, of course, had to share the costs of serving these new beneficiaries.

Not surprisingly, the outpouring of federal mandates prompted resistance by the states. In 1989 forty-eight of the nation's governors forwarded a request to Congress asking for a moratorium on Medicaid mandates. (Only Governor Cuomo of New York explicitly declined to sign the request and one governor could not be reached or did not respond.) Then-governor Clinton of Arkansas, a leader in the NGA, complained that "the poorest states in the country are going to have to pick up the biggest tab" for the mandates. "Nobody thought about what the practical impacts are." Governors from more affluent states also joined the chorus with Governor Celeste of Ohio, claiming that the mandates had "become a handy vehicle for people who have backed away from addressing the fundamental issue of what's wrong with our health-care system."[10] States that had had more restrictive eligibility policies expressed the most alarm at the expansion. As a top official in Florida's Medicaid program put it: "And I remember our Medicaid program growing, and we thought, 'When does it end . . . ? It was like Aliens IV. . . . Every time you thought you killed it, and it was slowing down, it knocked down the door, and you ran back, and Sigourney Weaver didn't have a shot.' It was terrible."[11]

States were not, however, without some means to take the bite out of the mandates. Many proved far from aggressive in working to ensure that newly eligible groups in fact signed up for Medicaid. As of 1994, for instance, over one-quarter of all children without any health insurance, nearly 3 million, belonged to families with incomes that made them eligible for

Medicaid. Moreover, nearly half of the QMBs eligible for benefits under the new mandates had not enrolled in Medicaid as of the early 1990s.[12]

The federal assertiveness of the late 1980s had a flip side, however. If the federal government pushed the eligibility floor upward, it also provided more subsidized options for states to cover new groups of citizens. For instance, 1987 legislation allowed states to place all pregnant women and infants with incomes below 185 percent of poverty on Medicaid. Many states seized this option. By early 1994 thirty-four states had expanded the categories of pregnant women eligible for Medicaid beyond those required by federal mandates.[13] Many states also began to receive additional federal funds under Medicaid's disproportionate share hospital (DSH) program, which provided payments to hospitals and mental institutions that served large numbers of Medicaid and other low-income recipients. Moreover, the Clinton administration proved quite willing to approve 1115 demonstration waivers for states that wanted to expand Medicaid coverage to the working poor. In doing so, HCFA went so far in accepting state claims that their projects would be budget neutral (a legal requirement) that the agency came under criticism from the General Accounting Office (GAO) and Congress. Most of the waiver requests submitted by the states promised to expand benefits to some groups that had previously been ineligible for Medicaid.[14]

The mandates and the federal government's new willingness to cover people with incomes above the poverty line contributed to significant growth in the number of Medicaid recipients in the late 1980s and the early 1990s. Table 2-1 provides summary data on different categories of Medicaid recipients from 1975 to fiscal 1994. In 1975, ten years after its birth, Medicaid subsidized care for 22 million recipients. (The number actually enrolled in Medicaid is somewhat larger because some who are covered by the program do not seek service in a given year.) During the 1975–85 period, the number of Medicaid recipients declined slightly. The next decade, however, witnessed a sharp growth in recipients—a 61 percent jump from 1985 to 1994; the period from 1990 through 1994 alone saw an increase of nearly 40 percent. Over the life of the program, the mix of program recipients changed slightly, with children under age twenty-one and the disabled becoming a larger proportion of Medicaid recipients by 1994. (The disabled amounted to over 95 percent of the "blind and disabled" category in table 2-1.)[15]

The expansionist period witnessed some decline in the degree of variation in eligibility policies among states, at least as measured by the ratio of Medicaid recipients to persons in poverty. Thanks in part to the federally

Table 2-1. *Medicaid Recipients according to Basis of Eligibility,
Selected Years, 1975–94*[a]

Basis of eligibility	1975	1980	1985	1990	1994
Number of recipients (*millions*)	22.0	21.6	21.8	25.3	35.1
Eligibility basis (*percent*)					
Aged (65 and older)	16	16	14	13	12
Blind and disabled	11	14	14	15	16
Adults in families with					
dependent children	21	23	25	24	22
Children under 21	44	43	45	44	49
Other	8	7	6	4	2

Sources: National Center for Health Statistics, *Health, United States, 1995* (Government Printing Office, 1995), p. 265; Health Care Financing Administration, *Medicaid Statistics: Program and Financial Statistics, Fiscal Year 1994* (Washington: HCFA pub. no. 10129, 1996), pp. 45–46.

a. Medicaid recipients are those who use program services during a given year. Medicaid eligibles include recipients as well as others enrolled in the program who did not use services. Columns may not equal 100 percent due to rounding.

mandated eligibility expansions, the variation among the states in these ratios fell by roughly half from 1979 to 1991.[16] It needs to be underscored, however, that the variation among states remains considerable; in 1994 Medicaid recipients ranged from a high of 171 percent of the poor in Vermont to 56 percent in Nevada.[17]

Welfare Reform and Devolution Options

The Republican initiative in the 104th Congress to devolve major responsibility for the Medicaid program to the states ran headlong into President Clinton's veto. But Congress and the president did reach accord on a related devolutionary measure—welfare reform. The Personal Responsibility and Work Opportunity Reconciliation Act of 1996 had the potential to affect the numbers eligible for Medicaid in three basic ways, among others.

First, the legislation struck a blow against the *Sullivan* v. *Zebley* ruling. Vowing to eliminate "incentives for coaching children to misbehave so they can qualify for benefits," Congress placed more hurdles in the way of children seeking SSI coverage on grounds of disability. Second, the welfare bill excluded certain categories of legal immigrants or aliens residing in the United States from Medicaid coverage. Third, the bill further severed the link between Medicaid eligibility and access to other welfare programs.

With some exceptions, the law froze into place the Medicaid eligibility standards for children, pregnant women, and adult caretakers of children that were in place for AFDC recipients as of July 16, 1996. Hence families that lose their eligibility for welfare under the new law may still preserve their Medicaid benefits. Calibrating the impact of these changes on the number of Medicaid beneficiaries is difficult. This is partly because so much depends on the vigor with which administrative agencies enforce the provisions (see the discussion of enrollment processes in chapter 8). It is also because Congress may well be inclined to soften the bite of these eligibility restrictions at least over the short term. The Balanced Budget Act of 1997, for instance, restored Medicaid coverage for certain disabled legal immigrants and certain children who had been adversely affected by the welfare bill of 1996. The 1997 act also authorized a new child health block grant whereby states will have the option of insuring additional children through their Medicaid programs.[18]

How much discretion should states have to determine Medicaid eligibility? The devolution proposals that became visible in 1995 and 1996 sharply differed in their responses. The Medigrant bill approved by Congress would have given states much more discretion. It asserted that states could provide Medicaid services to residents whose family income did not exceed 275 percent of the poverty line. It removed federal mandates requiring Medicaid coverage of poor children up to the age of nineteen. It allowed states to develop definitions of disability other than those promulgated by the federal bureaucracy for SSI. In contrast, President Clinton's plan preserved the categories of eligibles specified in existing Medicaid law, but allowed states "to expand or simplify eligibility, within certain parameters." These parameters "could be specified as either within a certain percentage of the federal poverty level (for example, 150 percent), or within a certain threshold level of enrollee expansion (for example, 30 percent)."[19] In turn, the NGA sought to forge a compromise by giving states the option of covering individuals or families up to 275 percent of poverty while sustaining mandates concerning the coverage of children and pregnant women. Whether these proposals or others subsequently garner support, the critical importance of eligibility issues for the devolution debate looms large.

Services: A Mixed Picture

The devolution menu also presents federal policymakers with choices about services. How much say should states have in defining the type,

amount, and quality of health care services delivered to Medicaid beneficiaries? Many proponents of devolution want to expand state prerogatives
at least marginally. Whatever the merits of these proposals, it would miss
the mark to view them simply as a response by the states to mounting pressures from the federal government to do more. The evolution of Medicaid
presents a mixed picture with respect to federal assertiveness along this
dimension. In terms of the service package, federal policymakers have done
little more than expand state choices. Only with respect to quality assurance have national policymakers become markedly more assertive about
program implementation.

The Service Options Expand

The range of required services that states must offer under Medicaid
has not grown appreciably over the life of the program. The original Medicaid legislation required participating states to provide such basic services
as hospital inpatient and outpatient care (excluding treatment for tuberculosis or mental disease), related laboratory and x-ray services, physician
care, and skilled nursing home care. By the mid-1990s the list of required
services for Medicaid beneficiaries had modestly expanded. The Health
Care Financing Administration formally listed thirteen services that states
had to provide AFDC and SSI recipients. These included care offered by
specific providers, such as rural health clinics, federally qualified community health centers, and pediatric and family nurse practitioners. They also
included nursing facility services for individuals age twenty-one or older.[20]

Although required to provide certain services, states have from the birth
of Medicaid possessed substantial freedom to determine the amount and
duration of these mandated benefits. Many states, for instance, set limits on
the number of hospital days and physician visits they will cover in a year.

States also have had latitude to pick from a steadily growing list of
optional services that the federal government will help reimburse. The original statute itemized eight of these options, including dental care, physical
therapy, and prescription drugs. The 1980s witnessed the approval of waiver
provisions that significantly expanded the choices on the service menu.
The Omnibus Budget and Reconciliation Act of 1981 allowed states to
apply for waivers (variously called 2176 or 1915c waivers) to provide a
multitude of home- and community-based services, including homemaker,
personal care such as help with bathing and shopping, and case management. By the early 1990s, all states except Alaska and Arizona had ob-

tained waivers to provide at least some of these services.[21] Some states, such as New York, excelled at "Medicaiding" services, thereby obtaining federal matching payments to deliver care that state and local governments had previously subsidized from their own treasuries.

Comprehensive 1115 waivers also cleared the path for more flexibility in service choices. The movement toward managed care encouraged some states to remove caps on the amount and duration of service they would cover. Under the TennCare program, for instance, Tennessee policymakers lifted prior restrictions on the allowable number of inpatient days, outpatient visits, home health visits, and prescriptions.[22] In contrast, another 1115 waiver state, Oregon, curtailed access to some services in order to expand eligibility for Medicaid. Through an elaborate process that mixed public forums with such methods of decision science as cost-utility analysis and modified Delphi techniques, Oregon's Health Services Commission developed a priority list of over 700 health conditions, each of which was paired with one or more appropriate treatments. Depending on the state budget picture in a given year, policymakers choose how far down the list of diseases they will go. In 1991, for instance, the legislature approved a Medicaid budget that funded the program through line 587 on the service list. Faced with budget pressures in 1995, the legislature actively considered cutting off Medicaid funding for the twenty-five services immediately preceding number 587.[23]

States' discretion to shape their service packages has yielded considerable interstate variation. According to HCFA, the number of optional services covered by the states as of October 1995 ranged from 15 in Alabama, Arkansas, and Delaware to 33 in Wisconsin. Ten states covered fewer than 20 optional services, while four provided 30 or more; the remainder offered from 20 to 29. Among the five most populous states, California led the way with 32 options, followed by New York with 26, Florida with 24, Texas with 23, and Pennsylvania with 21.[24]

Service choices by states as well as their compliance with federal requirements have led to a pattern of budget expenditures suggested by table 2-2. Among other things, it shows that as of 1994 payments for service in nursing facilities and for inpatient hospital care consumed nearly 50 percent of all vendor payments—a smaller percentage than in 1975. Expenditures for home health services rose sharply over that period, although they still made up only 7 percent of vendor payments in 1994. The limits to the data in table 2-2 deserve emphasis. The statistics do not, for instance, take into account the substantial Medicaid expenditures for the DSH program, to Medicare, or to HMOs.[25]

Table 2-2. *Medicaid Vendor Payments by Type of Service, Selected Years, 1975–94*[a]

Service	1975	1980	1985	1990	1994
Total vendor payments (*billions*)	$12.2	$23.3	$37.5	$64.9	$108.3
Type of service (*percent*)					
General hospitals					
Inpatient	28	28	25	26	24
Outpatient	3	5	5	5	6
Inpatient mental hospitals	3	3	3	3	2
Nursing facilities	35	34	31	27	25
Mentally retarded/intermediate care facilities	3	9	13	11	8
Physician	10	8	6	6	7
Home health	1	1	3	5	7
Prescribed drugs	7	6	6	7	8
Other[b]	10	6	8	10	13

Sources: National Center for Health Statistics, *Health, United States, 1995* (Government Printing Office, 1995), p. 266; Health Care Financing Administration, *Medicaid Statistics: Program and Financial Statistics, Fiscal Year 1994* (Washington: HCFA pub. no. 10129, 1996), p. 32.

a. The data exclude DSH payments as well as payments to HMOs and Medicare.

b. Other services include dental, laboratory and radiological, family planning, early and periodic screening, and clinic.

Federal Pressures for Quality

If the evolution of Medicaid featured only a modest increase in pressure on states to provide more services, it displayed a significant trend toward greater federal assertiveness with respect to quality assurance—especially in the case of long-term care. States, of course, have traditionally been responsible for ensuring that the health care delivered within their boundaries meets acceptable standards of quality. Among other things, they license health care providers and conduct investigations of malpractice claims.

The growth of Medicare and Medicaid prompted the federal government to become more involved in quality assurance efforts. In 1972 Congress passed legislation creating professional standards review organizations (PSROs). These entities, generally private nonprofit groups of physicians, were responsible for reviewing both the necessity for and the quality of treatment delivered to beneficiaries of Medicaid, Medicare, and related federal programs. By the early 1980s a new, somewhat more empowered set of entities, called peer review organizations (PROs) had succeeded the PSROs. Federal officials required state Medicaid agencies to exclude providers from the program who failed to meet quality standards.

Aside from establishing PSROs and PROs, the federal government pursued other means to enhance quality. In the case of managed care, for instance, Congress enacted two provisions in the 1970s aimed at counteracting any tendencies for HMOs to underserve or otherwise provide poor-quality care to Medicaid clients. First, it stipulated that managed-care plans could not serve Medicaid eligibles exclusively; at least 25 percent of the plan's enrollees would have to come from other sources. This 75/25 rule aimed at preventing these plans from becoming the managed-care version of Medicaid mills. Second, Congress sought to protect Medicaid enrollees by allowing them to terminate enrollment in a health care plan with very short notice. This threat of exit by beneficiaries would presumably keep these plans on their toes, encouraging them to meet the health care needs of those on Medicaid.

The 1115 demonstration waivers granted by the Clinton administration substantially freed states from both of these provisions, and the Balanced Budget Act of 1997 formally repealed them. HCFA has therefore sought other means to promote quality, including guidelines published under the banner of a quality assurance initiative. In this regard, the agency, in cooperation with the National Committee for Quality Assurance, issued a 374-page *Medicaid HEDIS* (Health Plan Employer Data and Information Set) in December 1995. This document detailed the data that managed-care plans involved in Medicaid should keep in order to establish report cards that could be used by the states and others to assess the level of access and service quality being provided to Medicaid enrollees by the plans.[26]

Although the federal government took these and other steps to encourage states to conduct utilization reviews and monitor medical care quality, state officials continued to possess considerable discretion in this area. In contrast, federal lawmakers proved to be much more exacting in their stance toward quality in long-term care. Historically state policymakers had paid much less attention to the quality of services in nursing homes as compared to that provided by physicians and hospitals. The quality of care in these facilities varied enormously, and critics frequently complained that many nursing homes were little more than warehouses.

Responding in part to these claims, Congress in 1987 approved detailed legislation aimed at ameliorating this deficiency. The requirements for nursing facilities cover almost fifty pages of the U.S. Code and are extremely specific.[27] The law requires, for instance, that each nursing facility maintain a quality assessment and assurance committee consisting of the director of nursing services, a physician designated by the facility, and at least three other members of the facility's staff. It prescribes that the committee must meet at least quarterly to identify any quality deficiencies and develop a written plan to identify and correct them. The statute also requires each facility to conduct "a comprehensive, accurate, standardized, reproducible assessment" of each nursing home resident's functional capacity. Each of these assessments has to be completed no later than fourteen days after the admission of an individual and must be conducted or coordinated and signed by a registered professional nurse. The statute not only assigns specific roles to physicians, registered nurses, and other professional staff but also devotes considerable attention to the definition of in-service education requirements for nurse aides who work in these facilities. It mandates that states establish and maintain a registry of all individuals who had satisfactorily completed a nurse aide training and competence evaluation program.

The statute also spelled out state responsibilities for conducting regular inspections of nursing facilities. Here, as well as in other spheres, the law called on the secretary of health and human services (HHS) to look over the shoulder of states as they implemented the law. For example, it required the secretary to "review each State's procedures for scheduling and conducting such surveys to assure that the State has taken all reasonable steps to avoid giving notice of such a survey through the scheduling procedures and the conduct of the surveys themselves."[28]

In placing more pressure on states to pay attention to the quality of long-term care, federal policymakers did not stop with nursing facilities. Other legislation addressed issues of quality for those providing home and community care to disabled Medicaid beneficiaries.

Devolution and Services

Although the federal government had grown more assertive about quality issues in long-term care and slightly ratcheted up the scope of the mandated service package, the fact remains that states possess considerable discretion concerning Medicaid services. Should their discretion be expanded further? Clearly some proponents of devolution believe so. For example, the Medigrant legislation approved by Congress but vetoed by

President Clinton would have removed many of the service requirements embedded in the existing program. The proposal allowed, but did not require, states to pay "part or all of the cost" of some thirty-one categories of services. It also granted the HHS secretary the authority to include other health care treatments not specifically excluded elsewhere in the law.

Other devolution proposals stopped far short of this posture, however. Neither the Clinton plan nor the one offered by the NGA espoused appreciable changes in Medicaid's mandated service package. As for quality assurance, even the more fervent devolutionists ran into strong sentiment against major change. Hence the Medigrant legislation continued to incorporate the elaborate process-oriented provisions targeted at promoting quality care in nursing homes.

Payment to Providers: Two Different Worlds

The efficacy of efforts to provide health care to the poor hinges not only on the jockeying of the federal government and the states over eligibility and service packages but also on payment practices. Which providers should be eligible for payment? How much reimbursement should they receive and based on what methodology—capitation, fee-for-service, or some other variant? The way in which federal and state players in the Medicaid program resolve these highly technical, yet fundamentally political, questions critically affects the balance that will be achieved in the program among access, quality, and cost.

From the dawning of Medicaid in 1965, the program has espoused certain payment principles. It has affirmed that payment rates to providers should be sufficient to ensure that Medicaid enrollees have adequate access to care. It has specified that, unlike Medicare, providers would typically have to accept Medicaid reimbursement as payment in full for their services and not bill beneficiaries for additional sums. It has emphasized that Medicaid should be the payer of last resort and not cover any expenses that a private insurer is obligated to pay.

State freedom to determine Medicaid payment practices can be seen in terms of two worlds. In the case of institutional providers, principally hospitals and nursing homes, state officials have often felt shackled. In the case of ambulatory, noninstitutional care, however, they have had vast discretion to determine payment levels.

Institutions: The Boren Boomerang

The initial Medicaid legislation vaguely specified that state payments to hospitals for inpatient services needed to reflect "the reasonable cost" of delivering that care. But it left the more precise definition of what this meant to the secretary of health, education, and welfare. By the end of the 1960s, federal officials had essentially imposed the same relatively generous payment practices on state Medicaid programs that they had adopted for Medicare. Officials in many states chafed under this federal requirement, believing that it led to excessive payment to hospitals. Despite resistance by the hospital lobbies, states won a modest victory in their efforts to gain more discretion. In 1972 Congress granted the secretary of health, education, and welfare the right to authorize alternative payment systems so long as the rates states approved did not exceed those authorized under Medicare and flowed from a conscientious assessment of a hospital's "reasonable costs." By the late 1970s the federal bureaucracy had approved ten alternative payment systems, including those in states with large Medicaid programs, such as California, New York, and Michigan.[29]

From the outset the federal government had not been nearly so assertive with respect to Medicaid nursing home payment as it had been with hospitals. As a result, state payment practices came to vary enormously. Rather than adopt the Medicare model of reimbursing nursing homes on the basis of the costs these institutions incurred in providing care to particular patients, many states paid a flat rate. Some adopted capitated systems. Calculations were often simple. In Pennsylvania, for example, officials took the welfare department's projection of nursing home utilization for the coming year, determined what funds would be available, and divided by the projected number of residents. Many states used this freedom to keep payment rates at a bare-bones level. Writing at the end of the 1970s, Bruce Vladeck noted that some states "kept rates uniformly low, accelerating the development of a 'dual market' in which private and Medicaid rates diverge substantially."[30] The results of state discretion made federal policymakers increasingly uneasy. By the late 1970s they adopted provisions limiting state discretion and pushing them toward a cost-based approach to nursing home reimbursement.

The arrival of the 1980s marked a major and ironic turning point for federal-state relations over Medicaid payment. The soaring costs of institutional care had increasingly soured Washington's policymakers on the retrospective, cost-based approach for paying hospitals and long-term care facilities. They became increasingly attracted to a payment methodology grounded in uniform, prospectively determined rates for various kinds of patients. In a move to tilt power back toward the states, Congress in 1980 and 1981 approved legislation that became known as the Boren amendments, named after the senator from Oklahoma. Amendments approved in 1980 granted more latitude to states to determine payment methodologies for long-term care facilities, and the 1981 provisions sought to do the same for hospitals.

While granting the states more discretion, the Boren provisions did mandate that state officials had to "make assurances" satisfactory to the HHS secretary that the rates were "reasonable and adequate to meet the costs which must be incurred by efficiently and economically operated facilities in order to provide care and services in conformity" with state and federal laws concerning quality and access in the Medicaid program. During the 1980s the federal bureaucracy proved quite willing to accept the assurances of the states that their approaches to Medicaid payment met this test. By the early 1990s the great majority of state Medicaid programs had instituted some form of prospective payment to hospitals and nursing homes.[31]

But if Congress and HCFA moved to give states more freedom, the federal courts proved less cooperative. Soon after passage of the Boren amendments, providers began to challenge state payment levels and practices in court. Their initial forays met with limited success. Gradually, however, the providers began to score some victories. They made particular headway in persuading some courts that a statute passed after the Civil War to protect the federal rights of those living in southern states also applied to hospital and nursing home payment under Medicaid. The law (Title 42, Section 1983 of the U.S. Code) created liability for anyone who, acting on behalf of state government, infringed upon the federally guaranteed rights of an individual.

With federal lower courts adopting conflicting positions on whether this Civil War legacy extended to the Boren provisions, the Supreme Court agreed to hear a case involving a challenge to the payment practices of Virginia's Medicaid program by the state hospital association. Virginia policymakers had devised a prospective payment plan that divided hospitals into peer groups based on their size and location. The state paid for particular services under a formula based on the median cost of medical care for that peer group. The HHS secretary had approved this plan in 1982 and again in 1986. Convinced that the approved payment levels were inadequate, the Virginia Hospital Association filed suit in federal court in 1986. The association wanted the courts to issue an injunction against the plan and in the interim reimburse Medicaid providers at more generous Medicare rates. A federal appellate court sided with the hospital association, and the state of Virginia appealed to the Supreme Court. Fearing that the Supreme Court might be about to open Pandora's box, forty-five states filed an *amicus curiae* brief expressing concern that a victory by the Virginia Hospital Association would expose them to protracted litigation over rates and a dual system of review—the existing one by the HHS secretary and one implemented by the courts.

The states' arguments ultimately fell on deaf ears. In *Wilder* v. *Virginia Hospital Association*, a five-to-four majority of the Supreme Court affirmed the ruling of the lower court and underscored that medical providers do have rights to sue state Medicaid officials under Section 1983 of federal law. In doing so the court dismissed claims that the judiciary lacked the expertise to fathom the enormous complexities of determining whether payment rates provided reasonable access to beneficiaries and met the standard of adequate reimbursement for "efficiently and economically operated facilities." Writing for the majority, Justice Brennan noted: "Although some knowledge of the hospital industry might be required to evaluate a State's findings with respect to the reasonableness of its rates, such an inquiry is well within the competence of the Judiciary."[32] Hence the added discretion that the states had won in 1980 and 1981 underwent serious erosion. State officials quickly learned that proposing major changes in rate methodologies would typically be an invitation to hand-to-hand combat in the courts.

The strictures placed on states by the Boren amendments heightened their interest in managed care. States that seized the opportunity that federal waivers provided to enroll Medicaid beneficiaries in HMOs and related organizations essentially left the burden of setting institutional payment rates to these large contractors. In this way state officials greatly reduced their exposure to legal action by providers under Boren.

Congress also took some of the sting out of Boren by giving states access to new federal dollars over which they had huge discretion. Initially approved by Congress in 1981, DSH payments were supposed to provide general financial support to institutions that served large numbers of Medicaid and other low-income patients. DSH funds were little used by the states in the early 1980s. In 1987 Congress established minimum criteria for the state allocation of these funds that went into effect on July 1, 1988. In general terms, a hospital became eligible for additional payment if (1) its

Medicaid utilization rate was more than one standard deviation above the average rate for all hospitals that participated in a state's Medicaid program, and (2) its rate of utilization by low-income persons was at least 25 percent. States soon began to take advantage of DSH. From 1989 through 1992, DSH payments for acute and mental health hospitals grew from slightly more than $500 million to more than $17 billion.[33]

States possessed enormous discretion to determine which hospitals got DSH funds. Policymakers in Texas, for example, adopted a formula that favored public hospitals, especially nine state psychiatric institutions that represented less than 10 percent of all qualifying hospitals but received about 40 percent of the DSH funds in that state.[34] Other states opted for different distributions. State discretion over DSH funding was so great that some analysts saw the program more as a vehicle for general revenue sharing than as a payment system for hospitals. The degree to which DSH actually prompted hospitals to provide more uncompensated care for uninsured people remains unclear.[35] Federal legislation approved in the 1990s sought to constrain the amount of DSH funds states could pay specific facilities; it also imposed an overall cap on DSH expenditures. Even with these changes, DSH continued to be a highly valued funding pipeline for many state Medicaid programs.

The Boren provisions and DSH funding did not mean that institutions invariably got compensated at rates they considered reasonable. For instance, the American Hospital Association estimated that as of 1990 Medicaid payments to hospitals fell short of covering the costs of treating program beneficiaries in forty-seven states (Maryland, Mississippi, and New Jersey being the exceptions). The amount of the shortfall ranged from 0.1 percent in Arizona to 5.7 percent in Illinois.[36] States also varied greatly in the extent to which they pursued DSH funds to subsidize hospitals. As of 1993, for example, only 2 percent of the Medicaid funds going to acute care hospitals in Arkansas emanated from DSH funds; mental hospitals in that state received no DSH monies. In contrast, over 60 percent of the Medicaid dollars going to acute care hospitals in Louisiana were funneled through DSH funds; mental health institutions in that state got 40 percent of their Medicaid support in this way.[37]

Ambulatory Care: The Unfettered States

In contrast to the constraints placed on them in paying hospitals and long-term care facilities, the states have from the start possessed much more discretion over reimbursement to individual physicians and other providers of ambulatory care. With a few exceptions, states have ample latitude to set rates for such providers—latitude they have used to traverse widely divergent paths. To be sure, states in general have been tightfisted about these payments, thereby depressing the level of provider participation in the program. As of 1993, for example, overall Medicaid fees for physicians approximated 73 percent of what Medicare paid. But states did vary substantially. Nine paid doctors more for treating Medicaid patients than these providers received from Medicare. The ratio of Medicaid to Medicare fees ranged from a low of .38 in New York to a high of 1.79 in Alaska.[38]

Although states possess ample freedom to set these payment rates, the federal government establishes some parameters. In the case of outpatient hospital and clinic services, for instance, the national government imposes an upper bound on payment. Aggregate Medicaid payments for outpatient services by a hospital may not exceed what Medicare would have paid for furnishing comparable services. Moreover, from the early stages of the program, states were required to cover the out-of-pocket costs for Medicaid beneficiaries who also qualified for Medicare coverage. These federally determined expenses include Medicare premiums, deductibles, and co-insurance. Over the last decade the national government has also mandated certain payments to safety-net providers. For instance, in 1989 Congress required state Medicaid programs to pay federally supported community health centers and rural clinics on the basis of their reasonable costs. In other instances federal policymakers attempted to help states lower the price they paid. In the Omnibus Budget Reconciliation Act of 1990, Congress sought to reduce Medicaid's prescription drug costs by insisting that drug manufacturers give state Medicaid programs rebates for outpatient drugs purchased with the program's funds. Compared to the world of inpatient institutional care, however, state payment practices to providers of ambulatory and home care are subject to much less federal regulation.

Devolution: More Freedom to Set Payment Rates

Proponents of devolution, from those favoring major shifts of responsibility to the states to those endorsing more incremental measures, all seem to agree that states should have more leeway to determine provider payment under Medicaid. The Medigrant bill approved by Congress affirmed that, with certain modest exceptions, "nothing in this title . . . shall be construed as requiring a State . . . to provide any payments with respect to any specific health care providers or any level of payments for any services."[39] This position won the endorsement of the NGA, which had long viewed the Boren amendments as a major barrier to cost control. The association proclaimed that states "must have complete authority to set all health plan and provider reimbursement rates without interference from the federal government or threat of legal action of the provider or plan."[40] The governors also explicitly called for ending the requirement that federally qualified health centers and rural health clinics be reimbursed at 100 percent of costs. The proposal of President Clinton essentially echoed these themes. This constellation of forces resulted in the repeal of the Boren provisions as part of the balanced budget agreement approved in August 1997. In general, the new law gave states appreciably more discretion to set provider payment rates, including those for federally qualified health centers and for providers of care to Medicaid recipients who are also enrolled in Medicare.

Financing: States as Entrepreneurs

The Medicaid dance between the national government and the states also involves financing. How free should a state be to determine the amount of money that it will contribute to Medicaid from various sources within its boundaries? The basic matching formula in federal Medicaid law has remained quite stable. The law specifies that the federal government's share of a state's Medicaid costs cannot be lower than 50 percent or higher than 83 percent. Each year HCFA computes the federal medical assistance percentage via a formula that compares a given state's per capita income with the national average and provides poorer states with a higher federal matching rate. Certain special funding categories have different matches. For instance, the federal government reimburses most of a state's administrative costs at 50 percent. The law authorizes higher matching rates for certain functions and activities, such as work by the states to develop the Medicaid management information system (MMIS).

The federal government has traditionally been concerned with regulating two sources of state funding for the program. First, it has sought to protect local governments by insisting that the state government pay at least 40 percent of the nonfederal share of Medicaid program costs. By the 1990s most state governments had removed the fiscal monkey from the backs of local officials, although twenty-one states required some contribution from their localities toward the costs of Medicaid.[41]

Second, the federal government has tried to prevent state Medicaid programs from shifting costs to beneficiaries via deductions, copayments, premiums, or other measures. The original law also restrained states from placing liens on the property of individuals to recoup their Medicaid costs. Over time the federal government has backed away from its blanket opposition to cost sharing. By obtaining waivers and through other means states as of the mid-1990s could impose nominal deductibles, co-insurance, or copayments on some Medicaid recipients for certain services. In some waiver states, for instance, program officials expected Medicaid enrollees with jobs to pay premiums. But many restrictions remained against shifting costs to beneficiaries. For instance, the federal government insisted that emergency and family planning services be exempt from copayments. It also ruled out cost sharing for such groups as pregnant women and children.[42]

Upping the Federal Match: Provider Taxes and Donations

Although constrained in several ways, states had by the late 1980s become increasingly creative in extracting more dollars from the federal purse. Some states proved adroit at "Medicaiding" services that they had previously subsidized purely from their own funds. In other instances, state Medicaid officials worked hard to help certain citizens, such as those with AIDS, become eligible for SSI and, hence, Medicaid. However, the most imaginative initiatives by states to shift more Medicaid costs to the national government involved special financing arrangements. Through the use of provider taxes and donations, as well as complex fund transfers between state and local governments or among state agencies, many states increased the federal share (or match) of Medicaid costs beyond that etched in law.[43]

Ironically, action by HCFA became the launching pad for these creative financing initiatives. On November 12, 1985, HCFA adopted a rule that expanded the funding sources states could use for purposes of determining federal matching payments. The issue at hand was the treatment of provider donations to the Medicaid program. Prior to 1985, HCFA had permitted states to finance their share of Medicaid training expenditures through donations to the program from hospitals and other providers. But these contributions would not count as the state match for the program in general. The new rule reversed this position, permitting states to count private and public donations as part of the state share of program expenditures.[44] In promulgating the rule, HCFA noted that in the past, "we wanted to prevent donations that could be conditional on some benefit to the donor. For example, we were particularly concerned that a 'kickback' situation could result from private donations made by a proprietary organization, such as a long-term care facility or data processing company, in return for Medicaid business." HCFA officials concluded, however, that the risk of conditional donations or kickbacks was slight and that the states should have "more flexibility in administering their programs."[45]

Financially strapped states wasted little time in taking advantage of the new rule. Action by West Virginia in 1986 set the pattern. Faced with acute budget problems, West Virginia officials persuaded hospitals to contribute some $22 million to its Medicaid program. Given the state's low per capita income—the critical factor in the federal formula—this donation became part of the state's Medicaid effort and generated over $60 million in federal matching payments. State Medicaid officials then found a way to return the $22 million to the hospitals that had made the donations and used the "profit" to pay for other Medicaid services. Awakening to the drain on the federal treasury that its new rule had created, HCFA moved to disallow West Virginia's Medicaid expenditures as an inappropriate interpretation of the 1985 rule. But West Virginia officials appealed and ultimately prevailed in a federal district court.

The practice spread. By 1990 all but six states operated a donation or provider tax program.[46] Estimates of the success states had in shifting program costs to the federal government vary, but clearly they made significant inroads. Under Medicaid law, the overall federal share of program costs approximates 57 percent of total Medicaid spending. By 1993 the federal government's proportion of the Medicaid bill had, by one estimate, risen to nearly 65 percent. Not surprisingly, some states proved to be more entrepreneurial than others. An analysis of three states, for instance, found that Michigan used special financing arrangements to increase the federal match from 56 to 68 percent in 1993; two other states, Texas and Tennessee, used creative financing techniques for more marginal improvements in the federal match rate—from 65 to 67 percent in the case of the former and from 68 to 71 percent in the latter.[47]

By the late 1980s the White House had become committed to stemming this flow of extra federal dollars to the states. But slamming the door on creative financing proved to be far from simple politically. State officials repeatedly stressed that efforts to dam the flow of money emanating from provider taxes and donations would hurt the poor; liberal allies in Congress, many of whom believed that the federal government ought to assume greater responsibility for providing health insurance to the nation, also resisted change. Others, however, viewed the state actions as a raid on the federal treasury. In 1991, for instance, Representative Norman Lent, a Republican from New York, likened claims that the poor would be hurt by changes in the 1985 HCFA rule to catching a bank cashier embezzling funds to support his wife and children: "Should he be allowed to do it for another year lest we lower the standard of living for his family?"[48]

The tension over state entrepreneurship played out in a series of skirmishes between the Bush administration and Congress. HCFA attempted to promulgate administrative rules that would curtail state opportunities to use provider donations and taxes for the federal match. These thrusts prompted Congress to insert provisions in the budget reconciliation acts of 1989 and then 1990, imposing a one-year moratorium on such rules. Despite congressional opposition, HCFA issued a rule placing broad restrictions on the states on October 31, 1991. Although Congressman Henry Waxman persuaded the House of Representatives to place another moratorium on this rule through September 30, 1992, the Bush administration and the NGA soon announced that they had reached an accord on legislation dealing with the subject. Their agreement broke the logjam and led to the passage of the Medicaid Voluntary Contribution and Provider-Specific Tax Amendments of 1991.

The new legislation, most of which became effective in 1993, contained three particularly important provisions. First, with a few exceptions, the law eliminated federal matching payments for provider donations. Second, it held out the possibility of a federal match for provider-specific taxes only if these taxes were uniform, broad-based, and did not in fact exempt providers from the costs of the tax. Broad-based implied that the tax would need to apply to an entire class of providers, such as acute care hospitals. The law also capped the revenue from such taxes for purposes of the state match at 25 percent of state Medicaid spending. Third, the new law constrained the main vehicle through which states had spent the monies generated through provider donations and taxes—the DSH program. Among other things, the legislation prohibited states from guaranteeing that DSH payments would exceed the tax payment for each hospital. As discussed earlier, it also capped DSH spending and the amount individual institutions could receive from the program.

The degree to which the new law will block fiscal entrepreneurship by the states remains to be seen. One legal analysis concludes that the 1991 act "creates as many questions as answers," leaving HCFA "to interpret vague, ambiguous phrases in the quickly-drafted legislation with little legislative history to guide its decisions."[49] Unquestionably, however, the amendments undercut state entrepreneurship. Moreover, the Balanced Budget Act of 1997 subsequently lowered the amount of federal Medicaid matching funds states could draw on for DSH payments. In the perpetual intergovernmental dance between the federal government and the states, the amendments affirmed the federal government's right to lead.

Devolution and Financing

The devolution debate will surely intersect with hard questions of whether to revise the formula currently used to distribute Medicaid funds among states. But from the perspective of state discretion, two general questions loom even larger.

First, how much funding effort should states have to exert for every federal dollar received? If the past is any guide, devolution proponents will differ considerably in their responses to this question. Not surprisingly, the NGA in 1996 pegged the maximum amount that any state should pay per federal dollar received at 40 cents (down from 50 cents). In converting Medicaid to a block grant, the Republican Medigrant bill echoed this perspective. In contrast, the Clinton proposal continued the current federal government match rate up to a spending cap per beneficiary.

Second, how constrained should states be in deciding the sources of their contribution to the program? Should federal policymakers continue to ensure that local governments and beneficiaries enjoy some protection from any state propensities to shift Medicaid costs to them? Should existing barriers to provider taxes and donations be retained? Again, the devolution debate in the period 1995–96 featured varying responses to these questions. For instance, the Medigrant bill approved by Congress gave states more freedom to shift costs to beneficiaries. Among other things it noted that states might wish to impose patient cost sharing "to discourage the inappropriate use of emergency medical services."[50] In contrast, the Clinton proposal affirmed the need to retain existing restrictions on copayments and other cost sharing unless they were reasonably related to the income of the beneficiary. For its part, the NGA proclaimed that federal laws limiting provider taxes and donations should be repealed and "current and pending state disputes with [the Department of Health and Human Services] . . . discontinued."[51] In contrast, the Clinton proposal sought to preserve existing prohibitions on provider donations and taxes. In these and other ways,

advocates for devolution raised and staked out a range of positions on financing. These issues seem likely to fuel additional debate in future considerations of Medicaid.

Administration: Reporting at Center Stage

The pushes and pulls of federalism also express themselves in the seemingly mundane matters of day-to-day administration at the state level—the
agencies that are involved, the procedures they use, and the information
they report to the national government. Although states have considerable
discretion under the current Medicaid program, the federal government does
impose on them a substantial volume of regulation. The Medicaid portion
of the U.S. Code (with annotations) runs to more than 500 pages. (In contrast, the original Medicaid legislation passed in 1965 was ten pages long.)
State Medicaid programs are also governed by more than 300 pages of
instructions in the *Code of Federal Regulations* as well as many other administrative directives and guidelines.[52]

Some of the rules HCFA imposes on the states target minute details.
For instance, HCFA regulations spell out circumstances under which state
agencies may substitute certified microfilm copies for original documents
to meet requirements for federal audit and review. An agency that wishes to
use this approach "must make a study of its record storage and must show
that the use of microfilm is efficient and economical." State agencies are to
obtain approval from the HCFA regional office for their microfilm plan.[53]

Other rules, of course, address much larger issues. For instance, the
federal government, in varying degrees of specificity, sets down requirements concerning state organization, personnel administration, fiscal administration, contracts, program integrity (systems for controlling fraud and
abuse), and utilization review of Medicaid services. Some of the rules provide for financial penalties to states if they make errors in implementing
Medicaid. For instance, federal regulations go into detail about systems
that states must have in place to detect claims-processing mistakes (for example, payment for a service not authorized under the state plan, or to a
provider who has not been certified for Medicaid participation) and eligibility errors (for example, reimbursement for services delivered to some-
one ineligible for program benefits). The rules also evince concern for due
process rights, spelling out how providers and beneficiaries can appeal if
Medicaid officials deny them access to the program.

The rules promulgated by the federal government to steer the states tend to be technical and soporific. But read carefully, they speak volumes about the balance of power and the level of trust between the federal and state governments. They intertwine with the interest of federal officials in ensuring accountability, efficiency, and effectiveness as defined by their understanding of the national government's objectives in sponsoring the program.

Consider, for instance, the requirement that each state delegate a single state agency to administer the Medicaid program and that personnel employed by the agency meet certain qualifications. This measure not only clarifies lines of communication and accountability in an otherwise fragmented and confusing political system, it also seeks to create an ally for federal officials. If the individuals who staff the state Medicaid bureaucracy and otherwise participate in the program have professional backgrounds similar to their federal counterparts, prospects improve that they will see eye-to-eye on issues of Medicaid implementation. Buttressing the authority and power position of the single agency in the state's policymaking process thereby becomes a vehicle for the federal government to get its own views taken seriously.[54]

The rules promulgated by the federal government impose some administrative uniformities on the states, but they do not stamp out state discretion and variation. New York State, for example, has a highly fragmented and decentralized administrative approach to Medicaid, while California's arrangements tend to concentrate authority and insulate state agencies from political forces.[55]

HCFA's Quest for Better Information

In considering the targets of federal regulation under Medicaid, data collection and reporting requirements loom particularly large in importance. HCFA's efforts to extract valid and reliable information from the states in part reflects a concern with compliance and accountability. Federal officials have an obligation to ascertain whether state Medicaid programs in fact play by the rules. The value of program information to the federal government goes much beyond this, however. It also intersects with the interest of federal officials in having states serve as laboratories for learning. Unless states provide a range of program data using the same format, federal policymakers stand little chance of comprehending the inputs, outputs, and outcomes of Medicaid in various states—let alone what accounts for these differences. Pitted against federal interests in this matter are, of course, the desire of many states to maximize their flexibility. State officials typically want to reduce the costs of collecting and reporting information. They want to assemble data that will be valuable to their program managers and state policymakers.

Medicaid law has given the HHS secretary substantial authority to require the states to provide certain information. On balance, the evolution of Medicaid has involved a steady effort by federal officials to improve the quality and comparability of the data that states provide. The Medicaid management information system (MMIS) has been the centerpiece of this initiative. Concerned about payment errors and other information deficits during the initial period of rapid program growth, Congress in 1972 approved legislation that authorized the federal government to pay state Medicaid programs 90 percent of the amounts attributable to the design, development, and installation of the MMIS. The legislation also provided another carrot by promising that the national government would pay 75 percent of the costs of operating the MMIS systems it found satisfactory. The 1972 provisions also authorized the federal bureaucracy to provide 90 percent of the funding needed by states to enhance their systems after they became operational. In 1974 legislation sought to empower the federal government still further by restricting the 90 and 75 percent funding rates to states that introduced systems that contained data elements determined by the Department of Health, Education, and Welfare. States that did not include all of these elements would find their federal match reduced to 50 percent.

Throughout the 1970s states made uneven progress in implementing MMIS. Many of the new systems had bugs that impeded their ability to produce reliable and valid information. By early 1979 less than half the states had managed to develop a federally approved MMIS.[56] Federal policymakers continued to apply pressure; in 1980 Congress passed legislation requiring states to acquire approved MMIS systems by the end of fiscal 1982 or have the federal match rate permanently reduced. (Five states with low population and enrollment costs were exempted.) By fiscal 1985 forty-five states had established MMIS systems that met HCFA standards.[57] Moreover, states proved aggressive in requesting the 90 percent federal match to upgrade their systems.

As a consequence of these efforts, states came to submit more valid, reliable, and comparable data to HCFA concerning expenditures and services provided to different clusters of beneficiaries. Nonetheless, complaints persist about the adequacy of HCFA efforts to gain comparable data about state programs. HCFA frequently finds statistical discrepancies and errors in the annual reports of the states. Noting this problem, GAO has criticized HCFA for being too deferential to the states in tolerating these errors. It has urged HCFA to demand more rigorously documented justifications from the many states that apply for federal funds to enhance their information systems and has chided HCFA for being weak in post-implementation reviews of these state enhancements.[58]

But if various players have pushed HCFA to be more assertive about MMIS, many states have found HCFA requirements to be onerous. The rise of managed care as a major vehicle for serving Medicaid beneficiaries—with its promise of capitated payment rather than the fee-for-service that MMIS emphasizes—has fueled discontent. As a top Medicaid administrator from the state of Wisconsin put it, "We have this awful MMIS that we're forced to operate that does us no good. And if you want to think one thing that should happen under a block grant, it's to dump that whole thing." Or as a state legislator from Minnesota involved in health care hearings in that state noted: "Whether it's the system or the process around it, one of the major concerns we heard was about MMIS. If everyone had had their way, everybody would have said 'Just blow it up.'" From the perspective of many state officials, MMIS does not "assist managers in making executive decisions or . . . assist program people in having their thumbs on the pulse of what is actually happening in terms of cost utilization trends and so on."[59] The tensions between Medicaid's traditional fee-for-service payment systems and the newer capitated managed-care plans have magnified the information challenges for HCFA.

The Information Options of Devolution

In a devolutionary period, how much freedom should the states have to design their own information systems? The considerations involved in responding to this question include those already discussed in the case of MMIS, but also extend to fundamental political issues. Those who see the devolution debate as an argument about which level of government can better deliver Medicaid services will tend to favor a strong federal hand in requiring the states to report comparable information. That way state failures can be detected and Medicaid policy recentralized if need be. But other devolution proponents harbor more fundamental ideological objections to government intervention in society. For this group the desirability of sustaining an ample flow of information may be less apparent. As a former legislative leader in New York State noted, "the one thing" certain advocates of devolution "don't want HCFA to do is to start to produce national numbers on what actually happens to people in this environment in terms of reductions in service and reductions in outcomes."[60] Such information can all too readily become a resource for those favoring reinvigoration of the federal government's attempts to deal with problems of the uninsured.

What does previous experience with the devolution of federal programs tell us about the propensity of the national government to continue to impose standardized reporting formats on the states? When in the early 1980s a number of categorical programs were converted to block grants, the federal government also relaxed data collection and reporting requirements. The result was predictable. States went different ways in deciding what to report; thus federal policymakers lacked comparable data about the state programs. Attempting to reduce this complexity and uncertainty while simultaneously respecting the principle of deference to state prerogatives, the federal government moved indirectly and slowly to encourage greater uniformity. Federal officials worked with various professional associations to develop model reporting forms that they urged, but did not require, states to adopt. Although many states responded by collecting the information in the manner suggested by the model, this approach failed to achieve the interstate standardization that had characterized the earlier categorical programs. In part for this reason, some impetus developed in Congress to chip away at the vast discretion built into block grants and to recategorize certain programs.[61]

Would these same dynamics apply in the case of Medicaid devolution? The answer remains unclear, in part because it is far from certain that devolution would bring a major relaxation of state reporting requirements. Neither President Clinton's proposal nor that of the NGA, for instance, called for greater state freedom in this sphere. For its part the Republican Medigrant bill required annual reports from each state concerning expenditures, beneficiaries, and utilization. It also called for independent evaluations of state programs every third year by an entity that would not be involved in the planning or administration of the state program. The bill gave the HHS secretary the authority to influence the information contained in annual reviews, the independent evaluations, and audit reports. The Medigrant proposal suggests that the importance of Medicaid for health and the sheer magnitude of its expenditures may drive even the more fervent devolution proponents to a relatively precise specification of reporting requirements.[62]

An Overview of State Discretion

Should pressures for Medicaid devolution be seen as a natural outgrowth of the steady erosion of state discretion over the program galvanized by an aggressive federal government? On balance, no. As one traces the evolution of Medicaid since its birth in 1965, a more complex picture emerges.

Figure 2-1 summarizes some of the principal findings with respect to each of the dimensions of devolution considered here—beneficiaries, services, provider selection and payment, financing, and administrative structure and reporting. It considers each of these dimensions in terms of the degree to which the federal government has constrained state discretion. In some areas the federal government has indeed moved to reduce state freedom. The number of pages of federal Medicaid law grew, as did the volume of rules contained in the *Code of Federal Regulations*. More specifically, the series of federal mandates approved by Congress in the 1980s unquestionably intensified pressure on the states to expand coverage to new groups of beneficiaries. In the case of services, the federal government forced states to pay more attention to quality, especially in the case of long-term care. Moreover, through much of the life of the program, the states chafed under federal restrictions on Medicaid payment for inpatient services.

In other spheres, however, figure 2-1 indicates that state discretion has grown. Federal waivers have freed states to try new approaches; the increasing acceptance of managed care has provided states with a golden opportunity to escape certain constraints, such as those imposed by the Boren amendments. As of the mid-1990s, therefore, it would be way off the mark to portray HCFA as the master puppeteer shaping the nuances of the Medicaid drama in the states. States have substantial discretion to shape program practices in each of the five areas explored in this chapter.

Nothing speaks more forcefully about the magnitude of this discretion than the great differences that characterize state Medicaid programs. No single summary measure can capture this variation and yield a parsimonious typology of these programs. However, as Donald Boyd documents in the next chapter, the juxtaposition of two indicators—Medicaid expenditures per enrollee and Medicaid enrollees as a proportion of all persons in

Figure 2-1. *The Dimensions of Devolution: Federal Constraints and State Discretion*

Dimension	Major federal constraints	Status of state discretion
Beneficiaries	Some erosion of state control beginning in the early 1970s with the nationalization of the SSI program. Supreme Court decision in 1990 opens the SSI gates to more children claiming disability, but 1996 welfare reform bill seeks to counteract Supreme Court ruling. The 1980s mandate benefits new groups of women and children as well as the elderly poor eligible for Medicare.	While reduced somewhat, state discretion remains substantial. States continue to vary greatly in the proportion of the poor and near-poor covered by Medicaid. Greater federal willingness to grant 1115 waivers provides states more freedom to extend Medicaid eligibility to new groups of citizens. Under the Balanced Budget Act of 1997, states acquire the option of obtaining additional federal funds to enroll new categories of children in their Medicaid programs (or alternative programs).
Services	The list of required services that states must provide grows slightly. The federal government imposes highly detailed regulations designed to bolster the quality of long-term care. Other regulations aimed at quality and utilization review also emerge.	State discretion is substantial. States define the amount and duration of services they provide. Through waiver provisions, the list of optional services they can cover grows markedly—especially with respect to home- and community-based care. Many states manage to "Medicaid" services that they had previously paid for out of state funds.

(Figure continues on the following page.)

Figure 2-1. (*continued*)

Dimension	Major federal constraints	Status of state discretion
Provider selection and payment	Throughout the life of the Medicaid program, payment to institutional providers is substantially regulated. Congress's efforts to provide greater latitude in this sphere via the Boren amendments backfire in the federal courts. Restrictions on state use of Medicaid managed-care plans persist into the 1990s. Legislation in the early 1990s places modest constraints on the state use of DSH funds; further limitations on DSH subsidies came in 1997.	States have great discretion to determine payment to physicians and other providers who deliver ambulatory or home care. They have modest discretion to set payment rates for inpatient care in hospitals and long-term care facilities. Developments in the late 1980s and 1990s expand their discretion. The DSH program gives states enormous latitude to provide extra payments to various hospitals and mental health facilities. Federal waivers have greatly expanded state discretion to use managed care and escape the constraints placed on them by court interpretations of the Boren amendments. The Balanced Budget Act of 1997 further enhances state discretion over managed care; through repeal of the Boren amendments and other provisions, the act significantly augments the authority of the states to determine provider payment rates.

poverty—yields important insight into the overall generosity of state programs.[63] States such as Rhode Island, Massachusetts, and Connecticut emerge from Boyd's analysis as relatively generous on both indicators; other states—such as Alabama, New Mexico, and Texas—spend relatively little per enrollee and trail other states in the percentage of poor citizens enrolled

Dimension	Major federal constraints	Status of state discretion
Financing	The federal government stipulates a matching formula and restricts the degree to which states can shift program costs to local governments and Medicaid beneficiaries. After a brief period of granting states vast discretion over the use of provider donations and taxes, the federal government imposes new regulations on state use of these tools.	States have substantial discretion to determine the level and sources of financing for their Medicaid program. Many manage to increase the federal share of program costs through the use of provider donations and taxes as well as other fund transfers. Through 1115 waivers, states gain more freedom to impose cost sharing on certain categories of Medicaid beneficiaries and at times extract additional funds from the federal government.
Administrative structure and reporting	Hundreds of pages of law and federal regulation target various aspects of program operations, including state organization, personnel administration, fiscal administration, contracts, and program integrity. Through generous subsidies the federal government makes strides in imposing more uniform reporting requirements on the states.	States have substantial discretion. The agencies responsible for implementing the Medicaid program and the procedures they use vary considerably from one state to the next. Many states chafe under the constraints imposed by the MMIS reporting format—especially in a period where managed care will play a larger role.

in the program. Still other states are hybrids. California and Tennessee score high in the proportion of poor citizens enrolled in their programs but low in expenditures per enrollee. Louisiana and South Dakota are above average in spending per enrollee but below the mean in the percentage of poor citizens they sign up for the program.

Boyd's typology drives home the point that efforts to devolve or otherwise change Medicaid will be likely to affect different states in different ways. It also highlights the need to consider two critical factors that markedly shape who gets what from the Medicaid program—state capacity and commitment.

Medicaid, Federalism, and Devolution

Basic questions concerning the appropriate division of labor between the national and state governments in providing health care to the poor and near-poor will occupy the country into the indefinite future. In the case of Medicaid, the dance between the national and state governments will persist over such issues as eligibility, services, provider selection and payment, financing, and general administration (especially reporting requirements). This dance will often fail to feature the dramatic gestures and flourishes that attract the media spotlight. But the technical politics that play out over program specifics may well yield changes that profoundly influence who gets what from Medicaid.

The chapters that follow focus on a range of important issues that intersect with questions of how far the country should go in devolving more responsibility over Medicaid to the states. By putting a particular facet of the Medicaid program under the microscope, each of the chapters captures the complexities and nuances of devolution. Yet in one form or another, all of the chapters intersect with two fundamental questions that the final chapter probes more extensively. First, how much capacity do states have to deal with the new burdens and opportunities that various types of devolution would pose for them? The concept of state *capacity* presents many daunting problems of definition and measurement. In general terms capacity denotes the potential for accomplishing some task—having the wherewithal in terms of resources, skill, and other intangible factors needed to do the job. Ample capacity does not, of course, mean that a state will creatively seize the opportunities offered by Medicaid devolution. But without adequate capacity, well-intentioned officials sincerely committed to "doing right" by Medicaid will tend to get sidetracked. Indeed failure to consider capacity in policy deliberations has often been a critical stumbling block to effective and accountable public programs. As two seasoned observers of state health care policy observe, "underinvestment in state management and implementation capacities [by policymakers] is penny-wise, pound-foolish, perverse, and predictable."[64] This observation highlights the need to consider whether any attempt to devolve more responsibility over Medicaid to the states would founder on the shoals of inadequate governing and fiscal capacity.

A second critical question about the states also looms large: to what degree are state policymakers and administrators committed to providing health care services of high quality to the needy? State commitment to Medicaid is, of course, a product of complex policy processes involving strategic interaction among a critical cast of players—governors, legislators, state administrators, local officials, interest groups, the media, and more. These political processes are shaped by a state's institutional configuration, ideology, and economy. The level of state program commitment is particularly important because major devolution proposals almost always embody plans to reduce the federal dollars that would otherwise flow to the states. In this regard, two competing scenarios have vied for attention in debates over Medicaid devolution—the race to the bottom and compensatory federalism.

The race-to-the-bottom scenario emphasizes that states vigorously compete with one another for economic development.[65] They do this in part by reducing their commitment to redistributive programs that tax the affluent to benefit the poor. At some threshold, higher taxes for such purposes tend to discourage firms and affluent individuals from remaining in or moving to the state, thereby eroding its revenue capacity. Simultaneously, generous redistributive programs may become a magnet attracting needy people to the state, thereby placing additional fiscal stress on that government. The validity of the race-to-the-bottom scenario rests only in part on whether firms, the affluent, and the poor actually respond in the predicted ways to state taxes and program benefits. What matters most is whether governors and legislators believe that redistributive policies motivate such behavior. To the degree that the race to the bottom holds sway, it fits the perspective of both conservatives and liberals who believe that devolution goes hand-in-hand with retrenchment. In this view rhetoric about devolution empowering the states masks its more fundamental purpose: less governmental involvement in addressing the needs of the poor and others.

In contrast, the perspective rooted in compensatory federalism asserts that policy retreat at one level of the federal system often spurs new activism at another level.[66] It hypothesizes that in response to Medicaid devolution, many states will rise to the occasion and compensate for diminished federal financial support through gains in efficiency and, possibly, increased provision of state dollars. The tension between the race-to-the-bottom and compensatory federalism perspectives undergirds much of devolution debate; the relative merits of each of these perspectives receives attention in the final chapter.

Notes

1. See John J. DiIulio Jr. and Richard P. Nathan, eds., *Making Health Reform Work: The View from the States* (Brookings, 1994).
2. Teresa A. Coughlin, Leighton Ku, and John Holahan, *Medicaid since 1980: Costs, Coverage, and the Shifting Alliance between the Federal Government and the States* (Washington: Urban Institute Press, 1994), pp. 116–17; Allen Dobson, Donald Moran, and Gary Young, "The Role of Federal Waivers in the Health Policy Process," *Health Affairs*, vol. 11 (Winter 1992), pp. 72–94; Nancy A. Miller, "Medicaid 2176 Home and Community-Based Care Waivers: The First Ten Years," *Health Affairs*, vol. 11 (Winter 1992), pp. 162–71.
3. General Accounting Office, *Medicaid Section 1115 Waivers: Flexible Approach to Approving Demonstrations Could Increase Federal Costs*, GAO/HEHS-96-44 (1995), p. 75; and direct communication from the Health Care Financing Administration, April 1997.
4. National Governors' Association, "Restructuring Medicaid" (Washington: unpublished document, February 2, 1996), p. 4.
5. National Center for Health Statistics, *Health, United States, 1995* (Hyattsville, Md.: U.S. Public Health Service, 1996), pp. 260–61.
6. John Holahan and David Liska, "Where Is Medicaid Spending Headed?" (Washington: Urban Institute Web Page [www.urban.org/entitlements/Forecast.htm], December 1996); Sally T. Burner and Daniel R. Waldo, "National Health Expenditure Projections, 1994–2005," *Health Care Financing Review*, vol. 16 (Summer 1995), pp. 239–41; Coughlin and others, *Medicaid since 1980*, p. 101.
7. Margaret W. Linn, Lee Gurel, and Bernard S. Linn, "Patient Outcome as a Measure of Quality of Nursing Home Care," *American Journal of Public Health*, vol. 67 (April 1977), pp. 337–44.
8. Coughlin and others, *Medicaid since 1980*, pp. 48–51, 81.
9. *Sullivan v. Zebley*, 493 U.S. 521 (1990); see especially at 540.
10. *Congressional Quarterly Almanac, 1989,* vol. 35 (Congressional Quarterly, 1990), pp. 173–74.
11. Nelson A. Rockefeller Institute of Government and the Brookings Center for Public Management, "Devolution and Medicaid: A View from the States" (Washington: unpublished conference transcript, May 23–24, 1996), p. 36.
12. See General Accounting Office, *Health Insurance for Children: Private Insurance Coverage Continues to Deteriorate*, GAO/HEHS-96-129 (June 1996), p. 3; and General Accounting Office, *Medicare and Medicaid: Many Eligible People Not Enrolled in Qualified Medicare Beneficiary Program*, GAO/HEHS-94-52 (January 1994), p. 6.

13. General Accounting Office, *Medicaid Prenatal Care: States Improve Access and Enhance Services, But Face New Challenges*, GAO/HEHS-94-152BR (May 1994), p. 12.

14. General Accounting Office, *Medicaid Section 1115 Waivers.*

15. Health Care Financing Administration, *Medicaid Statistics, Program and Financial Statistics, Fiscal Year 1994* (Department of Health and Human Services, HCFA pub. no. 10129, February 1996), pp. 64–65; see also HCFA 2082 reports.

16. Coughlin and others, *Medicaid since 1980*, pp. 72–73.

17. Analysis conducted by Donald Boyd, Center for the Study of the States, Nelson A. Rockefeller Institute of Government, from HCFA data. The computation of the poor in each state derives from a three-year average.

18. "An Analysis of Welfare Reform and Its Effects on Medicaid Recipients" (Washington: National Health Law Program, National Center for Youth Law, unpublished manuscript, August 12, 1996), pp. 13–16. For a general overview of the implications of the 1996 welfare law, see Jane Koppelman, "Impact of the New Welfare Law on Medicaid," *National Health Policy Forum Issue Brief No. 697* (Washington: George Washington University, 1997).

19. White House, "Medicaid" (Washington, unpublished statement, December 11, 1995), p. 5.

20. Health Care Financing Administration, *Medicaid Statistics*, pp. 5–6.

21. Miller, "Medicaid 2176 Home and Community-Based Care Waivers," p. 164.

22. General Accounting Office, *Medicaid: Tennessee's Program Broadens Coverage but Faces Uncertain Future*, GAO/HEHS-95-186 (September 1995), p. 6.

23. See Martin A. Strosberg and others, eds., *Rationing America's Medical Care: The Oregon Plan and Beyond* (Brookings, 1992); and Robert A. Crittenden, "Rolling Back Reform in the Pacific Northwest," *Health Affairs*, vol. 14 (Summer 1995), pp. 302–05.

24. Health Care Financing Administration, *Medicaid Services State by State* (Department of Health and Human Services, HCFA pub. no. 02155-96, 1996). The data did not include Medicare buy-ins, the early periodic screening and diagnosis treatment program, or special home- and community-based services provided by states under waivers.

25. See Coughlin and others, *Medicaid since 1980*, p. 18.

26. *Medicaid HEDIS* (National Committee for Quality Assurance, 1995).

27. *U.S. Code, Annotated, Title 42, Section 1396r* (1992).

28. *U.S. Code, Annotated, Title 42, Section 1396t* (1992).

29. Frank J. Thompson, *Health Policy and the Bureaucracy* (MIT Press, 1981), p. 123.

30. Bruce C. Vladeck, *Unloving Care: The Nursing Home Tragedy* (Basic Books, 1980), pp. 73, 77.

31. Paul Gurny, David K. Baugh, and Thomas W. Reilly, "Payment, Administration, and Financing of the Medicaid Program," *Health Care Financing Review* (1992 annual supplement), pp. 283–301.

32. *Wilder* v. *Virginia Hospital Association*, 110 S.Ct. 2510 (1990); see also Michael D. Daneker, "Medicaid State Cost-Containment Measures, and Section 1983 Provider Actions under *Wilder* v. *Virginia Hospital Association*," *Vanderbilt Law Review*, vol. 45 (March 1992), pp. 487–528.

33. Coughlin and others, *Medicaid since 1980*, p. 95.

34. General Accounting Office, *Medicaid: The Texas Disproportionate Share Program Favors Public Hospitals*, GAO/HRD-93-86 (March 1993).

35. Kaiser Commission on the Future of Medicaid, "Medicaid Special Financing Arrangements: Disproportionate Share Hospital (DSH) Payments, Provider Taxes, and Intergovernmental Transfers" (Washington, April 1995), p. 5.

36. Congressional Research Service, *Medicaid Source Book: Background Data and Analysis (A 1993 Update)*, Committee Print, House Committee on Energy and Commerce, 103 Cong. 1 sess. (Government Printing Office, January 1993), pp. 329–30.

37. Kaiser Commission, "Medicaid Special Financing Arrangements," table 1.

38. John Holahan and others, *Cutting Medicaid Spending in Response to Budget Gaps* (Washington: Urban Institute Press, 1995), pp. 26–28.

39. *Balanced Budget Act of 1995: Conference Report, Part 1* (Government Printing Office, 1995), pp. 211–12.

40. National Governors' Association, "Restructuring Medicaid," p. 3.

41. Kaiser Commission, "Medicaid Special Financing Arrangements," p. 3.

42. Health Care Financing Administration, *Medicaid Statistics, Fiscal Year 1994*, p. 8.

43. Coughlin and others, *Medicaid since 1980*, p. 89.

44. This description draws heavily on Michael O. Spivey, "Patching the Patchwork Quilt: 'Reforming' the Medicaid Program—The Medicaid Voluntary Contribution and Provider Specific Tax Amendments of 1991," *Annals of Health Law*, vol. 1 (1992), pp. 37–52.

45. *Federal Register*, vol. 50 (November 12, 1985), p. 46657.

46. *Congressional Quarterly Almanac, 1991*, vol. 37 (Congressional Quarterly, 1992), p. 358.

47. General Accounting Office, *Medicaid: States Use Illusory Approaches to Shift Program Costs to Federal Government*, GAO/HEHS-94-133 (August 1994), pp. 2, 13.

48. *Congressional Quarterly Almanac, 1991*, p. 358.

49. Spivey, "Patching the Patchwork Quilt," p. 49.

50. *Balanced Budget Act of 1995*, p. 203.

51. National Governors' Association, "Restructuring Medicaid," p. 4.

52. *U.S. Code, Annotated, Title 42, Subchapter XIX* (1992); and *Code of Federal Regulations, Title 42, Chapter IV, Subchapter C* (1995).

53. *Code of Federal Regulations, Title 42, Chapter IV, Subchapter C, § 431.17 (d)(1)*, p. 23.

54. See Martha Derthick, *The Influence of Federal Grants: Public Assistance in Massachusetts* (Harvard University Press, 1970).

55. Michael S. Sparer, *Medicaid and the Limits of State Health Reform* (Temple University Press, 1996).

56. Thompson, *Health Policy and the Bureaucracy*, pp. 136–37.

57. General Accounting Office, *ADP Systems: Better Control over States' Medicaid Systems Needed*, GAO/IMTEC-89-19 (August 1989), p. 10.

58. GAO, *ADP Systems*; and General Accounting Office, *Medicaid: Data Improvements Needed to Help Manage Health Care Program*, GAO/IMTEC-93-18 (May 1993).

59. Nelson A. Rockefeller Institute of Government and Brookings, *Devolution and Medicaid*, pp. 284, 447–48.

60. Ibid., p. 458.

61. General Accounting Office, *Block Grants: Federal-State Cooperation in Developing National Data Collection Strategies*, GAO/HRD-89-2 (November 1988); and General Accounting Office, *Block Grants: Characteristics, Experience, and Lessons Learned*, GAO/HEHS-95-74 (February 1995).

62. *Balanced Budget Act of 1995*, section 2102.

63. Greater expenditures per enrollee need not, of course, automatically indicate that Medicaid beneficiaries receive higher quality or more accessible care; it could also reflect inefficiency.

64. James R. Tallon Jr. and Lawrence D. Brown, "Health Alliances: Functions, Forms, and Federalism," in DiIulio and Nathan, eds., *Making Health Reform Work*, p. 58.

65. See, for instance, Paul E. Peterson, *The Price of Federalism* (Brookings, 1995).

66. See, for example, Richard P. Nathan and others, *Reagan and the States* (Princeton University Press, 1987).

3

Medicaid Devolution
A Fiscal Perspective

Donald J. Boyd

MEDICAID IS a huge program financed by the federal government and the states, exceeding $160 billion annually. Its costs have grown dramatically over time, and elected officials and policy analysts have called for reform for years. Much of the debate over Medicaid reform is couched in federalist principles. Devolution advocates say, Give aid to the states as block grants with no strings attached. States are closer to the people than the federal government, and they know their citizens' needs. They will know how to spend it wisely and efficiently. Advocates for national control over Medicaid say, Medicaid is a program for the poor, and it should be financed by taxpayers throughout the nation as a whole. Furthermore, we have to have rules. We cannot trust states to do the right thing; we have to set minimum standards and have federal oversight.

Medicaid reform, however defined, will shift money between the federal government and the states and among the states. To quote one state official, speaking about the 1996 National Governors' Association (NGA) Medicaid reform proposal:

> Most of this bill is about money, not about federalism . . . there is a column
> with every state by name, with a number next to it: . . . a large number of

states would fiscally be hundreds and hundreds of millions of dollars better off in the first two years or three years of this bill than they would be under current law. That kind of puts a different spin on the question of whether or not you support block grants.[1]

In other words, state governors and legislatures will not be for or against a particular Medicaid reform proposal solely on principle. Some states could come out hundreds of millions of dollars ahead in the short run, while others come out far behind. Whether one is for or against is not just about principle—it is about money.

This chapter tracks the enormous growth in Medicaid expenditures, which have placed fiscal pressure on federal and state budgets and created political pressure for reform. It examines the recent slowdown in expenditures and the extent to which fiscal pressures may have abated. It also analyzes how the federal and state governments share the cost of Medicaid. Under most reform plans the current formula will define in part how the federal government will share in future costs; this formula is sure to be a controversial issue in future Medicaid debates. The chapter then examines the tremendous variation in Medicaid spending across states that results from differing program designs and policy choices, differing needs, and differing economic conditions. This variation illustrates the broad flexibility states already have under Medicaid, even without further devolution. Past state policy choices will affect future federal reimbursement under most reform plans. Finally, the chapter analyzes the fiscal building blocks of devolution and how reform proposals might affect states differently.

National Trends in Medicaid Expenditures

Until recently, Medicaid expenditures have been explosive, growing at an average annual rate of more than 16 percent from 1966 to 1996, a rate far greater than the combined rate of growth in the population plus inflation, which was only 6.5 percent over this period.[2] At this rate expenditures double every four-and-one-half years on average. Growth was particularly rapid in 1991 and 1992, averaging 27 percent per year, but slowed to 11 percent in 1995.[3] In 1996 spending slowed even further, to a growth rate of 0.1 percent. Figure 3-1 shows recent Medicaid expenditure growth rates from 1982 through 1996. The rates of growth, and the reasons for growth, have varied over time.

Figure 3-1. *Medicaid Spending Growth Rates*

Percent

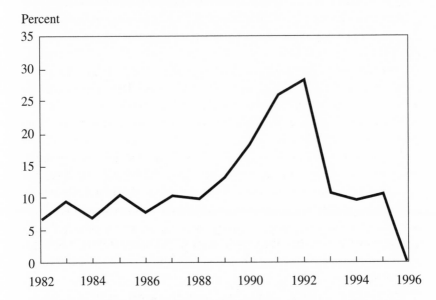

Sources: 1982–93 growth rates obtained from Health Care Financing Administration (HCFA), *Health Care Financing Review: 1996 Statistical Supplement* (Baltimore: HHS Office of Research and Demonstrations, 1996), table 109; 1994–95 growth rates obtained from HCFA, *Medicaid Statistics: Program and Financial Statistics Fiscal Year 1995,* table 1; 1996 growth rate based on growth in total computable expenditures for 1996 obtained from data file mfn96t01.xls, as compared with total expenditures for 1995 obtained from HCFA, *Medicaid Statistics,* table 1.

The Early Years

Growth from Medicaid's first full year in 1966 through 1974 averaged 25.5 percent annually.[4] This growth reflected rapid increases in both the number of beneficiaries and costs, with recipients nearly doubling and total costs increasing more than sixfold. According to the Congressional Research Service (CRS), the growth was driven primarily by (1) large increases in the number of single-parent families receiving cash assistance under the nation's primary welfare program, aid to families with dependent children (AFDC), as these families also were categorically eligible for Medicaid; (2) rapid growth in medical prices; and (3) the high cost of nursing home care.[5]

Between 1975 and 1981 expenditure growth slowed, averaging only 15.8 percent per year, but still was well above the combined growth in population and prices (10.1 percent), and still was placing increasing pressure on federal and state budgets. Growth in the number of recipients over this period was essentially flat, despite an approximately 25 percent increase in the poverty population. Much of the poverty increase was in two-parent households, which traditionally had not been eligible for AFDC and therefore would not be categorically eligible for Medicaid. Furthermore, AFDC benefit levels did not keep pace with inflation over this period, placing downward pressure on the number of families eligible for AFDC and therefore categorically eligible for Medicaid. The rise in costs over this period was essentially the result of increased costs per recipient, reflecting the dramatic general price inflation of the late 1970s, even more rapid medical price inflation, and intensified use of services—especially institutional services.[6]

Between 1981 and 1988 expenditure growth slowed substantially to an average annual rate of 9.0 percent. Growth in the number of recipients averaged only 0.6 percent per year, fluctuating between 21 million and 22 million over the period. The cost per recipient rose at an average annual rate of 8.2 percent.[7] This period reflects two important sets of policy changes: First, in response to the growing budgetary burden created by Medicaid, the federal government enacted the Omnibus Budget Reconciliation Act of 1981 (OBRA81). This legislation gave states a substantial incentive to slow program growth by reducing federal reimbursements to states whose spending growth exceeded targets tied to the medical care component of the consumer price index. OBRA81 also gave states flexibility to meet these targets, allowing them to impose cost-cutting controls, reduce some benefits, and establish new waiver programs. Many states took advantage of the waiver programs and also imposed cuts such as day limits for inpatient hospital services, reductions in prescription drug coverage, and limits on hospital and physician reimbursements. OBRA81 also made it more difficult for working mothers to qualify for AFDC cash assistance, and thus to qualify automatically for Medicaid. Largely as a result, program growth slowed dramatically, averaging 7.3 percent annually between 1981 and 1984, despite the recession of 1980–82 and the rise in poverty.[8]

The second set of factors affecting these years was that OBRA81 was followed in 1984 and later years by a series of enactments that either mandated or allowed states to expand eligibility, especially for pregnant women and for children. In addition, the number of disabled recipients, with expensive medical needs, grew much more rapidly than other beneficiaries. From 1984 to 1988 expenditure growth accelerated to nearly 10 percent per year. The Urban Institute attributes this acceleration in part to eligibility expansions, such as those for pregnant women and children, and service expansions, such as Early Periodic Screening, Diagnostic, and Treatment (EPSDT) services for children.[9]

The 1988–93 Cost Explosion

Medicaid expenditures skyrocketed between 1988 and 1993, growing at a compound annual rate of 19.3 percent that resulted in growth of 142 percent in only five years.[10] The Kaiser Commission on the Future of Medicaid divided this growth into major components: it concluded that 38 percent of the growth resulted from increases in recipients, 24 percent from medical price inflation, 22 percent from the ballooning growth of payments to hospitals serving a disproportionate share of the indigent (known as DSH payments), and the remaining 16 percent from a combination of increased service use, growth in reimbursement rates above medical price inflation, and increased premium payments for Medicare and HMOs. Of the growth attributable to increases in recipients, more than 60 percent resulted from increasing numbers of disabled and elderly recipients. The remainder was attributable to growth in the numbers of low-income adults and children caused by factors such as increasing numbers of single-parent households, the recession of 1990–91, and federally mandated expansions of aid to pregnant women and children. Although these mandated expansions accounted for a large share of the growth in *recipients*, they accounted for a small share of Medicaid *expenditure* growth—only 8.5 percent of the growth from 1988 to 1993—because average expenditures for these recipients are quite low.[11]

The conclusion that increased coverage of pregnant women and children accounted for only 8.5 percent of growth in total program costs between 1988 and 1993 runs counter to the common impression that federal mandates are driving program costs. For example, in its conference report on the proposed Medigrant legislation, the 1995 congressional majority stated:

> According to many State officials, the explosion of Medicaid spending is due in large part to Congressional and Executive directives. . . . Federally mandated eligibility changes over the last decade fueled the expansion of the Medicaid-eligible population and the cost of the program. Although States have the discretion of supplementing Medicaid's mandated cover-

age standards, the Federal government frequently expanded the scope of the standards. As a result, States have been compelled to increase their spending levels in order to receive their share of Federally matched Medicaid spending.[12]

To be sure, congressional and state complaints about the federal role in Medicaid go beyond mandated expansions to pregnant women and children, and the growth in costs related to these expansions may be more significant in some states than in others; in the overall national context, however, this growth was a relatively small element in the 1988–93 cost explosion.

What did drive costs in these years? According to analyses by the Kaiser commission and the Urban Institute, the key factors were:

Growth related to the elderly and disabled. Despite growth in the overall elderly population, the number of elderly Medicaid recipients had been declining for most years between 1975 and 1989, reflecting declining elderly poverty.[13] Beginning in 1990, however, the number of elderly Medicaid recipients began to increase. In addition, the number of disabled recipients, which already had been growing modestly, accelerated from 1990 through 1993. The growth in disabled recipients in part reflects a 1990 Supreme Court decision, *Sullivan v. Zebley*, that required retroactive SSI eligibility determinations for disabled children. The decision said that the law required disability determinations for children to consider not just medical impairment, but also whether a child was able to function independently in an age-appropriate manner based on individualized functional assessments. Other factors, including expanded outreach efforts also mandated by *Sullivan v. Zebley* and more extensive SSI enrollment of AIDS and HIV sufferers, also contributed to the growth in the Medicaid disabled population.

The average Medicaid costs for elderly and disabled recipients are much higher than for other groups, so growth in the number of these recipients resulted in large cost increases. The impact was especially acute in 1993, when growth in elderly and disabled recipients accounted for about half of the expenditure growth from 1992.[14]

Medical price increases, especially hospital inpatient care and nursing home care. Hospital inpatient and nursing home services account for about half of Medicaid spending. Although their prices grew much more slowly than prices for prescription drugs and physician services, they contributed more to overall cost growth.

Special financing programs. The Kaiser commission attributes more than one-fifth of the total increase in Medicaid costs between 1988 and

1993 to the growth of DSH payments. States had considerable discretion over these payments, and much of this growth may have been related to state efforts to maximize revenue from the federal government. They were able to do this by increasing their payments to hospitals to gain associated federal reimbursements, and then recouping some of their payments to hospitals in the form of taxes on those hospitals. Most of this increase occurred in 1991 and 1992.

The Recent Slowdown

After growing at an average annual rate of nearly 20 percent from 1988 to 1993, Medicaid expenditures slowed to about 10 percent annually from 1993 to 1995. Furthermore, expenditures in 1996 rose by only 0.1 percent. What happened?

First, the growth of DSH payments tailed off dramatically as a result of new federal limitations on this program. DSH payments grew enormously in two years, from $902 million in 1990 to $17.4 billion in 1992, and then stabilized. By 1995 DSH payments had grown only slightly more, to $19.0 billion, and in 1996 they declined to $15.0 billion.[15]

Second, the growth in costs for low-income children came to a screeching halt, and costs for low-income adults actually declined. In both cases the dramatic turnabout reflected a slowing in both the number of recipients and the average payment per recipient. The slowdown in the number of recipients no doubt reflects the combined impact of an improving economy and declines in AFDC caseloads resulting from improvements in the economy and stricter state welfare policies.[16] Between the 1994 and 1995 federal fiscal years, the number of AFDC recipients nationwide fell 4 percent, with declines in forty-two states. The number of recipients fell again in 1996. Through May 1997 AFDC caseloads had declined for twenty-six consecutive months.[17]

Third, there was some slowing in the growth of the number of elderly and disabled recipients and in their average costs, but the slowdown was nowhere near as pronounced as in the other categories. Furthermore, average payments in these two categories grew faster in 1995 than in any of the previous three years.

Relatively little data are available as of this writing to shed light on the 1996 slowdown. Recent data on program expenditures for the 1996 federal fiscal year show that some of the slowdown was related to a 21 percent decline in DSH expenditures; if not for this decline, expenditures would have grown 3 percentage points faster.[18] In other words, underlying growth in non-DSH expenditures was faster than the reported 0.1 percent growth in total expenditures. Many fee-for-service expenditures evidenced low growth, but expenditures for health insurance programs and home- and community-based services continued to grow at double-digit rates. One article offered, "The low 1996 growth probably, at least partially, reflects an acceleration of state spending in 1995 because of proposed legislation to restructure Medicaid that would have used 1995 data as the basis for distribution of block grants."[19]

The net result of recent shifts is that the elderly and disabled have accounted for a much greater share of Medicaid payment growth over the last few years than they have in earlier years: combined, these two groups accounted for 85 percent of the growth in payments to vendors between 1993 and 1995, even though they accounted for only 27 percent of recipients in 1993 and only 66 percent of payments to vendors. Table 3-1 shows

Table 3-1. *Summary of Medicaid Growth, 1966–95*

Years	Average annual growth (percent)	Driving forces
1966–74	25.5	— Recipients nearly doubled due in large part to AFDC growth (those categorically eligible for Medicaid) — Rapid medical price inflation, especially for nursing homes
1974–81	16.8	— Essentially no recipient growth, despite rise in poverty — Rapid general and Medicaid price inflation
1981–88	8.9	— OBRA81 allowed greater cost containment—especially affecting the early years of this period — Mandated and optional expansions began to take hold in later years
1988–93	19.3	— Increases in disabled and elderly recipients; disabled growth driven in part by Supreme Court decision and outreach efforts — Tenfold increase in DSH payments — Growth in AFDC caseloads due to increase in single-parent households and 1990–91 recession
1993–95	9.5	— New federal limits on DSH payments reduce payments to some states — Improving economy and AFDC declines — Slowing medical price inflation — Elderly and disabled account for 85 percent of growth in payments

the average annual growth rates in Medicaid spending for the periods discussed.

The Federal-State Split of Medicaid Funding

States share in most Medicaid costs according to a formula that requires a greater share from high-income states than from low-income states. The state share plus the federal share, known as the Federal Medicaid Assistance Percentage, or FMAP, add up to 100 percent.[20] Under this formula, as state per capita income rises relative to the national average, the federal share falls.[21] The formula sets a maximum FMAP of 83 percent and a floor of 50 percent, corresponding to state shares that range from 17 percent to 50 percent. In 1995 no state was at the maximum FMAP—Mississippi had the highest federal share at 79 percent. California, New York, and twelve other high-income states were at the 50 percent floor; ten were between 50 and 60 percent; sixteen were between 60 and 70 percent; and eleven were above 70 percent.[22] The average federal share of program expenditures in 1995, across all states and territories, was 56 percent. The other 44 percent—the state share—amounted to $66.3 billion.

States with income that is only 5.4 percent or more above the national average are subject to the maximum state share of 50 percent, while states must have income more than 38 percent below the national average to qualify for the minimum state share of 17 percent.[23] Clearly this asymmetric structure guarantees that a large number of states will be subject to the 50 percent maximum state share. The District of Columbia, Connecticut, New Jersey, and other high-income states, for example, would be subject to the 50 percent maximum state share even if their incomes were much lower.

One can think of the state share of Medicaid as the "price" a state pays for a dollar of Medicaid services received by its citizens. If high-income Connecticut wishes to purchase an additional dollar of Medicaid services, it must pay 50 cents, but if low-income Mississippi wants to buy an extra dollar of Medicaid services, it only pays 21 cents.[24] Therefore the price to Connecticut is nearly two-and-one-half times as great as the price to Mississippi. Because all states pay less than a dollar for a dollar of services, the FMAP encourages all states to spend more on Medicaid than they would under 100 percent state funding. Because the FMAP lowers the price to low-income states more than it does to high-income states, it provides an additional incentive for these states to broaden eligibility and expand services.

Medicaid analysts have long attacked the FMAP along two fronts: (1) it does not direct federal resources to states most in need, and (2) it does not require the greatest state share from states with the most resources. They argue, quite properly, that low per capita income is a bad measure of need for Medicaid services, and high per capita income is an imperfect measure of state resources.

Why Low per Capita Income Is a Bad Proxy for Medicaid Need

One of the primary goals of Medicaid is to provide medical care for those who cannot afford it, and so the poverty population provides a measure of Medicaid need. There is a general tendency for the poverty rate to fall as per capita income rises, however, so that income captures in an inverse fashion some of what a poverty measure might capture. The relationship is nevertheless weak and filled with exceptions. One can see from figure 3-2 that states with similar poverty rates may have very different

Figure 3-2. *Relationship between Average Poverty Rate and per Capita Income, 1994–95*

Percent unless otherwise indicated

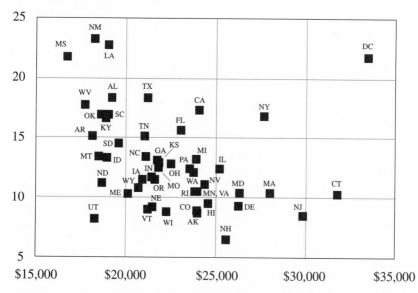

Sources: Per capita income is based on author's calculations from personal income data, U.S. Department of Commerce, Bureau of Economic Analysis [http://www.bea.gov] and population data from U.S. Department of Commerce, Bureau of the Census [http://www.census.gov].

federal Medicaid reimbursement under the income-based FMAP, and that states with similar Medicaid reimbursement rates may have very different poverty rates.[25]

New York and the District of Columbia both have very high poverty rates compared with other high-income states. New York's per capita income is roughly the same as that of Massachusetts, but its poverty rate is 62 percent greater; yet New York and Massachusetts receive the same 50 percent Medicaid reimbursement rate from the federal government.

Louisiana, Mississippi, and New Mexico are low-income states, but their poverty rates are much higher than those in other low-income states. At the other extreme are New Hampshire and Utah, which have much lower poverty rates than states with comparable incomes. The comparison between New Mexico and Utah is especially striking: per capita income in each state is about 22 percent below the national average, but New Mexico's poverty rate is 64 percent above the national average and Utah's poverty rate is 42 percent below the average. Despite clear differences in Medicaid need, each state pays the same price—about 27 cents per dollar of Medicaid services.

Other things being equal, at a given price high-income states would tend to purchase more of most goods or services than low-income states, and Medicaid is no exception. If high-income states paid the same price for Medicaid services as low-income states one would expect them to have greater total Medicaid expenditures per poor person. Although the price to high-income states can be nearly two-and-one-half times that to low-income states, high-income states tend to spend more on Medicaid in total (federal plus state share) per poor person than low-income states.[26] In fact, the state-share spending in some high-income states is so great that it outweighs the effect of a low *federal* share, and federal spending per poor person is actually greater than in low-income states.

Figure 3-3, which plots the federal contribution per poor person against state per capita income, illustrates this last point. The general tendency for higher federal spending in high-income states is clear. Federal expenditures per poor person in the District of Columbia, which has the highest per capita income, are about half again as large as federal expenditures in Mississippi, which has the lowest per capita income. Other examples are even more stark: New Hampshire's per capita income is about 41 percent higher than New Mexico's, and yet the federal government spends 241 percent more per poor person in New Hampshire than in New Mexico. Although the federal reimbursement formula favors low-income states, and narrows

Figure 3-3. *Relationship between Federal Spending per Poor Person and per Capita Income, 1995*

Dollars

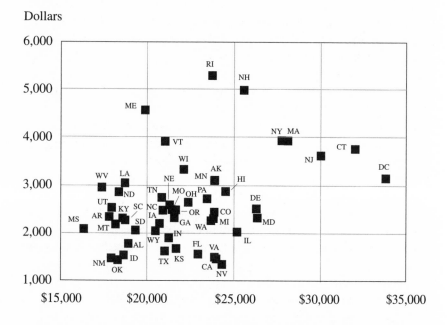

Sources: Federal spending amounts from *Medicaid Statistics: Program and Financial Statistics, Fiscal Year 1995,* HCFA-64 Report, Tables, table 1. p. 135.

the gap in spending on poor people, it does not begin to eliminate the gap arising from the large differences in need and preferences between high- and low-income states.[27] Naturally, some question the equity of an aid program that provides more federal money for poor people in high-income states than for poor people in low-income states.

Why per Capita Income Is an Imperfect Measure of State Resources

Analysts have opened a second front in the attack on the FMAP, arguing that per capita income is a bad measure of state economic or tax-raising resources. The main thrust of this argument is that personal income reflects only the income of a state's residents and thus does not reflect properly the role of interstate income flows. It understates fiscal capacity when income is produced in a state but paid to nonresidents (such as wages paid to in-commuters), because the income is counted in the nonresident's state. (States can and do tax this income.) Likewise, it overstates fiscal capacity when income received by residents is produced elsewhere, because both the producing and the receiving state may tax that income; when personal income is used as a fiscal capacity measure, it implicitly assumes that the receiving state can tax this income with impunity. These issues are especially important for states that have large numbers of in- or out-commuters or that have large amounts of business production that is exported to other states.

An alternative measure suggested by the General Accounting Office (GAO) in the past is "total taxable resources," estimated annually by the U.S. Department of the Treasury. It averages income received in a state (personal income) with a rough measure of income produced in a state (gross state product), implicitly assuming that receiving and producing states each have about a 50 percent claim to interstate income flows.[28] Total taxable resources is a misnomer, however, as it would not be practical for states to tax some elements of gross state product, and for states and the federal government to tax some kinds of income not found in this measure. The gross state product data on which this measure relies are slow to be released. As of this writing, the most recent year for which gross state product has been released by the U.S. Department of Commerce is 1994. While personal income is an imperfect measure of state resources, it is more timely than better data, and better than other equally timely data.

Alternatives to the Current FMAP

Over the years many analysts have suggested alternatives that might shift more federal Medicaid spending to poorer states, or otherwise improve the equity of funding in their eyes. GAO and the Kaiser commission have suggested changes such as:

—Using personal income per person in poverty rather than per capita, so that the FMAP takes into account the resources a state has per needy person;

—Using income per needy person, with the poverty measure and perhaps the income measure adjusted for cost-of-living differences across states, to recognize that a dollar of income does not go as far in a high-cost state as it does in a low-cost state;

—Using a more comprehensive measure of state resources, such as the U.S. Treasury's estimates of total taxable resources;

—Lowering the maximum state contribution from 50 to 45 or 40 percent; and

—Adding an incentive factor to reward states with lower-than-average spending.[29]

All of these changes would raise enormous political issues because they could rearrange billions of dollars of federal aid among the states. Furthermore, as policymakers examine alternatives, they have to confront the hard realities of soft data. There is a reason that many analysts examine spending per $100 of personal income despite its conceptual shortcomings: personal income is a reasonably broad measure of a state's resources, available in a reasonably consistent fashion across time and states, and available on a reasonably timely basis. The most important component of personal income—wages—is collected from a survey of several hundred thousand employers, and is of fairly high quality.

Poverty data, on the other hand, are collected as part of the Current Population Survey—a survey of households so small that poverty estimates for a single year generally are not reliable at the state level. Furthermore, official poverty data are not adjusted for cost-of-living differences across states. Everyone knows that it costs more to live in New York City than in Mississippi, and that an income sufficient to buy food and pay the rent in Mississippi may not be sufficient in New York; however, no government agency measures this difference in a consistent fashion on a regular basis.[30] Official poverty statistics therefore assume the same poverty level in all of the contiguous states.

Comprehensive measures of state tax capacity suffer from similar shortcomings. The conundrum policymakers face is that per capita income is a less-than-ideal measure of state resources, and of the need for Medicaid services, but conceptually better measures, such as total taxable resources, must either (1) rely on data that are several years old, (2) rely on less-reliable estimates of more current data, or (3) be made more current by investing additional money in data gathering and analysis.

Despite the enormous issues that changing the FMAP would raise, the issue would become more important under some of the Medicaid reform options put forward in recent years. Many Medicaid reform proposals have based initial federal aid to states on their current aid, which reflects the current reimbursement formula; future payments typically would be allowed to grow from this amount. Some of the issues that could arise in the context of Medicaid reform are:

—The current formula does not reflect the need for Medicaid services;

—High-income states frequently receive more federal aid per poor person than low-income states, in part as a result of state-level policy choices and in part as a result of differing price structures across states; and

—Changing the reimbursement formula is difficult because of data weaknesses; thus policymakers who wish to change the formula to better reflect Medicaid need or fiscal capacity must either accept the fact that the underlying data have significant weaknesses or are not timely, or that improved data will cost more money.

The Importance of Medicaid to State Budgets

Medicaid is important to not just the federal budget; it is the largest grants-in-aid program to state and local governments. In 1994 Medicaid accounted for 40 percent of all federal grants in aid to state and local governments, up from only 14 percent in 1975. Over that twenty-year period, Medicaid payments to state and local governments increased by 1,174 percent, while non-Medicaid payments increased by only 203 percent.[31]

Medicaid is a large and growing share of state budgets. Table 3-2 shows the share of state budgets spent on Medicaid and other major expenditure categories in selected years, for different fund types.

Medicaid Relative to State General Fund Budgets

One way of looking at Medicaid is to examine it as a share of states' general fund expenditures. States' general funds are not earmarked for any special purpose, and most state tax revenue is deposited in the general fund.[32] By looking at the general fund one looks primarily at the portion of Medicaid that is paid for with state tax revenue, excluding the portion that is paid for with federal funds.

In state fiscal years ending in 1994, Medicaid spending amounted to 14 percent of states' general fund expenditures, up from 12 percent in 1992 and from only 8 percent in 1987. State estimates for 1996 suggest that Medicaid increased its share of states' expenditures again. Medicaid is now the second-largest component of state budgets, edging out higher educa-

Table 3-2. *Medicaid and Other Programs as Percentage of State Budgets, Selected Years, 1987–96*

Percent unless otherwise indicated

State fiscal year	Fund type	Total ($ billions)	Medicaid	Elementary and secondary education	Higher education	Cash assistance	Corrections	All other
1987	General fund	212.6	8.1	34.2	15.5	5.3	5.0	31.8
	Other state funds	97.1	0.7	9.0	11.0	0.4	0.6	78.3
	Federal funds	89.7	26.0	11.5	6.4	10.3	0.1	45.6
	Total funds	405.3	10.2	22.8	12.3	5.2	3.0	46.7
1990	General fund	264.5	9.5	33.5	14.6	4.9	5.5	32.1
	Other state funds	110.8	1.4	10.6	15.3	0.5	0.8	71.4
	Federal funds	110.9	31.8	11.5	3.2	10.4	0.1	43.0
	Total funds	496.1	12.5	22.8	12.2	5.0	3.4	44.1
1992	General fund	293.4	12.1	34.0	13.5	5.1	5.6	29.6
	Other state funds	136.1	6.5	7.2	14.4	0.5	0.6	70.9
	Federal funds	149.0	40.9	10.2	2.6	8.9	0.1	37.2
	Total funds	592.2	17.8	21.5	11.0	4.9	3.2	42.0
1994	General fund	322.2	14.2	33.9	13.0	4.9	6.2	27.9
	Other state funds	159.5	6.5	6.7	14.3	0.4	0.7	71.4
	Federal funds	182.3	42.5	9.8	2.7	6.7	0.1	38.1
	Total funds	679.0	19.7	20.4	10.8	4.2	3.4	41.4
1996	General fund	356.0	14.8	34.1	12.9	3.9	6.8	27.4
	Other state funds	183.4	8.1	9.2	13.9	0.4	0.8	67.7
	Federal funds	194.4	43.0	10.0	2.8	6.0	0.3	37.8
	Total funds	746.2	20.3	21.3	10.7	3.5	3.7	40.5

Sources: National Association of State Budget Officers, *State Expenditure Report*, various years: 1987 numbers are from the 1989 report; 1990 numbers are from 1992; 1992 numbers are from 1994; 1994 numbers are from 1995. 1996 numbers are estimates by state budget officials. Bond funds (not shown) are included in total funds.

tion for second place behind elementary and secondary education. State spending on Medicaid is more than twice as large as spending on corrections, and larger by an even greater margin than state spending on cash-assistance programs such as AFDC.[33]

Medicaid's increasing share of states' general fund expenditures means that it has been growing faster than other programs, on average. In fact, between 1990 and 1992 non-Medicaid programs grew by 8 percent, while Medicaid grew by 42 percent. Between 1990 and 1992 Medicaid consumed fully 36 percent of the total growth in states' general fund expenditures. Although Medicaid growth slowed between 1992 and 1994, it still consumed 35 percent of growth in states' general fund spending.[34]

General fund numbers often are thought of as representing the portion of state spending that is a "burden" on a state's taxpayers. These numbers overstate Medicaid's importance in that sense: sometimes increases in state Medicaid spending occur because states have been creative in devising ways to maximize federal reimbursement. For example, states may shift costs into Medicaid that might otherwise be paid entirely from state funds, or they may make Medicaid payments from the general fund that are partly offset, on the bottom line, with Medicaid-related revenue such as taxes on hospitals and nursing homes. States sometimes use these devices to increase federal Medicaid reimbursement without increasing net costs paid by the state—actually saving taxpayers money, although the appearance is the opposite.[35]

There do not seem to be good data on the approximate magnitude of the first kind of Medicaid maximization strategy—shifting other state costs into Medicaid—but two examples drawn from work by the Urban Institute may be useful:[36]

—As Medicaid eligibility for pregnant women and children was expanded, states shifted related services from another federal funding source, the Maternal and Child Health Block Grant, to Medicaid, freeing up money from that grant for other uses.

—States have moved AIDS patients from state-funded general assistance programs to federally funded SSI, saving state cash assistance costs, while also making the patients categorically eligible for federal Medicaid reimbursement.

Both of these actions increased state Medicaid costs, but reduced other state costs.

The Urban Institute also has examined the second kind of maximization strategy—special financing programs. They note that between 1990 and 1992 states increased total DSH payments from $902 million in the

1990 federal fiscal year to $17.4 billion in 1992. The approximately $8 billion state share of this increase contributed to the large increase in states' general fund spending between 1990 and 1992. But states appear to have recouped most of the DSH-related increase through special provider taxes, donations, and intergovernmental transfers, which in aggregate increased from $403 million in 1990 to $7.7 billion in 1992.[37] Thus, although DSH payments caused a large increase in reported state general fund expenditures, their net impact on state budgets was much smaller.

Medicaid Relative to Total State Budgets

Although Medicaid maximization strategies can cause general fund expenditures to overstate the importance of Medicaid to state finances, in another sense the general fund understates the importance of Medicaid. Changes in the federal share of Medicaid—not reflected in general fund numbers—clearly have an impact on state budgets. If federal support for Medicaid were to disappear entirely, many states would replace some of the lost federal revenue with state tax dollars. Since the federal share of Medicaid is even larger than the state share, it is important to pay attention to total Medicaid expenditures as well as general fund expenditures. In 1994 state fiscal years, total state Medicaid expenditures, including the portion financed by the federal government, were 19.7 percent of total state expenditures, up from 17.8 percent in 1992 and only 10.2 percent in 1987.[38] State estimates for 1996 suggest that Medicaid increased its share of total state expenditures again.

No matter how the numbers are viewed, it is clear that Medicaid is of large and growing importance to states and has crowded out other government spending. Elected officials are well aware of this phenomenon and many have taken action to control Medicaid costs. To quote Governor Evan Bayh of Indiana in 1992: "If you want more money for education, you have to join us in fighting the exploding Medicaid budget. If you believe in holding the line on taxes, as I do, you have to be our ally in restraining these Medicaid costs. If you want jobs and economic growth, health care costs have to be brought under control."[39]

Outlook under Current Law

Now that Medicaid growth has been slowing for the past three years, is the fiscal crisis over? What would happen in the years ahead, absent changes in federal policy? Key factors that will affect Medicaid growth in the future include the number of recipients, the rate of medical price inflation, and the mix of beneficiaries.

Recipients

Growth in the number of recipients will be affected by state and federal policies, and by economic and demographic trends. The number of low-income adults and children will be subject to small upward pressure due to final stages of the mandated expansions. This upward pressure will be mitigated by downward pressure from continuing AFDC-related declines in the states. The net impact almost certainly will be small, given that this population is not expensive.

The number of aged recipients—an extremely expensive group—had been declining for most years until 1990 despite a growing elderly population, due to declining elderly poverty. However, elderly recipients have now increased for six consecutive years. As the baby boomers begin to age, the elderly population will grow more quickly than in previous years. The Census Bureau predicts that the sixty-five-and-over population will increase by 5 percent between 1995 and 2000, and about 10 percent between 1995 and 2005. Growth will accelerate after 2005, with total growth of 19.2 percent predicted between 1995 and 2010.[40] This growth will not lead to a near-term cost crisis, but it will place inexorable and accelerating upward pressure on program costs. The pressure will arrive sooner and be more intense in some states than in others. For example, the elderly population is expected to grow by more than 20 percent between 1995 and 2005 in Arizona, Arkansas, Colorado, Florida, Georgia, and Nevada. Between 1995 and 2010 the Census Bureau expects growth of more than 40 percent in Arizona and Nevada.

The disabled now are the largest Medicaid expenditure group, having surpassed the elderly in the late 1980s. Much of the growth in recent years was driven by retroactive disability determinations required by the *Sullivan* v. *Zebley* decision. Growth in this category will slow or even come to a halt over the next several years as a result of the 1996 welfare reform legislation, under which individualized functional assessments will no longer be used as a basis for determining SSI eligibility. Children who obtained benefits under this provision have had their SSI eligibility reviewed, and many may lose SSI benefits. Under the provision as originally enacted, children who lose SSI benefits also would have lost Medicaid benefits if they did not qualify for other reasons. As amended in the 1997 balanced budget agreement, children will not lose Medicaid solely because they have lost SSI.

Medical Price Inflation

In recent years, the medical price inflation premium has dropped dramatically. Inflation for medical commodities has dropped below the economywide inflation rate, and the premium for medical services above general price inflation has diminished. The Health Care Financing Administration (HCFA) predicted in 1996 that most prices for medical goods, medical services, and inputs will grow at rates averaging about 2.5 to 3.5 percent over the next six years—not much higher than overall price inflation.[41]

Shifting Mix

Although the growth in the number of recipients should be fairly slow over the next several years, the number of elderly recipients may grow more quickly than the number of children and low-income adult recipients. As elderly recipients are much more expensive than children and low-income adults, the average expenditure per recipient could continue to grow more rapidly than the rate of change in medical prices.

Implications

Forecasts prepared in 1996 by John Holahan and David Liska of the Urban Institute suggest that over the next five years, overall Medicaid expenditures will grow by about 7.4 percent annually, with beneficiary growth ranging from 1 to 3.5 percent, depending on eligibility group, and with average cost per beneficiary growing by about 5 to 6 percent annually, depending on category of service.[42] While these near-term growth rates are much slower than growth rates in the late 1980s and early 1990s, they still are likely to be faster than the growth in other state programs, and in state tax revenue, given an inflation environment of about 3 percent. Over the longer term (five to ten years out), Medicaid will grow more rapidly as the aging of the population accelerates. Selected states will feel this pressure in the near term, but for most states the aging of the population will not have a significant impact until 2005 or beyond. There will be no sudden fiscal crisis, just continuing upward pressure on program costs that will lead to continuing policy innovation and intervention to keep costs manageable. States will have an opportunity to plan rationally for growing Medicaid costs.

Underlying baseline growth in Medicaid is not the only factor that will determine how states will be affected by Medicaid reform. Current state Medicaid policies and economic and demographic conditions also will play a role in how states are affected by Medicaid reform.

Variations across States

Medicaid expenditures vary from state to state due to differences in state economic and demographic conditions and differences in policy choices. For example, states with high poverty, poor health conditions, an older population, or high costs of living might be expected to have higher Medicaid costs than other states. Also, some states may choose policies— either by exercising flexibility within Medicaid rules or seeking waivers to go beyond what the ordinary rules allow—that lead to higher costs by expanding eligibility or offering many services. Not surprisingly, the largest states spend the most on Medicaid. In 1995 the top three Medicaid-spending states—New York, California, and Florida—accounted for one-third of the nation's total Medicaid spending. New York, however, spent about 50 percent more than California, even though California's population is 78 percent larger than New York's.

Thus the enormous variation in Medicaid expenditures across states is not simply the result of differences in the degree of poverty; even on a per-poor-person basis, expenditures vary enormously across states.[43] Spending per poor person averaged $4,105 in 1995, ranging from $11,196 in New Hampshire to $1,974 in Oklahoma—a fivefold difference. Quantified explanations of why Medicaid spending varies across states are beyond the scope of this chapter, but this section delves into the extent of, and some of the apparent reasons for, variation.[44]

Depth and Breadth of Coverage

Total Medicaid expenditures per poor person can be divided into three components: (1) the amount a state spends on Medicaid services per enrollee (depth of coverage), (2) the breadth of coverage, measured by Medicaid enrollment as a share of the poverty population (this is greater than the share of poor people actually covered by Medicaid, as state Medicaid programs often allow some non-poor people to enroll); and (3) the amount a state spends through the DSH program—which cannot be tied to specific services or enrollees.[45, 46] DSH payments are highly concentrated among a few states that have been heavy users of the program, and the following analysis excludes these payments in order to concentrate on expenditures per enrollee and breadth of coverage.[47] Unless noted, subsequent discussion of expenditures in this chapter refers to non-DSH expenditures.

Table 3-3 lists states in descending order of spending per poor person, and indexes each state to the U.S. average for spending per poor person, spending per enrollee (depth), and enrollees as a share of the poor population (breadth).[48] A number greater than one means the state is above the average, and a number less than one means the state is below the average. The spending-per-poor-person index (within rounding error) is obtained by multiplying the depth index by the breadth index. States spending the most per poor person tend to be high on both dimensions, states spending the least tend to be low on both, and many states are high on one dimension and low on the other.

Figure 3-4 takes the same data and plots and categorizes the states according to depth and breadth of coverage.[49] The vertical and horizontal lines show average coverage and average expenditures per enrollee, respectively. States in the upper right quadrant have deep (high per-enrollee expenditures) and broad coverage; states in the lower left quadrant have shallow (low per-enrollee expenditures) and narrow coverage as a share of their poor population. States in the other quadrants are high on one dimension and low on the other.

The middle curve in figure 3-4 shows the combination of coverage and expenditures per enrollee that yields national average expenditures per *poor person*. States located near this curve have expenditures per poor person near the national average of $3,589.[50] States to the right of the curve have above-average expenditures per poor person, and those to the left have lower-than-average expenditures. The upper curve gives the combination of coverage and spending per enrollee that yields expenditures per poor person of

Table 3-3. *Indexes of Non-DSH Spending per Poor Person by State,*
1995

State	Spending per poor person	Spending per enrollee	Enrollees per poor person
Rhode Island	2.19	1.67	1.32
Massachusetts	1.99	1.72	1.15
New York	1.95	1.98	.98
New Hampshire	1.89	1.50	1.28
Hawaii	1.79	n.a.	n.a.
District of Columbia	1.73	1.99	.87
Connecticut	1.72	1.63	1.05
New Jersey	1.68	1.43	1.17
Maine	1.65	1.19	1.38
Vermont	1.59	.88	1.80
Minnesota	1.58	1.56	1.01
Wisconsin	1.54	1.20	1.28
Alaska	1.51	1.03	1.47
Delaware	1.36	1.17	1.16
Pennsylvania	1.23	1.15	1.07
Maryland	1.20	1.15	1.04
Nebraska	1.17	1.10	1.06
Tennessee	1.17	.70	1.66
North Dakota	1.14	1.32	.86
Ohio	1.09	1.07	1.01
Oregon	1.09	.90	1.21
West Virginia	1.08	.86	1.25
Illinois	1.06	.90	1.18
Washington	1.06	.91	1.16
Michigan	1.04	1.03	1.01
U.S. average	1.00	1.00	1.00
North Carolina	.99	.95	1.05
Colorado	.97	.98	.99
Iowa	.97	1.06	.92
Georgia	.91	.77	1.18
Wyoming	.90	.90	1.00
Arkansas	.88	.99	.89
Montana	.85	1.06	.80
Missouri	.84	.79	1.07
Kentucky	.83	.85	.98
South Dakota	.82	1.16	.71
Louisiana	.81	1.11	.73

State	Spending per poor person	Spending per enrollee	Enrollees per poor person
Virginia	.77	.81	.94
Florida	.73	.82	.88
Kansas	.72	.94	.77
South Carolina	.69	.88	.78
Indiana	.68	.81	.85
California	.67	.60	1.11
Mississippi	.65	.75	.87
Nevada	.62	.83	.74
Idaho	.60	.78	.76
Texas	.58	.77	.76
Oklahoma	.55	.74	.74
Alabama	.55	.76	.72
New Mexico	.55	.72	.76

Source: Federal spending is from HCFA, *Medicaid Statistics, 1995,* HCFA-64 report tables, table 1, p. 135. Number of persons in poverty calculated by author, using average of 1994 and 1995 poverty rates multiplied by 1995 populations; all data were provided by the Bureau of the Census (www.census.gov).

$6,000, and the lower curve gives the combination that yields $2,500. States near one of these lines have approximately the same expenditures per poor person, yet may arrive at this expenditure through different means. For example, the District of Columbia (upper left quadrant) and Vermont (lower right quadrant) are both near the upper line, so each spends close to $6,000 per poor person.[51] D.C. has high expenditures per enrollee but narrow coverage, however, and Vermont has broad coverage but below-average expenditures per enrollee.

Several observations are apparent from table 3-3 and figure 3-4:

—There is no clear relationship between depth and breadth of coverage. States with high spending per poor person can be high on one dimension and low on the other.

—Many northeastern states have deep and broad coverage.

—Many southern and western states have below-average depth and breadth of coverage, including the three states with the lowest spending per poor person—Alabama, Oklahoma, and New Mexico.

—Vermont covers far more people, relative to its poverty population,

Figure 3-4. *Breadth and Depth of Coverage for Non-DSH Spending per Poor Person*

Percent unless otherwise indicated

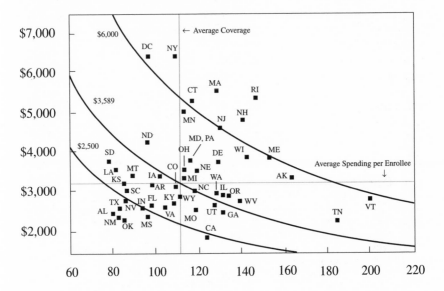

Source: Federal spending is from HCFA, *Medicaid Statistics, 1995*, HCFA-64 report tables, table 1, p. 135. Numbr of persons in poverty calculated by author, using average of 1994 and 1995 poverty rates multiplied by 1995 populations; all data were provided by the Bureau of the Census (www.census.gov).

than any other state. Tennessee also is a high-coverage state. Both have below-average expenditures per enrollee.

As figure 3-4 makes clear, there is no such thing as a typical state in any of the four groups. Each group has one or more states near the boundary of another group, a few states close to the center and therefore much like the U.S. average, and a diversity of states elsewhere in the quadrant. States in each group tend to have characteristics that distinguish them from states in other groups, although there are many exceptions. Generalizations about a group are most true for states that are far from the boundary lines, and least true for states close to these lines.[52] Small changes in data could move boundary states from one group to another. Figure 3-5 lists the states in each group.

Figure 3-5. *States as Categorized by Depth and Breadth of Coverage*

High	**Deep and Narrow** District of Columbia Iowa Louisiana Montana New York North Dakota South Dakota	**Deep and Broad** Alaska Connecticut Delaware Maine Maryland Massachusetts Michigan Minnesota Nebraska New Hampshire New Jersey Ohio Pennsylvania Rhode Island Wisconsin
Low	**Shallow and Narrow** Alabama Arkansas Colorado Florida Idaho Indiana Kansas Kentucky Mississippi Nevada New Mexico Oklahoma South Carolina Texas Virginia	**Shallow and Broad** California Georgia Illinois Missouri North Carolina Oregon Tennessee Utah Vermont Washington West Virginia Wyoming
	Low	High

Enrollees as percent of poverty population

Some of the factors that might influence a state's breadth or depth of coverage include (1) AFDC and medically needy income thresholds as a percentage of the federal poverty level, which are policy variables affecting breadth and potentially depth of coverage—a higher threshold means a state is likely to cover a greater number of people, all else being equal;[53] (2) the number of optional services covered, which might affect the cost of the program per enrollee; (3) average nursing home reimbursement rates, which might be considered a policy variable or a variable reflecting underlying market forces; (4) average wages in the hospital and nursing home industries, which reflect underlying market forces and also might reflect state policies; (5) per capita income and the poverty rate, which might be considered measures of resources and needs, respectively; and (6) the extent to which state residents consider themselves either liberal, moderate, or conservative, suggesting the degree to which residents would support a broad or deep Medicaid program (although such support is highly correlated with income).[54]

Broad and deep states tend to have relatively high eligibility levels for the categorically needy, and all but three of the fifteen such states have a medically needy program. They also generally offer more optional services than other states and have higher nursing home reimbursement rates. Massachusetts clearly fits the broad and deep mold: its breadth of coverage is 15 percent above the national average and its depth of coverage is 72 percent above the national average. Massachusetts's AFDC income eligibility threshold is 52 percent of the federal poverty level, as compared with a national average of only 41 percent; the state's income eligibility thresholds for medically needy coverage and for coverage of pregnant women and infants also are above the national average.[55] Factors that might influence spending per enrollee also are higher than the national average: for example, Massachusetts offered both its categorically needy recipients and its medically needy recipients twenty-seven out of thirty-four possible optional services, and its average nursing home reimbursement rate in 1992 was about 25 percent above the national average.

Broad and deep states, many of which are in the Northeast or Midwest, generally have lower poverty rates, higher per capita incomes, and view themselves as more liberal than the national average. Wages of hospital and nursing home workers in these states are higher than the national average. These states necessarily have higher-than-average Medicaid spending per poor person, given that they have higher-than-average coverage and spending per covered person. Finally, broad and deep states tend to have very high DSH expenditures per poor person, perhaps helping to finance their broad coverage.[56]

Narrow and deep states are more difficult to generalize about. Both New York and the District of Columbia combine extremely high spending per enrollee (98 percent and 99 percent above average, respectively) with coverage that is not far below average (2 percent and 13 percent, respectively). The combination of high spending per enrollee, a moderate number of enrollees relative to the poor population, and high poverty rates (extremely high in the case of D.C.) means that the District of Columbia and New York are by far the two highest-spending states in the nation on a *per capita* basis. They also score high on spending *per poor person*, with New York ranking third in the nation and D.C. ranking sixth.

Most other states in this group have spending per enrollee that is only moderately above average and coverage that is moderately below average. North Dakota is perhaps more typical of this group, with breadth of coverage that is 14 percent below average and spending per enrollee that is 32 percent above average. In August 1995, however, North Dakota expanded coverage for children ages thirteen to seventeen and for some adults with high medical expenditures, so its breadth of coverage should increase in future years.

New York and D.C. have very high per capita incomes, high poverty rates, liberal ideologies, and very high wages in the hospital and nursing home industries. Most other states in this group have below-average incomes, low poverty rates (Louisiana excepted), and relatively low measures of health care costs.

Broad and shallow states also are diverse. This is perhaps the most interesting category because these states manage to cover large numbers of beneficiaries relative to their poverty population at low cost per beneficiary. Most of these states are in the South or the West, but they tend to have relatively low poverty. Tennessee and Vermont cover far more individuals, relative to their poverty populations, than do other states in the group; Tennessee's breadth of coverage is 66 percent above the national average, and Vermont's is 80 percent above.

Tennessee's Medicaid program, known as TennCare, is a capitated managed-care waiver program implemented in 1994 that provides health care to Medicaid beneficiaries, uninsured state residents, and those with uninsurable medical conditions.[57] Under TennCare pregnant women and infants are automatically eligible if their income is below 185 percent of the federal poverty level; uninsured individuals may pay subsidized premiums to be covered by TennCare, with the subsidy phasing out by 400 percent of the federal poverty level. Vermont's Health Access Plan covers pregnant women up to 200 percent of the federal poverty level and infants up to 225 percent.[58] According to the Intergovernmental Health Policy Project, "as of May 1995, Medicaid had enrolled 84 percent of children below 225 percent of poverty level, about 12,000 children, one of the highest rates in the country."[59] The Vermont Health Access Plan was expanded further, effective January 1996, to include uninsured residents with income up to 150 percent of the federal poverty level. Vermont's program appears more comprehensive than Tennessee's, offering twenty-seven of thirty-four allowable services, while Tennessee's program offers eighteen services.[60]

Other states in this group generally have income eligibility thresholds that are more generous than states on average, but less generous than those in Tennessee and Vermont. California is notable because, although it has very broad coverage, it also provides a comprehensive array of services—more than any other state but Wisconsin. Michael Sparer argues in *Medicaid and the Limits of State Health Reform* that California keeps costs low in large part because its program administrators have considerable flexibility in implementing provider reimbursement systems, and interest groups have less influence than in New York.[61]

An important question—that is well beyond the scope of this chapter—is whether states in this group attain broad coverage at relatively low cost per enrollee because they are more efficient than other states, or whether their low costs result from tighter controls on usage, fewer services, poorer quality, beneficiaries that are less expensive to serve, lower costs of health care inputs (such as salaries of health care workers), or other reasons. It is worth noting that Tennessee's and Vermont's relatively low costs per beneficiary do not appear to be driven simply by a favorable age mix of their recipients—analysis discussed later in this chapter shows that neither state would have very different payments per recipient if it instead had the national age mix. Moreover, the average wages of hospital and nursing home workers are below the national average in these two states, thus low input costs may play a role in their low Medicaid costs.

Narrow and shallow states are found mostly in the South. Eight of the fifteen states do not have a medically needy program, and five of the other seven have income thresholds, as a percentage of the federal poverty level, below the national average. Although Texas has a medically needy program, it apparently does not cover the aged, blind, and disabled.[62] Choices to eschew or restrict the medically needy program limit not only the breadth, but also the depth of coverage, since medically needy recipients tend to be more costly to serve than other beneficiary groups. For every state in the group but Kentucky, AFDC thresholds for categorical eligibility were below the national average. Likewise nursing home reimbursement rates were below the national average for every state in the group but Florida, which was at the average. States in this group necessarily have lower-than-average spending per poor person, given that they have lower-than-average coverage and spending per covered person.

Most states in this category have high poverty rates, low per capita income, and conservative ideologies. Cost factors such as wages of hospital and nursing home workers tend to be well below the national average. Table 3-4 shows these characteristics. The ideology index reflects the extent to which state residents categorized themselves as liberal or conservative in telephone polls conducted by the Columbia Broadcasting System and the *New York Times* during the 1976–88 period. The index is calculated as the percentage answering "liberal" minus the percentage answering "con-

Table 3-4. *Key Characteristics of States as Grouped by Depth and Breadth of Medicaid Coverage*

Category	Deep and broad	Deep and narrow	Shallow and broad	Shallow and narrow
Depth: Non-DSH expenditure per enrollee	4,215	4,454	2,680	2,670
Breadth: Enrollees as percentage of poor people	130	93	138	92
Expenditures per capita (dollars)	625	774	504	420
Expenditures per poor person (dollars)	6,382	4,625	4,026	2,818
AFDC threshold as percentage of FPL	48	41	46	29
Medically needy threshold as percentage of FPL	45	37	42	15
Number of optional services	40	43	42	32
Nursing home per diem rate (dollars)	94	80	71	62
Hospital salaries (dollars)	28,401	26,778	27,538	25,721
Nursing home salaries (dollars)	17,065	14,954	14,502	13,981
1995 per capita income (dollars)	24,899	22,530	21,518	20,492
Poverty rate (percent)	10.1	16.0	12.7	15.4
Ideology index	(9.1)	(13.6)	(13.9)	(18.1)

Source: See note 54.

servative." A negative index indicates that a greater percentage of state residents consider themselves conservative rather than liberal. The more negative the index, the more conservative residents consider themselves.

Factors Leading to High Spending per Medicaid Enrollee

Variations in expenditures per enrollee and in coverage of the poor population are at the heart of interstate variations in cost, and it is worthwhile to investigate them separately, before recapping.

EXPENSIVE BENEFICIARIES. Perhaps some states spend more than others because their Medicaid populations are more expensive to serve? One way to examine this question is to control for the mix of beneficiaries by computing what each state would spend per recipient if it had the same recipient mix as the nation as a whole, but retained its state-specific costs. Table 3-5 shows the results of this exercise.[63] The first column shows actual vendor payments per recipient. The second column shows what these payments would be if each state's recipients had the nation's age distribution. A state whose actual payments are less than its age-adjusted payments has a favorable age mix (that is, its recipient mix is less expensive and probably younger than the national average). The third column shows actual payments per recipient indexed to the national average, and the fourth shows age-adjusted payments indexed to the national average. The national average, of course, does not change since it already reflects the average age mix.

The fifth column is the age-adjusted index minus the actual index. If it is positive, then the state has an unfavorable age mix. For example, Alaska's actual index is 1.07—its average payment per recipient is 7 percent above the national average. But Alaska has a favorable age mix, with a younger population than the rest of the country. If Alaska had the national age mix, its costs would be much higher: its index would be 1.33, so its payment per recipient would be 33 percent above the national average. Because Alaska has a much smaller elderly population than other states, its average costs are much lower than if it had to serve a greater number of elderly people, with the more expensive services they usually receive.

For about two-thirds of the states, their average payments—if adjusted to the national age mix—would be within 10 percentage points of their unadjusted average. Many deep-coverage (expensive) states have an unfavorable age mix, and many shallow-coverage states have a favorable mix.

For a few states, however, the impact is significant. Connecticut, Hawaii, Maine, Massachusetts, North Dakota, Rhode Island, and Wisconsin all are high-expenditure states and would have expenditures per recipient at least 10 percent lower, relative to the national average, if their Medicaid recipients had the national age mix.

REIMBURSEMENT RATES. The variation in reimbursement rates among states is enormous. For example, in 1992 average nursing home rates in deep-coverage District of Columbia and New York were $127 and $123 per day, respectively. In shallow-coverage California and Oklahoma, average rates were $73 and $46 per day, respectively.[64]

Payroll is a major expense of nursing homes. States with high nursing home rates have high wages in the nursing home industry, and those with low rates have low wages. For example, in 1993 the average nursing home wage in New York was $22,269, while the average wage in Oklahoma was $10,791.[65]

It might be that Medicaid also plays a role in high nursing home industry costs. Medicaid finances about half of all nursing home expenditures nationwide, so it clearly has an impact on the market for nursing home workers. In fact, in New York Medicaid finances more than 60 percent of all nursing home care.[66] Some analysts have suggested that high nursing home reimbursements may cause high nursing home wages rather than the other way around.[67]

STATE INCOME. It turns out that one can explain quite a bit of the variation in spending per poor person by the variation in incomes: richer states spend more on Medicaid, per poor person, than do poor states. This is not surprising: just as people with high incomes tend to buy more of almost everything than people with low incomes, states with higher incomes tend to purchase more Medicaid than low-income states. Other things being equal, wealthy states require less tax effort to support Medicaid than poor states.[68]

It is plausible to expect that states with high poverty rates will spend less per poor person than states with low poverty rates, all else being equal, since they have to spread their resources over a broader base of poor people. In general:

—States with low poverty rates tend to have lower expenditures per poor person than states with high poverty rates, although there are many exceptions to this general tendency.

—Northeastern states tend to spend quite a bit more per poor person

Table 3-5. *Medicaid Spending per Recipient as Adjusted for National Age Mix, 1995*

State	Vendor payments per recipient[a]	Payments if U.S. age mix[a]	Index of actual payments	Index if U.S. age mix	Impact of age mix
Alaska	3,698	4,570	1.07	1.33	0.25
Delaware	4,126	4,838	1.20	1.41	0.21
District of Columbia	3,843	4,545	1.11	1.32	0.20
Utah	2,895	3,518	0.84	1.02	0.18
Idaho	3,129	3,637	0.91	1.06	0.15
West Virginia	3,009	3,503	0.87	1.02	0.14
South Carolina	2,902	3,368	0.84	0.98	0.14
New Mexico	2,491	2,912	0.72	0.84	0.12
Wyoming	3,328	3,678	0.97	1.02	0.10
Texas	2,562	2,805	0.74	0.81	0.07
Nevada	3,322	3,554	0.96	1.03	0.07
Washington	2,285	2,492	0.66	0.72	0.05
Illinois	3,608	3,813	1.05	1.11	0.05
Michigan	2,918	3,095	0.85	0.90	0.05
Montana	3,300	3,474	0.96	1.01	0.05
Kansas	3,250	3,420	0.94	0.99	0.05
Indiana	3,359	3,526	0.97	1.02	0.05
Georgia	2,681	2,830	0.78	0.82	0.04
Vermont	3,210	3,356	0.93	0.97	0.04
Virginia	2,690	2,833	0.78	0.82	0.04
Colorado	3,619	3,734	1.05	1.08	0.03
Nebraska	3,609	3,723	1.05	1.08	0.03
Louisiana	3,449	3,537	1.00	1.03	0.03
Alabama	2,698	2,778	0.78	0.61	0.02
Ohio	3,644	3,706	1.06	1.08	0.02
California	2,097	2,144	0.61	0.62	0.01
Missouri	2,932	2,964	0.85	0.86	0.01
Florida	2,768	2,776	0.80	0.81	—
South Dakota	4,120	4,125	1.20	1.20	—
Tennessee	1,891	1,847	0.55	0.54	(0.01)
North Carolina	2,928	2,871	0.85	0.83	(0.02)
New Hampshire	4,880	4,820	1.42	1.40	(0.02)
Kentucky	3,035	2,969	0.88	0.86	(0.02)
Oregon	2,937	2,865	0.85	0.83	(0.02)
Mississippi	2,436	2,353	0.71	0.68	(0.02)

(Table continues)

Table 3-5. (*continued*)

State	Vendor payments per recipient[a]	Payments if U.S. age mix[a]	Index of actual payments	Index if U.S. age mix	Impact of age mix
Oklahoma	2,680	2,585	0.78	0.75	(0.03)
Iowa	3,406	3,302	0.99	0.96	(0.03)
Minnesota	5,386	5,220	1.58	1.51	(0.05)
Maryland	4,873	4,704	1.41	1.36	(0.05)
Arkansas	3,893	3,695	1.13	1.07	(0.06)
Pennsylvania	3,766	3,532	1.09	1.02	(0.07)
New Jersey	4,828	4,576	1.40	1.33	(0.07)
New York	7,276	7,016	2.11	2.04	(0.08)
Maine	4,965	4,602	1.44	1.34	(0.11)
North Dakota	4,839	4,441	1.40	1.29	(0.12)
Rhode Island	4,973	4,455	1.44	1.29	(0.15)
Wisconsin	4,118	3,561	1.19	1.03	(0.16)
Connecticut	5,588	4,908	1.62	1.42	(0.20)
Massachusetts	5,460	4,697	1.58	1.36	(0.22)
Hawaii	4,983	3,140	1.45	0.91	(0.53)
Sum of states	3,447	3,447	1.00	1.00	—

Source: Author's calculations based on data in Health Care Financing Administration, *Medicaid Statistics: Program and Financial Statistics, Fiscal Year 1995.*

a. Dollars.

b. Figure represents index of actual payments minus index if U.S. age mix.

than most other states. They also have lower-than-average poverty rates, with New York being the notable exception.

—Most southern and western states have lower-than-average expenditures per poor person.

IDEOLOGICAL LEANING. Another factor that might affect Medicaid spending is the willingness of a state's citizens to spend their resources to meet the need; that is, some measure of their ideological leaning. While it is difficult to measure the ideological leanings of a state's citizens, measures do exist, based on citizens' self-perceptions. In this chapter I have used an index calculated by subtracting the percentage of respondents who consider themselves conservative from the percentage of those who consider themselves liberal. It is clear from table 3-4 that residents of states with deep and broad coverage consider themselves less conservative than those from states with shallow and narrow coverage. It is difficult to separate the impact of ideology from the impact of income, as residents of high-income states tend to consider themselves less conservative than those from low-income states.

What Has Been Learned?

Medicaid expenditures per poor person vary enormously across states, but one must be cautious in drawing conclusions as to why. One cannot simply say that states with high Medicaid expenditures are generous and those with low expenditures are not. It is true that Medicaid expenditures reflect state policy choices about whom to cover, which services to offer, who can provide those services, and how much they should be paid—all of which can be considered related to state generosity. Yet Medicaid expenditures also reflect factors in part or wholly beyond state control, such as the health status and age distribution of the population, the condition of the economy, cost of living, the market power of health care providers, and the health care labor market. Furthermore, even the concept of state Medicaid expenditures can be hard to pin down. To the extent that states have been successful in "Medicaiding" services that otherwise would be financed from 100 percent state funds, and to the extent states have been successful in using provider taxes and other mechanisms to maximize federal reimbursement, high Medicaid expenditures may not reflect a generous commitment of state tax dollars, but rather success in minimizing the use of tax dollars.

Despite these caveats, one can explain a surprising amount of the variation in Medicaid expenditures across states based solely on our measures of resources (per capita income), need (poverty rate), and ideology. In fact, one can explain about 70 percent of the variation in state-only Medicaid expenditures using these three factors.[69] Of these three influences, income plays the greatest role, the poverty rate plays the next-largest role, and ideology, while important, is a fairly distant third.[70]

One can categorize states by depth and breadth of coverage, breaking down expenditures per poor person into expenditures per enrollee and enrollees relative to the poverty population, and draw the following conclusions:

—Depth of coverage (spending per enrollee) tends to increase as income rises, although the relationship is not very strong. Spending per enrollee tends to fall as the poverty rate rises.

—Breadth of coverage tends to rise as the poverty rate falls, but the relationship is not strong and there is no obvious relationship between breadth of coverage and per capita income.

—States with deep coverage do not necessarily have broad coverage— there simply is no apparent relationship between the two measures.

—Higher-income states tend to spend more per poor person, focusing on either high coverage or high expenditures, but not both.

—States with higher incomes spend more per poor person; for a given level of income, states with higher poverty rates must spread the same resources over more people, and thus spend less per poor person; and all else being equal, more liberal states spend more per poor person than conservative states.

In a Word, Flexibility

One clear conclusion from this discussion is that Medicaid is a different program in each state. States have enormous flexibility, and they use it. How can one summarize this flexibility neatly? One way is to look at how much money states spend on Medicaid above what they are required to spend. Two sources suggest that states choose to spend far more than they have to.

In a 1991 paper, Jane Sneddon Little, an economist at the Federal Reserve Bank of Boston, estimated how much California, Massachusetts, Minnesota, and New York spent on optional Medicaid programs and services in 1989. She examined the cost of medically needy programs and the cost of optional services. Because there is overlap between the two—some of the expense of optional services is for people who qualify for Medicaid under the medically needy option—it would be double counting to add the optional services and medically needy estimates together. Therefore Little did not come up with a single estimate for each state, but rather an estimate for the optional cost of the medically needy program and an estimate for optional services. Due to the overlap, the total cost states incur by choice is something more than the larger of the two numbers, but less than the sum.

Little's results are summarized in table 3-6. In two of the states optional costs were more than half of total costs, and probably an even greater share. In the other two states optional costs were at least a third of total costs:[71]

In a 1996 report on federal-state fiscal relations, Senator Daniel Patrick Moynihan estimated that of New York's $22.1 billion of 1995 Medicaid spending, $5.2 billion was mandatory and $16.9 billion, or 77 percent, was optional.[72]

While these numbers, with the exception of California, are for high-

Table 3-6. *Optional Medicaid Costs for Selected States*

State	Medically needy (percent)	Optional services (percent)
California	36	25
Massachusetts	54	44
Minnesota	39	42
New York	53	28

Source: Jane Sneddon Little, "Why State Medicaid Costs Vary: A First Look," Federal Reserve Bank of Boston, Working Paper 91-1, August 1991, p. 33.

expenditure states, it appears that states choose to spend a large share—perhaps even a majority of Medicaid spending—on programs and services that the federal government does not mandate.

With All This Flexibility, Who Needs Devolution?

Despite all this flexibility, states have found Medicaid restrictive in many ways.

Although states generally have great flexibility over who can obtain Medicaid services, in certain categories they have very little flexibility. For example, the blind and disabled consumed over 55 percent of the total growth in Medicaid vendor payments in 1994 and 1995, but states have almost no control over eligibility in this category: it is governed largely by federal SSI thresholds. Furthermore, states found their lack of control compounded by the *Sullivan* v. *Zebley* decision, which granted retroactive SSI eligibility for disabled children.

Where states do have flexibility over who can obtain services, Medicaid becomes an uncapped entitlement—in for a dime, in for a potentially unlimited number of dollars. Once states decide to cover the medically needy, for example, they must bear their share of services to eligible individuals without limit. This lack of control is one reason some states may choose to deliver some Medicaid-like services outside of the Medicaid system, forgoing federal matching money so that they can control eligibility and costs. States would like the flexibility to modify eligibility and benefits in a fashion that allows them to cap or limit costs.

Until recently states were required to offer Medicaid services in a statewide fashion and could not limit beneficiaries' freedom to choose providers, absent a waiver from HCFA. This runs counter to the whole concept of managed care, with gatekeepers and others deciding which providers beneficiaries can see, when, and for what services. States sought the flexibility to implement managed care without seeking federal waivers and received it in the Balanced Budget Act of 1997.[73]

States also have been frustrated with the requirement under the Boren amendment that reimbursement rates be "reasonably related" to actual costs for hospitals and nursing homes. This resulted in costly litigation and has limited states' ability to negotiate rates that the market will bear. States were able to circumvent the Boren amendment by obtaining waivers and using HMOs as intermediaries to negotiate with hospitals and nursing homes. In the 1997 budget agreement, however, they won their long-sought repeal of the Boren amendment.

States' new freedom in implementing managed care without waivers and in setting reimbursement rates will provide them with much greater flexibility than in the past. However, they still would like greater freedom to define eligible recipients and eligible services. States would also like to escape the HCFA bureaucracy, with its control over the waiver process and information-reporting requirements.

The Fiscal Implications of Devolution

With the new flexibility states gained through the Balanced Budget Act of 1997, is Medicaid devolution complete? CBO long-term budget projections show that although the federal budget may be balanced by 2002, the deficit will reappear in 2010 and beyond. Medicaid is an important contributor to this problem, due to the projected rapid growth in the expensive-to-serve elderly population. The federal government remains interested in devolution largely because it holds out the promise to slow growth in federal Medicaid costs. Any federal legislation to reform Medicaid will have several important elements that will determine how states fare from a fiscal perspective:

—*Initial level and distribution of funds:* How much will Medicaid be cut, and how severely will the distribution of funds be altered at the start?

—*Federal funding mechanism:* Will payments to states be capped and, if so, how? What sort of growth in total funding does the proposal allow, and how will it vary across states?

—*FMAP:* What share of costs will the federal government bear?

—*DSH payments and provider taxes:* Will states be allowed to continue DSH funding to hospitals? Will the current limitations of provider
taxes be repealed?

—*Provider reimbursements:* What flexibility will states have to negotiate payments to providers?

—*Beneficiaries:* Which categories will states be required or allowed to
cover? Will the program be an entitlement to beneficiaries?

—*Services:* Which services will states be required or allowed to offer?

—*Other flexibility:* Will states have flexibility to implement managed
care, for example, without requesting waivers from HCFA?

All of these issues are important, as is the interplay among them. This
section focuses on the first three questions, which have the most important
fiscal implications.

Medicaid proposals have varied greatly in the extent to which they
would cut the program. Medigrant, the block grant proposal passed by
Congress in 1995 and vetoed by the president, would have cut Medicaid
the deepest, reducing total spending by 28 percent by 2002 according to
the Kaiser commission. Congressional proposals in 1996 would have cut
total spending by about 22 percent in 2002, according to CRS, and the
president's proposal would have entailed somewhat smaller cuts.[74]

One of the most important *fiscal* questions for states probably relates
to the federal-state relationship: to what extent, and how, will the federal
government share in the cost of Medicaid? Current law provides an uncapped entitlement to states, with pro-rata federal cost sharing based on
each state's FMAP. The federal government shares in cost increases regardless of whether they are caused by (1) eligibility increases, resulting
perhaps from longer-term structural changes such as a growing population
and demographic shifts, shorter-term cyclical changes such as recession-
related poverty increases, changes in state policy such as an increase in the
medically needy income threshold, changes in federal policies, or changes
in judicial interpretation; (2) increases in services offered, service utilization, or the quality of service due to technological improvements; or (3)
increases in the cost of services due to overall price inflation or increases in
reimbursement rates above the general rate of inflation. Under the current
system, the effective price to states of a dollar of Medicaid services is less
than a dollar, depending on the FMAP. As discussed earlier, the effective
price is about 21 cents on the dollar in low-income Mississippi and 50 cents
on the dollar in high-income states such as California.

The current uncapped entitlement to states, with pro-rata federal sharing in all cost increases, is at one end of a continuum. At another extreme is a full block grant. A full block grant would provide a fixed dollar amount for each state, with no provision for future growth. Under a full block grant, states would have complete discretion in how to use their funds, and the federal government would have complete protection from fiscal risk. States would not have to spend any of their own funds to receive the grant, and the federal government would not have to provide any matching funds if a state chose to spend more than its block grant amount. Since state spending would not cause any changes in federal spending, the price to states of a dollar of Medicaid services would be zero for anything up to the amount of the block grant, and one dollar for anything above the block grant amount. The FMAP would be meaningless. States would bear the full risk of increases in enrollment—whether due to longer-term demographic shifts, recessions, or policy changes—and full risk for increases in the general price level, in medical prices, and in provider reimbursements. To date no proposal has been made to convert Medicaid to a full block grant.

In between the full block grant and the uncapped entitlement is a range of options that would provide varying degrees of state freedom and federal fiscal protection. Closest to the full block grant was the 1995 congressional Medigrant proposal, which was vetoed by President Clinton. This proposal provided block grants to states, with some strings attached. To receive their full block grant amounts, states would have to spend a corresponding amount, based on their FMAP. For example, a state with an FMAP of 60 percent and a block grant of $6 billion would have to spend $4 billion of its own money to receive the full block grant. If the state did not spend the full $4 billion, its block grant would be reduced. If it spent more than $4 billion, its grant would be capped at $6 billion. Thus the state price for one dollar of Medicaid services would be less than one dollar at spending levels below the block grant amount, and one dollar for state spending above the block grant. That is, states would bear the full cost of spending increases above the block grant amount, whether due to structural changes, cyclical forces, or policy choices. The Medigrant legislation provided for growth in block grant amounts, at rates of less than one-half the baseline growth forecasted by CBO.

Closest to current law was President Clinton's 1997 Medicaid budget proposal. The proposal provided for per capita growth caps—caps on the allowable increase in spending per beneficiary based on growth in the economy. This provided protection to states for cost increases due to growth in the number of beneficiaries, but not for those resulting from unanticipated price or utilization changes.

In between Medigrant's block grants with growth and the president's per capita spending caps, congressional proposals would have provided a block grant amount, with growth, plus a supplemental allotment that gives additional funds to states with enrollment growth that exceeds specified amounts.[75] These proposals shift less fiscal risk for program growth to the states than the Medigrant plan, and they appear to shift more fiscal risk to states than the president's plan.

Another important element of the federal-state fiscal relationship is the treatment of the FMAP. Here the range of likely options is straightforward: Congress proposed increasing the minimum FMAP from 50 to 60 percent in the Medigrant proposal and also in the 1996 House and Senate bills. The NGA also would have increased the minimum FMAP to 60 percent, as would the 1996 congressional bills. The president's past proposals would have retained current law.

The Urban Institute and others have proposed modifying the FMAP calculation to take into account differing degrees of poverty in the states and to lower the minimum FMAP from 50 to 40 percent. Given that no legislators are discussing the former changes, and that the latter change goes in the opposite direction of what Congress wants, these proposals seem unlikely to succeed.

Winners and Losers

If Medicaid is reformed, with the intent of slowing its growth, most, if not all, states are likely to wind up with less federal support for Medicaid than under current law. But this does not necessarily mean that all states would consider themselves losers. First, some states may be willing to accept cuts in Medicaid in exchange for greater flexibility in program design and implementation. Second, if current law is unsustainable over the longer term—as many think it is given the aging of the population, the growing support for balancing the federal budget, and the growing anti-entitlement sentiment—then the question is how would states fare under one proposal versus another, and how would they fare in comparison to other states?

It is not possible to predict how states will fare under future legislation—that will depend on the overall level of cuts in Medicaid; the degree of flexibility granted to states; the initial distribution of funds; the provision for future growth in funding; and the complex interplay between the floors, caps, growth rates, indexes, and other factors that enter into proposed Medicaid funding formulas.

In general, pure block grants based on the existing distribution of funds, and uniform growth caps that allow the same growth rates for all states, would tend to benefit high spending and slow growth states. High-spending states would benefit from having the existing distribution of federal funds, which works in their favor, frozen. Slow-growth states would benefit, relative to high-growth states, under uniform growth caps that would limit all states to the same annual growth rate in costs.

There have been a few specific analyses of prior proposals that shed light on possible outcomes. According to an analysis by the Kaiser commission, the Medigrant legislation allowed federal spending growth at about half the rate of baseline Medicaid growth. Federal Medicaid spending would have been cut by 28 percent in the year 2002, with eighteen states experiencing reductions of more than 30 percent. The reductions relative to baseline spending ranged from 9 percent in Tennessee to over 50 percent in Louisiana and New Hampshire. The states with the largest reductions generally were heavy users of DSH funding, which would have been eliminated by Medigrant. Southern and western states tended to have smaller-than-average reductions, while high-spending northern and eastern states tended to have above-average reductions.[76]

In 1996 CRS analyzed Medicaid reform proposals (H.R. 3507 and S. 1795) that would eliminate the entitlement to coverage; limit base federal Medicaid funding to a specific amount each year that would not vary with enrollment, prices, or other variable factors; and provide uncapped "umbrella" aid to states that have unexpectedly rapid growth in enrollment. The base allotment would be distributed to states according to a formula that would give a greater proportion of aid to states with growing populations or relatively large numbers of people in poverty. According to the CRS analysis, "States that would gain federal funds *relative* to other states under H.R. 3507/S. 1795 tend to be located in the South or West. States that would receive fewer federal dollars not only in absolute terms, but also relative to other states, tend to be those in the Northeast and the Midwest, the regions of the country where population is growing more slowly."[77]

One feature common to many recent proposals is that, at least over some potential range of spending, the federal government would no longer share in increased costs. Under Medigrant, essentially all spending above the block grant amount would have been 100 percent state financed. Under the Clinton 1997 plan, expenditures per beneficiary that exceed the allowed growth rates would have been 100 percent state funded. Under H.R. 3507, spending above the base allotments that is not funded with a supplemental allotment would have been 100 percent state financed.

Thus for expenditures above certain levels the state price of a dollar of Medicaid services could increase substantially—doubling in the case of states like New York, Connecticut, and California with 50 percent FMAPs, and quintupling in the case of Mississippi with its 79 percent FMAP. A price change of this magnitude is likely to lead states to cut back on Medicaid spending. A recent review suggested that AFDC block grants might lead to as much as a 20 percent decline in basic cash grants. The same review suggested that Medicaid could be more responsive to price changes than AFDC.[78]

The Timing of Medicaid Cuts

States and the federal government have different planning horizons. States must strive to balance their budgets on an annual basis, and they generally do not enact multiyear plans that are meaningful from political or planning perspectives. When states have multiyear plans or projections, it is common for the first year to be balanced, and for outyears to be unbalanced. In an annual budget-balancing environment, without requirements to balance the outyears, decisions that take effect in the near term are the most important. By contrast, the federal government enacts multiyear plans. Frequently the first year is the most out of balance, with projected budget gaps narrowing as the time horizon lengthens and potential future policies are assumed to take effect.

The difference in planning horizons and constraints creates opportunities for the federal government to further its longer-term budget balancing objectives while enhancing states' short-term budget balancing objectives and quieting state opposition. A good example of this is the welfare reform legislation enacted in 1996. This legislation restructured the nation's primary cash welfare program and cut welfare aid to the states, generating federal budget savings over the federal government's seven-year planning horizon. Much of the savings to the federal treasury will come at the expense of state treasuries. But Congress structured the bill so that it actually cost the federal government money in the first few years by giving block grants to states based on older, higher state spending levels (before the recent caseload reductions lowered state costs), and thus generating payments to states greater than they would have been under the old system.

These additional payments, for some states, were several hundred million dollars in 1997–98. But because the block grants will not grow in any meaningful fashion, over the longer term states could lose money and the federal government could save money. Thus states, with their short-term budget balancing goals, make out in the short term while the federal government, with its longer-term budget balancing goals, makes out in the longer term.

The federal government has a similar, if less straightforward, opportunity with Medicaid reform. Medicaid caseloads and expenditures are unlikely to fall the way AFDC expenditures have fallen, but Medicaid expenditures have slowed significantly. If the federal government were to enact block grants with growth, and if the growth allowed in the early years were generous, then states would reap a short-term windfall at the expense of longer-term losses, much in the way they have with the welfare reform legislation. This might be of interest to the federal government only if significant budget-balancing pressures return.

Conclusions

For much of the past decade Medicaid has been a budget buster for state governments—especially in the early 1990s, when it consumed more than a third of general fund spending growth. Although growth has slowed dramatically in the last few years, some of the slowdown is due to temporary factors. Without policy changes, Medicaid would be likely to outstrip growth in tax bases over the near and middle term. It will continue to place pressure on state budgets, although growth is unlikely to accelerate to rates seen in the late 1980s and early 1990s. Actual expenditures, after reflecting state policy actions, could be flat or even decline in some states. The longer-term prognosis is for accelerating growth when the aging of the population picks up early next century.

Given that Medicaid is the second-largest state spending program, even moderately fast growth will lead to continued state pressure for more control over Medicaid policy and costs. Even without new efforts to balance the federal budget, federal spending on Medicaid would be subject to similar trends and pressures. If the 1997 federal budget agreement holds—if, for example, there is no recession in the next few years—then Medicaid may escape significant federal budget cutting in the near term. Over the longer term, however, CBO budget projections suggest the need for sizable federal cuts, and Medicaid is likely to be targeted.

In the near term, administrative devolution seems likely to continue, with waivers giving states more and more flexibility. Significant federal budget cutting in the longer term would require legislation. The following are possible elements of any future Medicaid agreement:

—The entitlement to states might be limited, but not eliminated. Federal fiscal risk may be reduced by placing caps on growth in average cost per beneficiary. States and the federal government seem likely to share in the risks and costs of extraordinary enrollment increases that might occur, for example, as the result of a recession.

—The entitlement to individuals may be limited, but not eliminated. States may gain greater flexibility to determine who is eligible and who is not. They still will be required to offer some guarantees of service, especially for pregnant women and young children.

The details of each element would determine which states could face the greatest reductions in federal Medicaid reimbursement, and which states might face the smallest cuts. The changes probably would be structured to make the transition as easy as possible for states: they might receive greater aid in the near term than they would receive under current law, and cuts relative to baseline growth could be phased in gradually in successive years.

A new Medicaid fiscal structure might be unstable politically, however. A capped entitlement, or a block grant with growth, probably would give dramatically more federal aid, per person in poverty, to high-income states than to low-income states—just as current law does. Because this policy distribution of federal spending would result solely from federal rather than state choice, as is the case now, the distribution of funds would be under constant attack. This would be likely to lead over the longer term to changes in allowable growth, or in the FMAP, that favor low-income states.

Although states share a common interest in controlling Medicaid costs, they may find themselves pitted against one another if and when the federal government seeks to cut the program. High-spending states, such as many northeastern and midwestern states, could be relative winners under an approach with block-grant features, at the expense of lower-spending but faster-growing southern and western states. At the other extreme, if the federal government allows for growth in spending per enrollee, southern and western states could be relative winners at the expense of slower-growing northeastern and midwestern states. State opinions on Medicaid devolution will be influenced at least as much by these fiscal effects as by general attitudes toward devolution and public assistance.

Notes

1. Nelson A. Rockefeller Institute of Government and the Brookings Center for Public Management, "Devolution and Medicaid: A View from the States" (Washington: unpublished conference transcript, May 23–24, 1996, pp. 23–24).

2. For 1966 spending, see Congressional Research Service, *Medicaid Source Book: Background Data and Analysis (A 1993 Update)*, Committee Print, House Committee on Energy and Commerce, 103 Cong., 1 sess. (Government Printing Office, January 1993), p. 83. 1996 total computable spending (including administration) obtained from http://www.hcfa.gov.

3. 1991 and 1992 growth rates obtained from Health Care Financing Administration, *Health Care Financing Review: 1996 Statistical Supplement* (Baltimore, Md.: Department of Health and Human Services, Office of Research and Demonstrations, 1996), table 109. 1995 growth rate obtained from Health Care Financing Administration, *Medicaid Statistics: Program and Financial Statistics, Fiscal Year 1995*, table 1.

4. Congressional Research Service, *Medicaid Source Book*, p. 83.

5. Congressional Research Service, *Medicaid Source Book*, pp. 85–86, based on total computable expenditures including administration. See Teresa Coughlin, Leighton Ku, and John Holahan, *Medicaid since 1980: Costs, Coverage, and the Shifting Alliance between the Federal Government and the States* (Washington: Urban Institute Press, 1994), pp. 87–99.

6. *Medicaid Source Book*, Committee Print, pp. 85–86.

7. Calculated from Health Care Financing Administration, *Health Care Financing Review: 1996 Statistical Supplement* (Baltimore: Department of Health and Human Services, Office of Research and Demonstrations, 1996), pp. 400, 402.

8. Congressional Research Service, *Medicaid Source Book*, p. 83.

9. Coughlin, Ku, and Holahan, *Medicaid since 1980*, p.14.

10. HCFA, *Health Care Financing Review*, table 109.

11. David Liska and others, "Medicaid Expenditures and Beneficiaries: National and State Profiles and Trends, 1984–1993," report prepared for the Kaiser Commission on the Future of Medicaid, July 1995, p. 104.

12. *Balanced Budget Act of 1995*, H. Rept. 104-350, 104 Cong. 1 sess. (GPO, November 16, 1995), p. 1056.

13. HCFA, *Health Care Financing Review*, pp. 373, 385, 386, 402; *1996 Green Book*, Committee Print, House Ways and Means Committee, 104 Cong. 2 sess. (GPO, 1996), pp. 1225–26.

14. Liska and others, "Medicaid Expenditures and Beneficiaries," p. 104.

15. The source for the 1995 DSH number is HCFA, *Medicaid Statistics 1995* (1995), table 3, HCFA form 64; the source for 1996 is the computer-readable version of same, obtained from http://www.hcfa.gov.

16. In addition, as more and more children are covered under mandated expansions, the growth rate slows, because each additional one-year age group is a smaller percentage of a now larger base of covered children.

17. Department of Health and Human Services, Administration for Children and Families, *AFDC Flash Report: September 1996* (November 27, 1996).

18. Based on HCFA, *Medicaid Statistics 1995*, tables 1, 3; and HCFA, *Medicaid Statistics 1996*, tables 1, 3.

19. John Holahan and David Liska, *Where Is Medicaid Spending Headed?* (Washington: Urban Institute Press, December 1996).

20. Some states require local governments to pick up a portion of Medicaid costs, although the local share is quite small in most of the twenty-one states that do this. Except where noted otherwise, this section includes local costs in the definition of state costs.

21. Technically, the FMAP varies inversely with the *square* of the ratio of state per capita income to the national average, but squaring this ratio has little importance.

22. HCFA, *Medicaid Statistics: Program and Financial Statistics, Fiscal Year 1995*, HCFA-64 report tables, table 1, p. 135.

23. The state share, under the FMAP calculation, is the ratio of state per capita income to the national average, squared, multiplied by 45, and subject to a minimum of 17 and maximum of 50. Setting 50 equal to the squared ratio times 45 and solving for the income ratio yields 1.054. Setting it equal to 17 and solving yields 0.615.

24. One should not think of this as the price for an extra unit of medical services— a dollar of Medicaid might buy more or less medical service in one state versus another, depending on relative costs, quality, and other factors.

25. Leatha Lamison-White, "Poverty in the United States: 1996" (Bureau of the Census, September 1997), p. ix.

26. One can easily think of at least four reasons why this might be so, despite the higher price for high income states: (1) the influence of higher incomes might be very strong, and more than enough to offset the impact of a higher price, (2) high-income states tend to be more liberal than low-income states and so might prefer to spend more on aid to the poor, (3) high-income states tend to have lower poverty rates, and so it is easier for them to spend more per poor person than low-income states, and (4) prices in high-income states tend to be higher than in low-income states, so that high-income states may have to spend more dollars to receive the same amount of medical services.

27. State spending is more variable than federal spending. The standard deviation of state spending per poor person in 1995 was 63 percent of mean state spending. This measure, known as the coefficient of variation, was only 35 percent for federal spending per poor person. For total federal and state spending, the coefficient of variation was 45 percent. In other words, total Medicaid spending per poor person varies less across states than does state-only spending.

28. Max B. Sawicky, "The Total Taxable Resources Definition of State Revenue-Raising Ability," *Federal-State-Local Fiscal Relations, Technical Papers Volume II* (U.S. Department of the Treasury, Office of State and Local Finance, September 1986).

29. See General Accounting Office, *Changing Medicaid Formula Can Improve Distribution of Funds to States*, GAO/GGD-83-27 (March 9, 1983); John Holahan and David Liska, "Expenditure Caps and the Distribution of Federal Medicaid Payments," report prepared for the Kaiser Commission on the Future of Medicaid, September 1995.

30. Some analysts outside of government have constructed state price indexes for selected years.

31. HCFA, *Health Care Financing Review*, p. 396.

32. Taxes on Medicaid providers such as hospitals and nursing homes may or may

not be deposited in state general funds, depending on the state and year in question. This section, however, is focused on Medicaid spending, not revenue.

33. National Association of State Budget Officers, *1994 State Expenditure Report* (April 1995), p. 94; National Association of State Budget Officers, *1995 State Expenditure Report* (April 1996), p. 47. Note that the numbers are for state fiscal years, which for forty-six states run from July 1 to June 30. The exceptions are Alabama (October 1), Michigan (October 1), New York (April 1), and Texas (September 1).

34. National Association of State Budget Officers, *State Expenditure Report*, various years. 1987 numbers are from the 1989 report; 1990 numbers are from 1992; 1992 numbers are from 1994, 1994 numbers are from 1995.

35. These numbers also overstate Medicaid's importance in another sense. State general funds often do not include highway-related spending and certain other functions that nonetheless are a burden on state taxpayers.

36. Coughlin, Ku, and Holahan, *Medicaid since 1980*, pp. 87–88.

37. Ibid., pp. 27–31, 81–97.

38. National Association of State Budget Officers, *1994 State Expenditure Report*, p. 94; National Association of State Budget Officers, *1995 State Expenditure Report*, p. 47.

39. Susan Hanafee, "Medicaid Putting Squeeze on State, Bayh Says," *Indianapolis Star*, December 18, 1992.

40. Bureau of the Census, *Current Population Reports, P25-1111, Population Projections for States, by Age, Sex, Race, and Hispanic Origin: 1993 to 2020*, by Paul R. Campbell (GPO, 1994), table 5.

41. Health Care Financing Administration, *Health Care Financing Review*, vol. 17 (Summer 1996), pp. 245–51.

42. Holahan and Liska, *Where Is Medicaid Spending Headed?*

43. The number of poor people in a state is only a rough indicator of the need for Medicaid services or expenditures, in part because (1) the Medicaid program serves many non-poor, (2) it does not serve all of the poor, (3) costs vary due to factors not necessarily related to poverty, such as the age and health status of recipients, (4) the prices of services vary across states, and (5) measures of poverty are imperfect.

44. Throughout this section on variation, unless otherwise noted, analysis will focus on states, excluding Arizona, plus the District of Columbia. As in many other Medicaid analyses, Arizona is excluded because of the unique, noncomparable nature of its program, which has operated under a waiver since 1982. Possessions and territories also are excluded. Unless noted otherwise, references to the nation or to national averages refer to the forty-nine included states plus the District of Columbia.

45. Expenditures per enrollee multiplied by enrollment as a share of the poverty population yields expenditures per poor person.

46. Jerry Cromwell and others, *Examining the Medicaid Fiscal Crisis* (Waltham, Mass.: Center for Health Economic Research, October 20, 1994).

47. Five states accounted for more than half of the $18.9 billion of DSH expenditures in 1995: New York, California, Texas, New Jersey, and Louisiana. Relative to overall Medicaid expenditures, DSH was most important to New Hampshire (39 percent), Louisiana (31 percent), Missouri (27 percent), New Jersey (24 percent), Colorado (23 percent), South Carolina (22 percent), and Alabama (21 percent).

48. Hawaii is missing data because it did not report enrollment figures in 1995.

49. States do not always fall neatly into categories. Some states are close to the boundary between groups, and small changes in data could shift them into another group. Nonetheless, the depth and breadth division is an interesting way to look at state Medicaid programs.

50. Arithmetically, the percentage of the poverty population covered (x axis) multiplied by spending per enrollee (y axis) and divided by 100 equals $3,589 for each point on the line.

51. D.C. spent $6,205 per poor person in 1995 and Vermont spent $5,692.

52. In general, the discussion that follows is based on data for the 1995 federal fiscal year, and for state policies in effect during that year. To the extent that policies have changed, some states may no longer have the characteristics they had in 1995.

53. AFDC has since been converted to temporary assistance to needy families (TANF). It is no longer an entitlement, and state income thresholds may change considerably.

54. The AFDC and medically needy thresholds are based on a family of three and are from National Governors' Association, *State Medicaid Coverage of Pregnant Women and Children—Summer 1996*, September 10, 1996, table 2. The number of services is from Health Care Financing Administration, *Medicaid Services State By State*, October 1, 1995. Nursing home reimbursement rates are from Health Care Financing Administration, *Extramural Report: State Data Book on Long-Term Care Program and Market Characteristics*, 1994. The ideology index is the mean index from Robert S. Erickson, Gerald Wright, and John P. McIver, *Statehouse Democracy: Public Opinion & Policy in the American States* (Cambridge University Press, 1993), pp. 12–16.

55. *State Medicaid Coverage of Pregnant Women and Children*, table 2.

56. DSH expenditures are not included in the spending figures discussed in this section on state variation.

57. See Health Care Financing Administration, *State Medicaid Demonstrations*, July 1996, p. 5; *State Medicaid Coverage of Pregnant Women and Children*, table 1.

58. *State Medicaid Coverage of Pregnant Women and Children*, table 1.

59. Intergovernmental Health Policy Project, "Fifty State Profiles: Health Care Reform," report prepared for the Henry J. Kaiser Family Foundation, October 1995.

60. HCFA, *Medicaid Services State by State*.

61. Michael S. Sparer, *Medicaid and the Limits of State Health Reform* (Temple University Press, 1996), pp. 189–95.

62. Health Care Financing Administration, *Medicaid spDATA System: Characteristics of Medicaid State Programs* (Washington: HCFA pub. No. 10130, December 1993), p. 80.

63. These calculations are based on recipients rather than enrollment because an age breakdown of enrollment was not available. Enrollment is so highly correlated with recipients that even if enrollment data were available, the results of the calculations almost certainly would not be different in a meaningful sense.

64. HCFA, *Extramural Report*.

65. Bureau of Labor Statistics, *Employment and Wages, Annual Averages, 1993* (Department of Labor, October 1994), p. 494.

66. Katherine R. Levit and others, "State Health Expenditure Accounts: Building

Blocks for State Health Spending Analysis," *Health Care Financing Review*, vol. 17, no. 1 (Fall 1995), pp. 243–44, 249–50.

67. Jane Sneddon Little, "Why State Medicaid Costs Vary: A First Look," Working Paper 91-1 (Federal Reserve Bank of Boston, August 1991).

68. This ignores an important complication: that the "price" of Medicaid changes as income changes; the federal reimbursement share is lower in high-income states than in low-income states. If income could be held constant, one would expect states with a higher "price" for Medicaid to buy less of it. It also ignores a complication that cuts in the other direction: that higher-income states also tend to be higher cost-of-living states; a dollar does not necessarily buy as much health care in New York as it does in Iowa.

69. Based on a regression of the log of state Medicaid expenditures per poor person against the log of per capita income, the log of the poverty rate, and the ideology index from *Statehouse Democracy*. The R-squared from such a regression is approximately 0.80, and all three coefficients are significantly different from zero at the 95 percent confidence level and have the expected signs—spending per poor person increases as income increases, decreases as the poverty rate increases, and is greater in states that view themselves as ideologically liberal.

70. As noted elsewhere, this equation is intended to add to our ability to understand state variation. Many important variables are left out, and I do not present it as the best equation for explaining how states decide on Medicaid policy, or for predicting Medicaid expenditures.

71. Little, "Why State Medicaid Costs Vary," p. 33.

72. Daniel Patrick Moynihan and others, "The Federal Budget and the States, Fiscal Year 1995" (Taubman Center for State and Local Government, Harvard University, September 30, 1996), p. 7.

73. H.R. 2015.

74. John Holahan and David Liska, "The Impact of the 'Medigrant' Plan on Federal Payments to States," report prepared for the Kaiser Commission on the Future of Medicaid, December 1995; and Patrick Purcell, *Medicaid Reform: Estimates of the Distribution of Federal Funds under H.R.3507/S.1795* (Congressional Research Service, July 24, 1996).

75. See S. 1795, *Congressional Record*, June 27, 1996, p. S7171-2.

76. Holahan and Liska, "The Impact of the 'Medigrant' Plan," pp. 10–11.

77. Purcell, *Medicaid Reform*, p. 1.

78. Howard Chernick, "Fiscal Effects of Block Grants for the Needy: A Review of the Evidence," paper prepared for the 1995 National Tax Association Annual Conference, pp. 30–31.

4

Managed Care and Devolution

James W. Fossett

THE DIFFUSION of managed care has been perhaps the most significant change in the organization and financing of care to Medicaid clients in the last decade. Medicaid enrollment in various forms of managed-care arrangements has increased almost fivefold since 1990, with the largest increases coming in more aggressively managed full capitation plans. A number of states, including several with very large Medicaid populations, are contemplating even larger expansions of managed care by mandating enrollment of a broader range of Medicaid clients into managed care, including such expensive and difficult-to-care-for populations as supplemental security income (SSI) clients and patients with AIDS and severe and persistent mental illness.

Recent changes in Medicaid relating to managed care present strong apparent incentives for states to expand and accelerate these trends. While falling short of earlier proposals to change Medicaid to a block grant, impose per capita caps on federal Medicaid spending, or to drastically curtail federal controls over state Medicaid programs, the Balanced Budget Act of 1997 appreciably lessened federal control over state managed-care programs by effectively eliminating past requirements that states seek waivers from the Health Care Financing Administration (HCFA) to mandate enrollment, with fewer regulatory requirements, of almost all Medicaid recipients in managed care. Medicaid clients in many states have become more attractive to commercial managed-care organizations as a result of increased competition in the private market, and this increased flexibility may offer states the opportunity to move Medicaid clients into better-quality care in the medical mainstream by devising arrangements that are, at least in principle, more responsive to the realities of local institutions and markets.

This chapter examines the major political, managerial, and implementation issues likely to arise around managed care as a result of the devolution of Medicaid under the Balanced Budget Act of 1997. It first examines recent trends in the size and scope of Medicaid managed care, then reviews the political and legal controversies that have arisen around managed care that may affect its attractiveness, feasibility of expansion, and extension to new groups. It next describes the changes made by the Balanced Budget Act compared to those in earlier devolution proposals and evaluates the likely effects of these changes on the further diffusion of managed care across states and its extension to new groups. Finally, it examines the most likely effects of expanded use of Medicaid managed care under devolution on the accessibility and quality of care available to Medicaid clients.

My conclusions are mixed. While Medicaid managed-care enrollments have expanded dramatically in recent years, the proportion of Medicaid dollars spent through various forms of managed care remains small, as does the amount of savings attributable to managed care as compared to total Medicaid expenditures. Achieving major savings from managed care will require large expansions in the scale and scope of managed care to more expensive populations.

The prospects for continued dramatic expansion of Medicaid managed care, however, appear more problematic than in the immediate past. A number of states have made major political and managerial commitments to managed care and might be expected to take full advantage of the increased discretion now available to them. Others may elect to move managed-care clients out of less aggressive forms of managed care and into full risk capitation programs, where the potential budget savings are appreciably larger. Other states, however, may be less aggressive. Managed care has become a controversial legal and political issue in many states, and a variety of management problems and occasional scandals associated with Medicaid managed care in some states, as well as a broader recognition of managed care's consequences for providers and clients, may have made managed care a harder political sell than in the past. Selling managed care may be particularly difficult in states that envision expanding managed care to the elderly and the disabled. The provider and advocacy groups associated with these client groups are more geographically dispersed and politically powerful than those associated with the aid to families with dependent children (AFDC) population, providing them with the resources to contest managed-care rates or policies that they deem unsatisfactory. Finally, other states may rely more on alternative cost-cutting methods also made available under the Balanced Budget Act and less on managed care.

These developments suggest two factors worthy of considerable attention in debates as state implementation of managed care proceeds under the enhanced flexibility made possible by the Balanced Budget Act. One is the change in the politics surrounding state debates over the size and form of managed care that allowing states greater discretion over managed care will most likely produce. The elimination of the federal presence in negotiations over the size and shape of Medicaid managed-care programs is likely to make these negotiations resemble other legislative debates in which long-standing geographic and partisan cleavages are prominent. Eliminating or diminishing federal supervision over state managed-care activities is likely to enhance the political position of long-term care and other Medicaid providers with significant political resources at the expense of inner-city providers and clients, who are less powerful. The advocacy groups for this population have typically invested more effort in developing contacts and influence in Washington than in state capitals and might be expected to be less effective in these negotiations than in those involving waivers.

This redistribution of political advantage is of particular concern given the likelihood that the future political appeal of Medicaid managed care in many states will be centered on its potential to provide budget savings. The primary circumstances most likely to produce large-scale movement toward managed care in the future are dramatic declines in state financial conditions, whether as a result of economic downturns or of sharp increases in Medicaid spending in the rate of health care inflation. Under these circumstances there is likely to be considerable pressure from governors and budget offices to build up enrollments rapidly and sharply reduce capitation rates. Given the relative balance of power between providers and client groups in most states, plans and providers serving the urbanized AFDC population would bear a disproportionate share of Medicaid spending reductions.

A second concern relates to the strong incentive that states have to underinvest in managed-care oversight under these conditions. The record seems clear that implementing large-scale managed care is a complex and demanding management task that requires considerable upfront investment in information systems, staff, and oversight on the part of both managed-care plans and state agencies as well as considerable changes in practices and internal culture inside state agencies. Potential management problems are most likely to be systematically understated and measures to address them systematically underfunded in the financially stressed environments that are likely to furnish the major pretext for future large-scale expansions of managed care. Political and budget officials are likely to be interested in managed care primarily as a means of realizing large, short-term budget savings and are unlikely to be receptive to requests for additional support to add staff, develop new management information systems, or provide support for patient education programs to aid in choice of plans and the appropriate use of the managed-care system. Managed care is likely to be seen by political and budget officials in most states as solely a cost-containment device. The political need to reduce expenditures by moving clients into plans as rapidly as possible is likely to take precedence over considerations of quality, access, and accountability; and the investments in staffing, information systems, and other oversight elements necessary to realize the advantages of managed care as a delivery system may not materialize.

These arguments suggest that the reduced federal oversight of managed care envisioned in the Balanced Budget Act carries some appreciable risks. Federal review and oversight of state managed-care initiatives appears to have served to maintain accountability for the federal funds paid to managed-care organizations and to provide a counterweight to the incentives present in many states to focus cuts on more politically vulnerable populations in urban areas. Reducing federal oversight may reduce the administrative overhead associated with implementing managed care and allow states to devise programs that are more responsive to local conditions, but it also creates the potential for states to manage managed care primarily as a means for realizing short-term budget savings and underinvest in oversight of managed-care plans. Under these conditions, managed care might very well reduce the accessibility and quality of care available to Medicaid clients by concentrating them in plans with a strong financial incentive to underserve and eliminating or restricting access to traditional safety net providers.

Medicaid Managed Care—The Current Context

Enrollment in Medicaid managed care has increased sharply in recent years. While the form and scale of state programs varies widely, forty-six states were reported in 1995 (the most recent year for which data are currently available) to have at least some portion of their Medicaid populations enrolled in some form of managed care.[1] As shown in table 4-1, enrollment in managed care increased by a factor of six between 1991 and 1996, from 2.7 million to more than 13.3 million, so that 40 percent of Medicaid recipients are now enrolled in some form of managed-care arrangements. Managed-care enrollment more than doubled between 1993 and 1995, largely as the result of large expansions stemming from the approval of major waiver proposals in eight states, which accounted for more than 70 percent of enrollment growth over this period.[2]

This recent growth in enrollment has been accompanied by a marked shift in the form of managed-care arrangements in which Medicaid clients are enrolled. Earlier Medicaid managed-care programs were frequently operated as primary care case management (PCCM) programs, which are less aggressive forms of managed care. Under these programs, Medicaid clients were required to designate a primary-care physician who received a small monthly fee for acting as a case manager, providing primary-care services and authorizing all other care the client received. In most cases services continued to be reimbursed on a fee-for-service rather than a capitated basis, and case managers were not at any financial risk for the care provided to their clients.[3]

Recent enrollment growth, by contrast, has been concentrated in more aggressive forms of managed care, in which payments are capitated and managed-care organizations are at risk for the care provided to their members. The percentage of enrollees in entities classified by HCFA as health

Table 4-1. *Enrollment in Medicaid Managed Care as Percentage of Total Medicaid Enrollment, 1991–96*

Year	Managed care enrollment (millions)	Total Medicaid enrollment (millions)	Percent enrolled in managed care
1991	2.7	28,3	9.5
1992	3.6	30.9	11.8
1993	4.8	33.4	14.4
1994	7.8	33.6	23.2
1995	9.8	33.4	29.4
1996	13.3	33.2	40.1

Source: http://www.hcfa.gov/medicaid/trends1.htm.

maintenance organizations (HMOs) increased from 41.7 percent of all enrollees in 1992 to 48 percent in 1995, while the percentage of enrollees in PCCM programs increased from 33.3 percent in 1992 to 36 percent in 1995.[4] Two-thirds of managed-care recipients in 1995 were enrolled in plans classified as full risk, although these enrollees are concentrated in a limited number of states.[5]

While enrollment in managed care has increased sharply in recent years and might be expected to continue to grow—as a result of both continued expansion in existing plans and the recent approval of new large-scale waivers in Illinois and Maryland—much of this expansion has been concentrated in the AFDC population, which accounts for a small share of Medicaid's expenditures relative to its size. As of mid-1994 thirty-six states had some form of managed-care program for the AFDC population, primarily for pregnant women and children, while less than twenty enrolled other Medicaid populations, such as SSI enrollees, in managed care of any form.[6] While a number of states are developing separate "carve-out" programs to enroll SSI populations, particularly the severely and persistently mentally ill, these programs under managed care are typically less aggressive in form than those for the AFDC population, and typically continue to pay for a variety of expensive services heavily used by these clients—such as inpatient care at state psychiatric facilities, supervised residential programs, and substance abuse services—on a fee-for-service basis outside the capitated payment.[7]

This concentration of managed-care enrollment among the AFDC population rather than less numerous, but more expensive, Medicaid enrollees such as the elderly and SSI populations is the result of several factors. First, existing managed-care "technology" can be more easily adapted to the AFDC population than to other Medicaid enrollees. The AFDC population more closely resembles the private managed-care population demographically and uses the same types of providers. Almost all AFDC enrollees are either relatively young women or their children, so that they are typically younger and healthier than other Medicaid recipients and hence incur smaller health care bills than older or more disabled recipients. They also make much less use of nursing homes, other long-term care services, and mental health and other "nonmedical" services than other recipients. This closer similarity in demography and usage to the private managed-care population has meant that existing private managed-care models have been more readily adaptable to the AFDC population than to others. There is considerably less experience with applying managed care for the elderly, who make extensive

use of nursing homes and other long-term care, or to the severely and persistently mentally ill or the developmentally disabled, whose usage profiles
differ dramatically from those of the private managed-care population. Second, the AFDC population and the providers that typically serve them (which
will be discussed at some length in a later section) are more geographically
concentrated and less politically powerful than other Medicaid populations
and providers, which has made it more difficult for them to resist state
efforts to mandate enrollment in managed care.

As a result, the proportion of Medicaid expenditures accounted for by
managed-care premiums is much smaller than the proportion of enrollees
in managed-care plans. AFDC enrollees account for approximately 70 percent of Medicaid enrollees nationally, but less than 30 percent of Medicaid
expenditures.[8] Table 4-2 displays recent trends in the size of Medicaid
managed-care capitation payments as compared to vendor payments under
traditional fee-for-service arrangements. The capitation payments exclude
fee-for-service payments made under primary care case management programs and payments to health insurance organizations in Texas and California, and hence are not complete counts of the money spent through all
forms of managed-care arrangements.[9] In spite of these qualifications, these
data indicate that managed-care premiums remain small when compared to
total Medicaid expenditures. Managed-care premiums were equivalent to
only slightly more than 6 percent of vendor payments in 1995. The bulk of

Table 4-2. *Managed-Care Premiums as a Proportion of Vendor
Payments, 1990–95*

Millions of dollars unless otherwise specified

Year	Medicaid managed-care premium payments	Medicaid vendor payments	Percentage
1990	2,064	64,900	3.18
1991	1,919	77,000	2.49
1992	3,995	91,500	4.37
1993	4,219	101,700	4.15
1994	6,153	108,300	5.68
1995	7,500	120,500	6.22

Source: 1990 and 1991: Health Care Financing Administration form 64; 1992–95: HCFA
form 2082. 1992–95 data exclude payments to health insuring organizations (HIOs) in Texas and
California.

premium payments are also made in a limited number of states. In 1994, for example, only eight states paid more than 10 percent of program expenditures as capitated payments in any form, with five states accounting for two-thirds of total capitated payments.[10]

In addition, there is evidence that Medicaid clients enrolled in managed care are healthier than those who remain in traditional fee-for-service arrangements. Risk selection, or the disproportionate enrollment of healthier individuals into managed care, has been widely noted in other managed-care settings,[11] and the available evidence indicates the presence of this phenomenon in Medicaid programs as well. While some states have attempted to mandate enrollment in order to minimize selection bias, exemptions of potentially high-cost groups are common and mandatory enrollment for all groups covered by managed care is relatively rare. In addition to the elderly and disabled, most states exclude the medically needy and other potentially expensive groups, such as those in institutions and residential long-term care, and allow individuals, frequently those with chronic conditions, to seek exemptions from mandatory enrollment.[12] Mandatory enrollment is frequently required for less aggressive PCCM programs, but participation in capitated programs is more commonly voluntary.[13] Many large states, including California and New York, mandate enrollment only in particular geographic areas.[14] As a result of these practices, as well as possible "cream-skimming" of healthier patients by plans, there is both formal and informal evidence of risk selection.[15]

This combination of small expenditures and relatively healthy clients suggests that the potential budget savings from Medicaid managed care as currently constituted are relatively small. At least some states, particularly those with traditionally high Medicaid hospital payment rates, have been able to realize appreciable premium savings by taking advantage of increasing competition in the private managed-care market, which has led to appreciable declines in the premiums paid by private employers. Because Medicaid managed-care premiums in many states were initially calculated based on Medicaid fee-for-service experience, which incorporates relatively high hospital rates and greater use of hospital and emergency services than by the population as a whole, Medicaid premiums in these states were frequently as high as, if not higher than, those available from private employers. These high initial rates made Medicaid managed-care clients more attractive to managed-care organizations. As premiums have declined in the private managed-care market as a result of competition, states have been able to reduce Medicaid premiums without reducing access or making Medicaid clients unattractive to managed-care plans.[16] These savings have been small as compared to total Medicaid expenditures, however, and fall well below the savings required for states to adjust to reductions in Medicaid of the magnitude envisioned in some devolution proposals. Achieving large-scale savings from managed care will require shifts toward mandatory, rather than voluntary, enrollment of greater numbers of AFDC clients as well as the less numerous, but more expensive, disabled populations such as those afflicted with AIDS and severe and persistent mental illness. As will be argued in detail in later sections, managing managed care on this scale for these populations is a complex and difficult task with which most states and managed care organizations have little experience. This suggests that realizing significant short-term budget savings from a rapid expansion of managed care is unlikely.

In similar fashion, the political conditions that motivated recent increases in managed-care enrollment have shifted appreciably. Much of the initial political appeal of Medicaid managed care stemmed from (1) the high Medicaid growth rates of the early 1990s, which created severe budget pressures in many states to which managed care appeared to be a ready solution, and (2) the political climate preceding the defeat of national health reform, when many state politicians saw health reform, frequently involving Medicaid, as a means of both expanding coverage for the uninsured and achieving national political visibility.

The impetus provided by both of these forces has largely dissipated. Medicaid growth rates have declined sharply in recent years, from 20-plus percent growth rates between 1990 and 1993 to less than 1 percent in 1995-96.[17] Much of the initial political impetus for health reform and the large-scale waivers, which have produced the largest expansions in Medicaid managed-care enrollments, was generated by rapid increases in Medicaid expenditures, which roughly doubled between 1988 and 1993.[18] The recent decline in Medicaid growth rates may be explained largely by the recovery from the recession of the early 1990s, which has reduced growth in caseloads and in federal legislation that had curtailed growth in disproportionate share hospital (DSH) payments and the creative use of provider taxes as state match. It also seems likely that many states that have aggressively "Medicaided" previously state-funded human service programs in the past have curtailed these efforts, in part to forestall major federal cuts in Medicaid. Together with the revenue growth that has resulted from economic recovery, this decline in Medicaid growth has lessened pressures on state budgets and reduced the intensity of complaints in legislatures and other public forums that had likened Medicaid to a budgetary Pac-Man that crowded out spending on education and other public programs.[19]

A closely related set of factors that also gave considerable impetus to managed care in many states were the opportunities perceived by many state politicians to achieve national visibility by mounting large-scale health reform in the political climate surrounding the debate over national health reform in the period 1992–94. As noted by numerous commentators, the widely held perception during this period was that the American health care system was in serious trouble, if not crisis, and that there was widespread public support for major restructuring of the system that had not been seen previously as politically feasible. Health expenditures, both public and private, had increased rapidly through the late 1980s and early 1990s, as had the number of uninsured, and there were widespread reports of public concern over the loss of health insurance and diminished access to health care. The perceived political possibilities for health reform were further enhanced by the election in 1991 of Harris Wofford from Pennsylvania to the U.S. Senate on a platform that stressed health care reform.[20] Under these conditions governors and state legislative leaders were more receptive to major reforms than they might otherwise have been, and a number of states put forth ambitious proposals that included managed care as part of larger-scale restructurings of state health care systems, typically as a source of Medicaid savings that would finance insurance coverage for previously uncovered groups.[21]

Managed care, either for Medicaid or private patients, was not a major point of controversy in public debates over these proposals.[22] While not large or widespread, experience with Medicaid managed care in most states gave little support for concerns that managed care would reduce access to care for Medicaid clients, and most statewide hospital and physician groups—the bulk of whose members generally are not major Medicaid billers—did not see themselves as having major financial stakes in managed care. In states where Medicaid expenditures had grown particularly rapidly or fiscal conditions were particularly severe, managed care could be presented as a responsible means of slowing Medicaid growth that did not require arbitrary and onerous cuts in services or eligibility or restrictions on service use.[23] Some states also found managed-care-based waivers, which could commit the federal government to at least what they would have spent under a continued fee-for-service program, to be a prudent hedge against the possibility of future Medicaid cuts.

The political environment around health care in general and managed care in particular has shifted appreciably in recent years. First, the defeat of health reform nationally and in several states, such as Vermont, as well as changes in the partisan composition of many state legislatures after the elections of 1994 have lessened the appeal of large-scale health reform as a potential political issue in most states. A number of states that had begun major reform initiatives have been compelled to reduce the scale or pace of these initiatives as legislative support has diminished and state politicians have been drawn to other less controversial issues.

Second, managed care has become a controversial political and legal issue in many states as the economic consequences for providers have become better defined and broad concerns have emerged over potential compromises in the quality of care that many fear have accompanied a widespread move to managed care by private employers. Large numbers of stories in both local and national media have highlighted managed-care payment practices that give physicians financial incentives to reduce care, gag rules that prohibit physicians from informing patients either of uncovered treatment alternatives or their payment arrangements, and a wide range of "casualties of the day"—patients who have been denied services by managed-care companies.[24] When combined with widespread media coverage of the high salaries paid to executives in managed-care companies, these concerns have produced a backlash of widely varying scope and consequence among both the general public and disenfranchised providers against managed care in many states.

This backlash has had a wide range of political and legal manifestations. One is the increasing visibility of proposals to establish medical savings accounts, which have attracted considerable support from organized medicine and indemnity insurance companies as a means of competing with managed-care organizations for healthy clients.[25] A second are frequently successful attempts in both Congress and state legislatures to limit or eliminate a wide range of practices by managed-care companies pressed by historically unusual alliances between provider groups, particularly physicians and nurses, and consumer groups. By one count, over 1,000 bills restricting managed-care practices were introduced in state legislatures in 1996, up from 250 in 1995.[26] Perhaps the most successful proposals have been those mandating minimum lengths of stay for particular procedures. By one recent count, thirty-four states and the federal government have enacted legislation mandating minimum lengths of stay for delivery,[27] and the American Association of Health Plans (AAHP), the trade association for managed-care organizations, has recently urged its members to permit hospitalizations for mastectomies, a position widely interpreted as an attempt to forestall minimum-stay legislation for this procedure.[28]

Legislation has also been passed or introduced in a number of states to restrict or eliminate a wide range of physician payment and other contractual practices inside the managed-care industry, provide patients with information and procedures to challenge denials of care, limit the circumstances under which particular services can be denied or providers denied entry to or eliminated from managed-care networks, mandate disclosure-of-payment arrangements and clinical criteria for judging the appropriateness of care for particular conditions, and in some cases mandate minimum medical loss ratios or limit the profits managed-care organizations can realize.[29] By one recent count, twenty-one states had passed reasonably comprehensive consumer rights legislation by mid-1997, and similar bills were pending in thirteen others.[30] Physician groups have also pressed demands to be allowed to own and operate networks of providers, variously labeled as "integrated delivery systems" or "physician-hospital organizations," that can compete with licensed HMOs for managed-care contracts. In other states efforts have been made to limit or prohibit the operation of for-profit plans or providers. These initiatives have not been universally successful; coalitions of managed-care companies and large employers have frequently defeated or weakened proposed restrictions on managed care, and ballot propositions that would have prohibited financial incentives to physicians have been overwhelmingly defeated in California and Oregon.[31] It is quite clear, however, that managed care is likely to remain a controversial issue nationally and in many states. Arguments that managed-care plans are more interested in profits than health care and that widely used payment arrangements are "bribes" to withhold needed care appear to have considerable popular appeal, and demands for legislation to protect consumers or providers can be expected to continue.[32] AAHP has also urged plans to limit the use of so-called gag clauses in physician contracts and disclose both financial incentives and procedures and standards for denying or approving care, positions that, again, could be interpreted as attempts to forestall legislative attention to these questions.[33]

In addition to legislative controversy, managed care has become the subject of increasing litigation by customers challenging—on a wide range of grounds, including malpractice—decisions by managed-care plans that deny them care; physicians appealing exclusion from managed-care networks or seeking relief from the corporate practice of medicine; and managed-care organizations claiming that state legislation limiting their activities is preempted by the Employee Retirement and Income Security Act (ERISA).[34] Established regulatory doctrines in a number of areas—including antitrust, fraud, malpractice, and licensure—have proven difficult to apply unambiguously to managed-care arrangements, and further litigation and legislation is likely to be required to establish regulatory regimes appropriate to changed organizational and financial circumstances.[35]

While these political and legal controversies have only rarely been the direct result of the operation of Medicaid managed care, they have appreciably complicated its political and managerial environment. Debates over the role of for-profit health care in the larger system, for example, have frequently spilled over into debates about the type of plans that should be eligible to compete for Medicaid managed-care contracts. Particularly in debates over the design of Medicaid mental health managed-care programs, provider groups and their legislative allies have argued against allowing firms from other states to make profits from state taxes and that preference should be given to locally based provider networks, which do not currently exist in appreciable numbers and whose precise status under state laws is frequently unclear.[36] In similar fashion, state and federal minimum treatment and consumer protection statutes and judicial rulings frequently cover Medicaid as well as private patients. If, for example, a recent federal district court decision that HMOs serving Medicare clients are government agents and thus subject to the due process requirements of the Administrative Procedures Act were extended to plans serving Medicaid clients, plans would be required to provide clients with full notice of adverse rulings and the opportunity for formal hearings. Such requirements would appreciably increase plans' administrative costs and might be expected to limit the budget savings from managed care if plans' denial of care is frequently overruled in the hearing process or curtailed because plans wish to avoid lengthy appeals.

In addition to being affected by debates and developments in the larger system, Medicaid managed care has also acquired a distinctive set of horror stories and political controversies. A number of larger states, particularly those that have attempted to achieve rapid increases in managed-care enrollment over a short period of time, have experienced substantial, well-reported implementation problems—ranging from chaotic and confused start-ups and enrollment and marketing problems in such states as California, Tennessee, and New York to large-scale scandal and fraud in Florida—and frequently publicized problems with the quality of care and state oversight of plan operations.[37] In contrast to other states, recent enrollments have declined significantly in Tennessee and New York as a result of a variety of implementation problems in Tennessee and the suspension for several months of direct enrollment by plans in New York.[38] In addition to complaints about the use of state tax dollars by for-profit managed-care companies and the political embarrassment of adverse publicity surrounding enrollment, marketing, and quality-of-care problems, state programs have also frequently had to deal with the political problems raised by public hospitals and other safety net providers about the potential loss of revenue and jobs from managed care, as well as complaints from advocates and specialized providers seeking carve-outs independent of other managed-care arrangements, designation as "essential community providers" with whom managed-care organizations are required to contract, and other provisions affecting particular groups.[39]

These political difficulties seem likely to intensify as the stakes in Medicaid managed care become better defined. While consumer influence over Medicaid managed care has been limited to date, the expansion of managed care to the more expensive disabled and elderly populations required to generate extensive state budget savings will most likely require potentially expensive concessions to neutralize opposition from these groups and their service providers, who are typically more geographically dispersed, better organized and funded, and more politically powerful than the lower-income women and children who have constituted the majority of enrollees in managed care to date.[40] Quite clearly, states' ability to transfer the political blame to managed-care agencies for making unpopular cuts in Medicaid services and payments has declined significantly, and the political opportunity cost to state legislators and governors of major expansions of Medicaid managed care has increased appreciably.

These arguments suggest that the demand for large-scale, reform-oriented managed-care expansions of the type that have driven managed-care enrollments through the early 1990s may well have peaked. Medicaid growth rates have slowed dramatically in recent years, and state revenues have largely recovered from the recession of this same period, lessening the immediate political need to make major efforts to reduce Medicaid growth rates. In addition, managed care in many states has lost its political appeal as a "silver bullet" and become a potentially controversial issue around which winners and losers are much better defined.

How Devolution Affects Managed Care

In current parlance, "devolution" proposals contain two general elements that affect the programmatic and political feasibility of managed care for many states. One is the amount of both federal and state money that devolution takes out of the Medicaid program and the precise form in which it comes out. If the argument presented previously is correct, the major continued political appeal of managed care rests on its perceived ability to produce budget savings while shifting financial risk and political blame for spending reductions to private agencies. States that experience major deterioration in their financial positions as a result of large reductions in future federal Medicaid revenues, economic downturns, or major alternative political priorities for spending state funds may continue to find large-scale movement toward aggressive forms of managed care worthwhile.

The appeal of managed care to a particular state is also likely to be heavily influenced by its fee-for-service spending levels. Large, high-benefit states in the Northeast and Midwest are more likely to find managed care appealing as a response to fiscal stress than low-benefit states in the South and West. High-benefit states have historically low physician fees under Medicaid but higher-than-average rates for hospital care, while low-benefit states' payment patterns have been the reverse. Managed care's penetration into the private health market is also higher in the larger industrial states, which has frequently meant sharp declines in use, particularly of inpatient hospital care. Under these circumstances Medicaid agencies can frequently realize considerable savings through managed care without dramatically affecting access because of the sharp declines in private rates.[41] In contrast, states that have historically paid low hospital rates are not in a position to save large amounts of money from a major investment in managed care, and may even have to make sizeable upfront investments in order to develop adequate capacity to treat managed-care enrollees.[42]

Alternatively, if states are allowed to reduce their own contributions to Medicaid considerably without any reduction in federal support, the potential for large-scale savings may make a large-scale investment in managed care more attractive, particularly if state financial conditions deteriorate appreciably. Smaller reductions in Medicaid funding, or those that limit reductions in state support to levels proportionate to federal reductions, could most likely be absorbed by less dramatic and more traditional changes in provider payments, or in the "amount, duration, and scope" of care, particularly as the Boren amendment and other mandates are weakened or eliminated.

The spending reductions enacted in the Balanced Budget Act of 1997 are appreciably less onerous than those in earlier devolution proposals. The Medigrant proposal passed by Congress in 1996 would have reduced federal payments to states by some $133 billion over seven years and contemplated reductions in federal support of almost $50 billion, more than 25 percent below the Congressional Budget Office baseline, in 2002. States would have been completely responsible for any additional expenditures required by increases in caseload or increases in the cost of health care. The Clinton administration's proposals would have reduced federal support by lesser amounts and provided some protections for states against unanticipated expenditure growth, but would still have produced a reduction of federal support in the tens of billions of dollars over a seven-year period. Either of these proposals would have required states to adjust to significant reductions in the level of federal funding in a relatively short period of time.

The Balanced Budget Act, by contrast, reduces federal support by an appreciably smaller amount and gives states considerable flexibility to reduce their own Medicaid spending in a variety of areas. The act reduces federal support by an estimated $17 billion over five years, largely through a reduction in payments to disproportionate share hospitals (DSH), which serve large numbers of Medicaid and uninsured patients, and limited use of DSH reimbursement to support state psychiatric hospitals. It also increases state Medicaid spending by sharply increasing the premiums charged to recipients under Part B of Medicare, which pays for physician care and other services outside the hospital. States are required to pay these premiums for low-income Medicare recipients, whose numbers are projected to increase by 20 percent over the next five years. The act also restores Medicaid eligibility and state financial responsibility for certain disabled legal immigrants and disabled children who had lost eligibility in the welfare reform act of 1996.

While the largest reductions enacted in Medicaid since 1981, these changes are significantly smaller than those proposed in earlier devolution packages and present few incentives for states to expand managed care as a means of adjusting to major cuts in federal support. DSH payments are concentrated in a limited number of states, and increased premiums for Medicare recipients may be more than offset by a variety of additional changes in the Balanced Budget Act that gave states considerable flexibility in setting payment rates for a variety of services and providers. States can now limit or effectively eliminate payments for Medicare co-payments and deductibles for a large number of low-income elderly. The Balanced Budget Act also eliminated the Boren amendment, which provided hospitals and nursing homes with grounds for suing states in federal court for "reasonable and adequate payment" and removed requirements that states pay federally qualified health centers at 100 percent of the cost of providing care. While states will thus lose DSH funds that they would have received under prior legislation and will be required to spend additional funds to cover Medicare premium increases, they have also been provided with considerable flexibility to offset this added financial burden.

A second major devolution feature that has obvious bearing on the future of managed-care arrangements is the amount of flexibility that states are provided in alternative versions of Medicaid reform, both with respect to managed care and other features that affect managed care's political opportunity cost. Elimination of the requirement that states seek waivers from the HCFA to engage in large-scale, mandatory managed care or the removal of restrictions on types of acceptable plans or other particular issues may decidedly increase the attractiveness of expanding managed care in many states; but state decisions about managed care may also be affected by the opportunity to realize savings in other areas. Part of managed care's current political appeal has been the insulation that it provides states from litigation, under the Boren amendment, over hospital payments as well as requirements governing payments to federally qualified health centers, so that the elimination of these requirements in the Balanced Budget Act reduces the comparative advantage of managed care by offering states the opportunity to realize savings in other ways. The current Medicaid statute also mandates coverage of a variety of services for a variety of population groups and imposes payment requirements on other services. The elimination or limitation of these mandates would broaden the range of permissible responses states could make in light of large-scale reductions in federal support and might lessen the appeal of a major investment in managed care.

The Balanced Budget Act of 1997 expands state flexibility in several ways. As noted above, it increases state flexibility in setting payment levels in several areas. Perhaps more important, it considerably expands states' ability to mandate enrollment in managed-care programs without detailed federal scrutiny and reduces federal oversight of the conditions under which Medicaid managed-care programs operate. Previously, states that wished to enroll Medicaid recipients in managed-care programs were required to seek any of several different types of waivers from HCFA to eliminate a variety of standards and conditions required under the fee-for-service version of Medicaid.[43] As part of the process of applying for these waivers, states were required to offer a variety of assurances that managed-care arrangements would maintain quality and access and to show that waiver proposals would be budget neutral or would not produce a higher level of spending than the state would have incurred under a continuation of the fee-for-service program.

While requests for waivers were rarely denied outright, the application process was lengthy and frequently contentious. Individual state waiver requests were on occasion the subject of considerable local debate that spilled over into the review process, and at least one, proposed by Oregon, became the subject of considerable national controversy.[44] State officials complained bitterly that HCFA reviews of waiver requests have typically taken too long, required too much additional information and too many re-estimates of spending to demonstrate budget neutrality, been too detailed and too responsive to the complaints of advocates. Approval of waiver requests has frequently been accompanied by extensive terms and conditions that frequently mandate detailed reporting on the provider capacity of individual plans, the individual encounters between providers and clients, and a variety of other detailed matters. State officials complained that this level of scrutiny and distrust constituted overly invasive micromanagement, hostility to innovation, and a major obstacle to the improvement of health care to Medicaid recipients. These officials repeatedly argued for a greatly diminished level of federal review as well as an increased federal focus on outcome standards and other measurement tools to permit improved assessment of Medicaid's effectiveness.[45] Supporters of the greater federal oversight attached to the waiver process argued in their turn that the federal government, as the largest payer under Medicaid, has an obligation to ensure the quality of the service it receives in return for its expenditures.[46] They note that some states have experienced considerable implementation problems and been found to have violated the budget neutrality requirements,[47] so that skepticism about state claims was not entirely unfounded. They also contended that outcome standards and other less intrusive means of holding states accountable are still at a primitive stage of development and are unlikely to be viable alternatives for a number of years.[48]

The states largely won this argument, which culminated in the Balanced Budget Act of 1997. The act dramatically expands state ability to mandate enrollment in managed care without prior federal approval and enhances state control over the types and numbers of plans with which contracts can be drawn.[49] States can now mandate the enrollment of any Medicaid recipient, except so-called special-needs children, Medicare beneficiaries, and American Indians, in managed care without a waiver. States are still required to file an amendment to their state plans, a process that requires nominal federal approval, to implement mandatory managed care, but this process has been widely treated as pro forma by both HCFA and states.[50]

The act also allows states to mandate a minimum enrollment, or lock-in, period for Medicaid clients and to restrict the plans in which clients can enroll. Recipients had previously had the ability to disenroll from a managed-care plan on 30-day notice; the Balanced Budget Act allows states to lock in clients to a particular plan for up to one year unless they can show cause for the change. It also allows states to limit clients to a choice of two plans, or only one in rural areas, and to restrict enrollment to plans that contract exclusively with Medicaid and have no other clients. Previously, plans that contracted with Medicaid were required to draw at least 25 percent of their enrollees from sources other than Medicaid and Medicare. Both the 75/25 requirement and the short notice for disenrollment requirements have been held by advocates to provide some minimal checks on the quality of care offered by plans. By allowing states to restrict the ability of Medicaid clients to vote with their feet and eliminate the requirement that plans attract some number of commercial enrollees, the act permits states to eliminate or restrict market competition between plans as an incentive to maintain quality and access for clients.

The Balanced Budget Act also imposes a variety of administrative requirements intended to ensure adequate quality and protect Medicaid clients against the arbitrary denial of care. States are required to develop strategies for quality assessment and improvement that specify standards for access to care, the collection of data from plans to monitor the quality of care provided to recipients, and to make provision for an annual review of the operations of individual managed-care organizations by an organization independent of the state. It also requires that states establish sanctions short of contract termination, such as allowing disenrollment and suspending payments or further enrollment, to apply to plans that fail to provide adequate care or discriminate among enrollees on the basis of health status.

These provisions make it significantly easier for states to institute managed care and appreciably lessen federal oversight of state managed-care operations. The Balanced Budget Act establishes significant procedural safeguards against the provision of inadequate care but leaves much discretion over the implementation of these safeguards to states. Given that major future expansions of managed care appear likely to be driven by fiscal stress, whether induced by recession or political demands to produce budget savings for other purposes, it is appropriate to consider what major political and implementation issues are likely to arise in the event that states make major attempts to expand managed care to the size required to generate appreciable budget savings.

Limiting Federal Oversight

The consequence of eliminating or greatly diminishing federal involvement in the review of state managed-care proposals is to magnify the role of state legislative and other politics in determining the shape of state efforts. While states were required to gain legislative as well as federal approval for the terms of waivers, legislative consideration of waiver terms was frequently less than exhaustive and heavily influenced by arguments about what HCFA was and was not likely to approve. Some states made political decisions to push for major waivers with only the most limited involvement of either legislature or state advocacy groups—New York, for example, prepared its waiver request in only six weeks with little or no consultation with either the state legislature or the state's large and vocal advocacy community,[51] and was not able to gain legislative approval to implement the waiver until more than a year and a half after it was submitted.

Eliminating or dramatically reducing the federal role in negotiations over managed care seems likely to amplify the role of state legislative politics in debates over these questions. The client groups that are likely candidates for inclusion in expanded versions of Medicaid managed care and the providers who serve them are not evenly distributed geographically across most states, but instead are disproportionately concentrated in areas that overlap and reinforce other long-standing political cleavages in state legislatures.

Low-income households in general—and the poor, female-headed households with children who constitute the bulk of the AFDC population in particular—are disproportionately urban.[52] On average, cities have much larger concentrations of their state's AFDC recipients, poor individuals, poor children, and female-headed households than of the state's overall population. This urban concentration of low-income groups is particularly pronounced in the large states in the Northeast and the Midwest, where AFDC recipients are up to seven times more concentrated than the relevant population as a whole. While these groups are typically less urbanized in southern and western states, southern cities such as Atlanta, Miami, Birmingham, New Orleans, and Richmond also have heavy concentrations of low-income populations. While more fragmentary, available evidence also suggests that the severely and persistently mentally ill are also disproportionately concentrated in urban areas as well.[53]

This urban concentration of the AFDC population, which has been the major Medicaid client group enrolled in managed care to date, has meant that managed care currently serves a poor, minority, inner-city clientele. Because Medicaid fee-for-service rates have historically been low relative to those available from other carriers or private-pay patients, providers have financial incentives to discriminate in favor of non-Medicaid patients, from whom they can receive higher fees, and accept Medicaid patients only when other patients are not available. As a result, Medicaid patients have been concentrated in a small number of providers who are disproportionately located in inner cities and have little professional prestige.[54] Organized provider constituencies such as state medical societies have thus been lukewarm supporters of Medicaid at best, because the bulk of their members have had few Medicaid clients and hence no strong financial stake in program decisions. The program's major provider support has historically come from such agencies as public hospitals, community health centers, and other providers that more or less exclusively serve a poor, minority, inner-city clientele. These providers are generally lacking in prestige, numbers, and other political resources and have frequently been unable to attract legislative support from outside central cities.

A similar pattern has emerged in many state managed-care programs, in spite of strong financial incentives for managed-care organizations to become actively involved in the Medicaid market. Increased competition in the private health care system and relatively rich Medicaid capitation payments have made Medicaid patients attractive to mainstream managed-care organizations in many states. Some states have created even stronger incentives for mainstream organizations to enroll Medicaid clients. Several states link access to managed-care contracts for state employees to enrollment of Medicaid clients,[55] and New York exempted managed-care organizations that meet specified Medicaid enrollment targets from its hospital rate system and allowed them to pay negotiated rates rather than the rates set by the state.[56]

In spite of these strong financial incentives, Medicaid managed-care enrollment in many states remains concentrated in a small number of organizations that disproportionately enroll Medicaid clients, particularly in urban areas, and have few commercial clients. Medicaid managed care is less common and less well developed in rural areas, so managed care largely remains an urban phenomenon. In Massachusetts, for example, 60 percent of the managed-care clients in the state's large primary-care case management program are enrolled in two managed-care organizations, with the remaining 40 percent divided among six organizations that have large commercial bases and only a small proportion of Medicaid clients.[57] More than one-half of the capitated clients in Medicaid managed care in Florida and Tennessee are in one HMO,[58] and the bulk of managed-care clients in Illinois's recently concluded waiver were in one large HMO, which is expected to be the major actor under the state's recently approved mandatory enrollment program in Chicago. In similar fashion, while twenty-three plans participate in New York's voluntary enrollment program in New York City, more than 50 percent of the enrollment are in only four plans,[59] and the bulk of enrollment in Minnesota is concentrated in three plans in which Medicaid clients make up more than three-quarters of total enrollment.[60] As noted in Michael Sparer's chapter in this volume, many states have also authorized the creation of so-called safety net plans composed of networks of public hospitals, community health centers, and other public and nonprofit providers, which are also heavily concentrated in urban areas.

In contrast to the urbanized managed-care population, less visible, but more expensive, elderly and disabled clients and the institutional providers that serve these clients are more geographically dispersed across smaller urban areas, suburbs, and rural areas, which in many states are more typically represented by Republicans. Nursing homes and nonprofit providers of services to the developmentally disabled and the elderly are typically more geographically dispersed, particularly in traditionally Republican suburban areas, and state institutions for the mentally ill and the mentally retarded and developmentally disabled (MR/DD), which in many states rely heavily on Medicaid support, are typically located outside major urban areas. In addition, many individual legislators retain strong political ties to nursing homes and hospitals, which are major employers and purchasers in many suburban and rural districts; state associations of these providers have typically found congenial receptions in many state legislatures.

These differences in client and provider demography suggest that the legislative politics around Medicaid managed care without federal controls will become increasingly partisan. Frequently heated, geographically based partisan debates about how to distribute spending reductions are common features of state budget processes, and similar cleavages have been prominent in past debates over Medicaid growth. In New York, for example, suburban Republican legislators were among the most vocal critics of

Medicaid's rapid growth in the early 1990s, which they argued crowded out spending in other state programs, particularly in elementary and secondary education, which is of prime political importance in suburban areas. Republican proposals for Medicaid reductions were heavily focused on those parts of the program whose recipients and providers are concentrated in New York City and much less on long-term care and other parts of the program from which their constituents benefited.[61]

The need to "sell" federal officials on the waiver process as well as state legislatures and interest groups on the size and form of managed care may have allowed urban interests that were not well represented at the state level to get a better deal than they otherwise might have if managed-care decisions were made at the state level without any further review. The advocacy groups for this population, which have been major actors in the waiver process in some states, have typically invested more effort in developing contacts and influence in Washington and with HCFA than with state legislatures and executive agencies,[62] and have been more effective in negotiations around waivers than they might be expected to be in negotiations limited to state actors. During the extended debate over the recently approved New York waiver, for example, New York City's advocacy community, which had largely been excluded from the process of developing the state's waiver request, was able to raise its concerns with allies in the federal bureaucracy and in Congress. Media reports have also highlighted the role of the head of the private hospital workers' union in New York City, who has strong ties to national Democratic politicians, in securing considerable transitional funding to allow city hospitals to develop primary-care clinics that would allow them to compete more effectively for Medicaid clients.[63]

The significant reduction of the federal presence in negotiations over the size and shape of Medicaid managed-care programs as a result of the Balanced Budget Act is likely to make these negotiations resemble other legislative debates in which long-standing geographic and partisan cleavages are prominent. The increased flexibility provided to states by the Balanced Budget Act of 1997 to restrict Medicaid clients' choice of plans and to contract with plans without commercial members seems likely to increase the concentration of Medicaid clients, particularly women and children, in a small number of plans centered in urban areas that have few, if any, non-Medicaid clients. It might be expected that suburban and rural representatives, as well as representatives of many provider groups, would press for large-scale buildups of managed-care enrollment of AFDC clients and reducing capitation rates to plans enrolling these clients as a primary means of limiting expenditures. Because of their lack of political resources, these clients and the providers that serve them are unlikely to be able to resist these demands effectively. Under these circumstances it seems likely that plans and providers serving urban residents would bear a dispropor-tionate share of spending reductions. The possible consequences of this diminished federal role were stated by one Medicaid director:

> In urban areas particularly, it's all going to play out the same way . . . with cost pressure, we're going to ratchet down our capitation rates. We are no longer going to be a profitable market for the private, traditional, main-stream providers. . . . And the only plans that will bid in urban areas will be the safety-net created plans. And we will capitate them so low that there will be de facto rationing within them. . . . Because it will be to the same providers with the same relatively low standards for provision of service, with an acceptance of queuing and denial of care.[64]

The effects of diminished federal supervision over state managed-care activities, in short, seem likely to enhance the political position of long-term care and other providers with significant political resources at the ex-pense of inner-city providers and plans, which are less powerful. If states are under pressure to reduce Medicaid spending growth by large amounts in a short period of time, there is likely to be considerable pressure from governors and budget offices to build up plan enrollments rapidly and sharply reduce capitation rates. We now turn to an examination of the management and implementation issues likely to arise around such a large-scale buildup.

Managing Managed Care—States as Prudent Purchasers

Medicaid managed care represents a major change from traditional fee-for-service Medicaid in the management requirements it places on states. Under fee-for-service, clients are responsible for finding providers who are willing to treat them, and providers are responsible for defining appropriate treatment and submitting a bill. The state is responsible primarily for pay-ing the bill under a set of closely defined rules governing the eligibility of clients, providers, and services and, for some types of providers and ser-vices, the rates they are obligated to pay. The management information and other systems states are required to maintain in order to receive Medicaid reimbursement from the federal government are largely designed to verify eligibility of clients, providers, and services; detect fraud, waste, and abuse; and document payments for particular services. Most state Medicaid agencies have historically defined their role primarily in terms of this passive bill-paying function and have not seen themselves as having any affirmative responsibility for setting or enforcing standards for gauging the appropriateness of care, improving access to care for Medicaid clients or improving the quality of care Medicaid clients receive.

Implementing Medicaid managed care requires significant changes in this orientation. Rather than paying bills for individual services to individual clients by individual providers, states are now required to award, negotiate, and implement contracts with managed-care organizations for packages of services to large populations covered by a single payment for each enrollee. Among other new tasks, this process requires that states develop standards for networks of providers required to care for large populations, set premiums appropriate to the benefits package, define procedures by which clients will be enrolled in managed-care plans, and develop methods for monitoring and evaluating the quality of care provided to Medicaid clients in managed-care plans.

Managed-care advocates argue that these changes present states with potential opportunities for improving access and quality of care to Medicaid clients in ways unobtainable under a fee-for-service payment system. By creating one organization that accepts payment for the entire range of services to Medicaid clients, managed care creates a means of defining standards for the adequacy and quality of care to which plans can be held accountable and sanctioned if they fail.[65] One state Medicaid official has put this perspective in strong terms:

> The leveraging power that you have from a contract truly makes all the difference because we can demonstrate with data through annual reports . . . [that] we have totally turned around the perception of managed care. . . . We have a report that we produce every year with 52 utilization and outcome indicators that reports, by HMO, . . . how they are doing compared to each other and compared to our Medicaid fee for service. This report when it started was truly embarrassing. Now it's truly positive. I can't emphasize enough how you can leverage this fish bowl environment to really change things. . . . [Medicaid] contract standards and requirements do become the norm in HMOs, even those that are providing care to private purchasers. . . . When they have to change their systems for Medicaid,

they change it for everybody. . . . [Advocacy groups] have pushed us to expand [these] programs as fast as we are able . . . because they are seeing that they can have more of a role in identifying what consumers need and want through managed-care plans than they can with 10 million disparate fee for service providers.[66]

While there is evidence that managed care can represent an appreciable improvement over the fee-for-service system, there is also an increasing amount of evidence that achieving these improvements is a complex, difficult, and, at least in the short run, expensive process. At least in theory, managed care provides states with opportunities to influence the way care is delivered to Medicaid recipients and to hold managed-care organizations and providers to standards of care that were not available under fee-for-service, but it also requires that states develop the administrative capacity to exercise this influence. As a method for purchasing and managing health care for low-income populations, managed care requires more attention to the education of patients, plans, and providers on how to deal with each other; the development of procedures to govern plans' marketing to enroll-ees and the process of enrollment; the development and enforcement of standards for network capacity, access, and the quality of care; the creation of management information and other systems to monitor how plans implement these standards; and the creation of means to feed back plan performance into the contracting process—in a word, more management—than fee-for-service. The experience of states that are widely agreed to have performed these tasks well suggests the need for considerable upfront investment of both time and money to develop systems, provide technical assistance to plans unaccustomed to dealing with this population, enhance the capacity to oversee plan performance, and reorient the operations of Medicaid agencies toward a more aggressive management style. One Medicaid official in a state with considerable experience with managed care has commented at some length on the magnitude of the management tasks associated with effective implementation of managed care:

What we really need in Medicaid is to talk about managed purchasing where, from procurement to evaluation, you have a hands-on partnership with the plans you contract with and the local communities to identify standards for getting a contract, for performance, for reporting on that performance, [and] for sharing the results of that performance. . . . This requires an enormous amount of staff resources, time, and knowledge, all things that most Medicaid programs really have to totally re-engineer to become capable of doing. . . . We need people in our programs that are capable of identifying health care outcomes that are appropriate to these different populations. . . . We need people who . . . can go out and talk to these HMOs about what their quality assurance programs ought to be doing with some knowledge and experience. . . . Managed care means that Medicaid really has to change its operational focus and administrative structure. It's very resource intensive and . . . very, very difficult. . . . We are moving from the old fashioned insurance model to something much more aggressive and proactive [and] we will end up . . . reorganizing our organization with more and more people dedicating more and more of their time to the management of our managed-care contracts.[67]

While precise comparisons between administrative costs in fee-for-service programs and managed care are not currently possible, because most states do not separate the operations of the two types of programs and give existing units additional tasks associated with the operation of managed care, the available anecdotal evidence suggests strongly that Medicaid managed care is appreciably more expensive and time-consuming to oversee than fee-for-service Medicaid. Some states have felt compelled to increase, in some cases dramatically, the resources they spend on managed-care oversight and increased the frequency with which they review plan performance and operations. Florida, for example, almost quintupled the size of its managed-care staff after a well-publicized marketing and enrollment scandal.[68]

Conversely, the difficulties experienced in some states can be traced in many cases to the failure to give sufficient consideration and resources to these management concerns. Many states appear to have made unrealistic assumptions about the ease and speed with which managed care could be instituted, underinvested in both planning and oversight structures, and experienced considerable controversy, administrative difficulties, confusion among both clients and providers, and, in some cases, scandal in implementation.[69] While these problems may have been transitory in some states, in others they have been more lasting. As noted earlier, for example, enrollment in New York and Tennessee has fallen sharply as a result of marketing problems and underfinancing, and there is evidence in a number of states of continuing difficulties with such managerial problems as "cream-skimming" and other enrollment difficulties, obtaining payment for services out of plan, and providing adequate physician supply and access to care.[70]

These potential problems are likely to be systematically understated and measures to address them systematically underfunded in the financially stressed environments that are likely to furnish the major pretext for future large-scale expansions of managed care. Under these circumstances, political and budget officials are likely to be interested in managed care primarily as a means of realizing large, short-term budget savings and are unlikely to be receptive to requests for additional support to add staff, develop new management information systems, or provide support for patient education programs to aid in choice of plans and the appropriate use of the managed-care system. Under conditions of financial stress, managed care is likely to be seen by political and budget officials in most states solely as a cost-containment device. The political need to reduce expenditures by moving clients into plans as rapidly as possible is likely to take precedence over considerations of quality, access, and accountability; and the investments in staffing, information systems, and other oversight elements necessary to realize the advantages of managed care as a delivery system may not materialize.[71]

In addition, past experience or expansion of existing systems already in place for the smaller geographic, voluntary programs centered around the healthier portions of the AFDC population, which have constituted most states' experience with Medicaid managed care to date, are unlikely to be particularly useful precedents for states attempting large-scale expansions of mandatory enrollment to the AFDC population or extensions of managed care to elderly and more disabled populations. Large-scale expansions or extensions of managed care are likely to exacerbate several existing management problems and create several new ones stemming from the extension of managed care to previously uncovered populations. Four such problems are likely to prove particularly difficult.

Financing

One of the more complex logistical problems likely to accompany attempts to extend managed care outside the AFDC population, particularly to the disabled, is the complex manner in which public services to these populations have historically been financed. In contrast to health care services to the AFDC population, which have primarily, if not exclusively, been financed through Medicaid, services to the severely and persistently mentally ill, the MR/DDs, and other more expensive groups have been financed from a more variegated set of sources, including state general funds,

a variety of categorical federal programs, and, in many states, significant
local funding. Medicaid has historically covered only a portion of the services provided to these populations, and attempts to consolidate them into
single funding streams that can be distributed via a capitated payment—
either as part of an integrated plan that covers all services or separately
through a carved-out benefit—are likely to be administratively and politically complicated.

Mental health financing provides one example of this complexity. Medicaid has historically covered drugs, case-management expenses, inpatient
hospitalization at community hospitals, and the costs of professionally provided therapy common in licensed outpatient settings. For adults, however, it
does not cover the cost of hospitalization at state psychiatric facilities, which
has historically been financed with state general fund revenue.[72] In similar
fashion, Medicaid does not cover a variety of community-based services that
have been argued to be particularly successful in reducing the need for extended hospitalization among the severely and persistently mentally ill. For
example, it does not cover the costs of housing, whether mortgages or rent
subsidies, or much of the self-help agenda, such as psychosocial clubs or
peer counselors favored by mental health consumer groups. In many states
these sorts of programs are not well developed, so that expansion to a level
where they could provide viable alternatives to hospitalization for a sizable
number of clients would require considerable amounts of new funds. In other
states where such programs are larger and better developed, they are also
likely to have providers and other constituencies who are likely to resist the
incorporation of their funding base into managed-care premiums. The financial politics of managed care in disability program areas is complicated further by the fact that state and other public agencies are much larger components
of the delivery system in these areas than in the health care system. In some
states, state psychiatric or developmental facilities are prohibited from accepting risk in the same manner as a private facility or from competing with
private facilities for clients, and hence may be unable to be incorporated in
networks; in others, state civil service or work rules or the terms of pre-
existing state contracts with providers may make treating state providers the
same as others difficult; in still others, budget bureaus or local officials may
object to the loss of control over state funding implied by incorporation of
general funds into a premium.

Many states have dealt with these difficulties by excluding large numbers of services, even expensive ones from which managed care might be
expected to realize savings, from managed-care benefit packages and con-

tinuing to pay for these services on a fee-for-service basis. Most states, for example, exclude hospitalization at state psychiatric facilities from capitation, and some, such as New York, exclude the most expensive community residence programs as well. Many states also exclude other services, such as substance abuse, which are heavily used by the severely and persistently mentally ill. This exclusion of expensive services from capitation limits the direct savings that can be realized from managed care and provides an incentive for managed-care organizations to shift the cost of expensive patients outside the premium.

The financial politics of disability programs, in short, are likely to be appreciably more complicated than those surrounding the AFDC population, which may make the task of extending managed care to the disabled appreciably more complex. As argued previously, providers and client groups in these areas are also better organized and more geographically dispersed than those associated with the AFDC population, which may limit states' ability to realize appreciable savings in this area.

A second financing issue that is likely to become more visible if managed care is dramatically expanded to more expensive populations is risk adjustment, or the payment of higher premiums for the disabled or chronically ill in order to prevent "cherry picking" of healthier and less-expensive populations and "dumping" of more expensive patients by managed-care organizations.[73] While this issue has been a matter of academic concern for some time, its practical consequences for Medicaid managed care to date may have been muted by the prevalence of voluntary enrollment and the limited number of plans participating in managed care in most states. Many states have also instituted adjustments for age and sex, which may have offset some of the incentives for plans to select among the healthier portions of the AFDC population, which have been the largest enrollees in managed care to date. If mandatory enrollment for both AFDC and more disabled populations becomes widespread, however, more expensive populations will be drawn into managed care, making the need to adjust payments more critical.

While a variety of proposals, some quite complex, has been made to address this problem, there is no particular evidence of convergence or clear agreement on the most appropriate means of either recognizing differences in risk or in the adjustment of payments to plans that incorporate these assessments, or much experience with the use of any of these schemes in practice.[74] Concern with risk selection has been a commonly cited justification in some states for carving out the severely and persistently mentally ill into plans separate from the ones for the AFDC population, with separate premiums, and in structuring the selection process for plans to select exclusive rather than multiple competing vendors, but the effectiveness of these procedures in reducing risk selection remains to be assessed.

Enrollment

Management of large-scale enrollment buildups has been perhaps the most persistent and visible, if not the severest, management problem in Medicaid managed care to date. Much of the recent adverse publicity around the implementation of managed care in such states as Florida, Tennessee, New York, and California has resulted from problems connected with attempts to enroll large numbers of clients in a short period of time, but similar problems have been noted by the General Accounting Office and others in managed-care programs since the early 1980s.[75] While the most visible abuses have been associated with direct marketing practices by plans in low-income areas, many states have experienced considerable difficulties associated with poor or limited educational material being available to clients on what enrollment in managed care means with regard to how they should seek care or what providers were affiliated with particular plans; the lack of information for clients who are illiterate or not native English speakers; higher-than-expected volumes of calls to information numbers; confusion about assignments; and a variety of other related logistical difficulties. These states have also typically experienced high rates of "auto assignment," under which clients fail to select a plan and are assigned to one automatically according to plan price, proximity to the client, unfilled capacity, or simply at random. The few states that have been successful in avoiding these problems have typically phased in enrollments over extended periods of time, required recipients to enroll in person at a welfare or plan office rather than allowing direct marketing or enrollment through the mail, and provided educational sessions to clients about managed care and the choices of plans available to them. Such states have typically had fewer logistical problems associated with the enrollment process and appreciably lower auto-assignment rates than states that invested fewer resources in managing the enrollment process.[76]

Such problems seem likely to persist or even intensify under large-scale expansions of managed care to the balance of the AFDC or disabled populations. Many states and plans appear to have systematically underinvested in client education or enrollment efforts, and anecdotal reports of auto-assignment rates of over 50 percent in many areas are common. The persistence of large-scale efforts to increase enrollment rapidly in spite of the extensive history of problems associated with this pace suggests that most states are unlikely to make the expensive investment in phased enrollment or client education that would lessen these difficulties. Gold and Sparer's explanation of the persistence of such efforts is persuasive:

> A key problem is that many states try to implement managed-care initiatives quickly. The speed is generally prompted by two factors. First, many state officials hope that their initiatives will produce significant short-term savings. And second, the cost containment goal is particularly appealing because the alternative ways to generate needed savings usually involve more explicit (and unpopular) cuts.
>
> In this situation [policymakers and career administrators] may be tempted to discount past experience and their own judgment, assuming a "can-do" attitude. Particularly in these situations, resources to effectively confront the administrative challenges also tend to be lacking or absent, since support for administrative staff and spending may be hard to generate in an environment in which human service programs are being cut. . . . As a result, problems sometimes are underestimated or ignored.[77]

Provider Capacity

A third persistent management problem that seems likely to become more acute under large-scale expansions of Medicaid managed care is ensuring adequate provider capacity or that a sufficient number of physicians, social workers, or other appropriate providers are affiliated with managed-care organizations to provide adequate care to the Medicaid clients they enroll. This issue was a particularly contentious one in waiver negotiations between several states and HCFA, and the terms and conditions attached to some waiver approvals have required states to regularly collect and evaluate lists of providers affiliated with individual networks on a regular basis and monitor such variables as the number of practices that are no longer accepting new patients.

This problem of inadequate capacity has historically been a particularly severe problem in the depressed inner-city communities where many Medicaid clients, particularly AFDC clients, reside. As a variety of studies have indicated, physicians typically find these areas unattractive ones in which to practice, so that there are relatively few office-based physicians in these areas. Recent research in Chicago, for example, found dramatic disparities in the availability of maternal and child health physicians between inner-city and more prosperous residential areas. Relative to population, there are almost three times as many obstetrician/gynecologists in more prosperous areas as in Chicago's inner city.[78] Similarly, there are almost twice as many children per office-based pediatrician in inner-city residential areas than in the most prosperous areas, and 60 percent more children per child health physician in Chicago's poorest areas than in its best-served residential areas.[79] While there are no recognized standards for determining the adequacy of supply of obstetric care, the ratio of child health providers to children in Chicago's inner-city communities is only half that recommended by the American Academy of Pediatrics.[80] Similar disparities in the availability of physician care between white, upper-income communities and minority, poor communities have been reported for other large cities.[81]

It is far from clear that current managed-care plans provide an adequate incentive for managed-care organizations to address this deficiency. Managed care does not alter any of the factors that give rise to undersupply in the inner city, but simply transfers jurisdiction over the supply problem from Medicaid programs to managed-care organizations. Inner cities remain low-prestige, unpopular areas that do not appeal to physicians for a variety of reasons, and inner-city patients still retain the characteristics that cause providers to label them as uncompliant and difficult, so that plans would have to pay a very large premium to attract providers into these locations. A variety of research indicates that Medicaid fees would have to be nearly doubled to induce physicians who currently limit their Medicaid practice loads to accept all Medicaid patients. The size of the fee increase required to produce increased Medicaid participation among physicians who are already participants suggests that plans would have to pay well above prevailing salaries to make inner-city locations attractive to providers. While detailed evidence on the financial relationships between plans and providers is lacking, the analysis of Rosenbaum and her co-authors of more than one hundred provider contracts found that more than 40 percent of plans pay fee-for-service rates to providers, frequently with considerable withholds of payment at levels that in many cases are not appreciably different from existing Medicaid fees.[82]

There is also little systematic evidence on the types and numbers of providers who have been included, excluded, or recruited into Medicaid managed-care networks, and the anecdotal evidence is decidedly mixed. In some cities there are reports that managed-care organizations have in fact taken steps to expand capacity in previously underserved areas; in other areas Medicaid clients have been segregated into separate lines of business with different rosters of providers than those available to other groups.[83] Most, if not all, of the providers in these arrangements have been physicians who were large billers under fee-for-service Medicaid and who have been enrolled with multiple plans.[84] Because plans and most (though not all) states have taken the existing inner-city provider system as a given and made few efforts to expand the supply of care in these areas, the capacity of most networks active in inner cities to absorb the large number of new patients that would accompany mandatory enrollment is small to nonexistent.[85]

States anxious to expand managed-care enrollment for budgetary reasons have few incentives to inquire closely into the adequacy of provider supply available in individual plan networks or in inner-city areas as a whole. States typically require plans to submit lists of physicians and other providers affiliated with their network, which state agencies can then compare to any of several widely promulgated staffing standards for primary care and other specialties. States may be less likely, however, to inquire closely into such matters as the appropriateness of the specialty mix represented in the plan's network, how many physicians belong to other plans' networks, the number of providers who are actually accepting new patients, or the travel time required to get to providers' offices.[86] Establishing the reporting systems to collect and analyze such information is time-consuming and expensive, and the potentially negative information such an effort might provide would only interfere with the process of certifying plans and enrolling members. Under these conditions, states are unlikely to look behind plan assurances of adequate capacity.

Even more pronounced problems of network capacity and capability are likely to accompany attempts to expand managed care to the disabled, particularly the severely and persistently mentally ill. While there are no broadly prescribed standards for judging network staffing patterns or service adequacy, at least some systematic evidence suggests that there may be insufficient capacity outside hospitals and state facilities to absorb the numbers of clients with severe and persistent mental illness who are likely candidates for inclusion in managed care. Estimates by the New York State Office of Mental Health, for example, indicate shortfalls in excess of 25 percent, as compared to estimated need for outpatient services and almost

50 percent for supported housing units.[87] These deficiencies were particularly large in New York City, where the shortfall approached 30 percent in outpatient services and 60 percent in housing units. Shortfalls of this magnitude in a state that has spent large amounts of money on developing community capacity and would be widely agreed to have a relatively large and well-developed community structure suggests that capacity may be a particularly severe problem in the larger number of less aggressive states.[88]

A potentially more severe management problem in the large-scale implementation of managed care for mental health rests in the limited integration of the public mental health system in most states. The large-scale consolidation and integration of the health care system and the increased use of managed care in the private health care system have been under way for some time in most states, so that Medicaid agencies proposing to expand managed care for AFDC populations are frequently dealing with providers and plans that have some experience in dealing with capitated payments and the organizational and information demands associated with managed care.

This basis of experience, for the most part, does not exist in the public mental health system. Managed care has become increasingly prevalent in the private mental health care system in recent years.[89] Behavioral health firms have become increasingly active in the management of mental health benefits for private employers, and office-based mental health practitioners such as psychiatrists, clinical psychologists, and social workers are increasingly consolidated into large multispecialty group practices that compete for managed-care contracts with these firms.

These developments have not, for the most part, penetrated the public mental health system. Behavioral health firms have little experience with public sector clients, who are typically much more severely disabled and expensive than the private patients that have formed their major clientele to date. In similar fashion, those providers with the most experience in dealing with the severely and persistently mentally ill have been largely unaffected by the advent of managed care in the private sector. Private office-based psychiatrists and other mental health providers have historically provided very little care to Medicaid clients, so that care for the severely and persistently mentally ill has largely been the province of a separate complex of independent public and quasi-public agencies. This system is very decentralized, with few organizational and contractual ties between hospitals and the large numbers of independent public and quasi-public agencies that provide service to public patients and are hence competing with others for patients and income. Inpatient care for mental health has largely been exempted from the shift in both Medicare and, in some states, Medicaid,[90] to prospective payment based on diagnosis and continues to be paid on a per-diem basis, while other services are reimbursed by Medicaid on a fee-for-service basis. There has thus been little incentive for providers to form the integrated networks that are becoming increasingly common in medical care, that provide a broad range of services, and that can be held accountable for all the services provided to a given individual. Providers have been unwilling to cede any authority over the clients they accept or discharge or over how long and through what methods they are treated to outside agencies. Referral structures exist in most areas, but they are typically small, ad hoc, and informal and not suited in scale or process to deal with the large numbers of clients produced by a large-scale move to managed care. Until recently, for example, all referrals to intensive case management programs in New York City for the several thousand individuals discharged each year from psychiatric centers were handled by a single staff member in the city's department of mental health. Establishing links to outpatient treatment and other community services for inpatient discharges has been a severe and persistent problem for both public and private hospitals, in spite of court cases mandating such linkages for public hospitals[91] in some areas and attempts to develop financial incentives in some states for private hospitals to place clients in outpatient programs.[92] In similar fashion, there are few organizational antecedents or models to follow in the extension of managed care to the mentally retarded and developmentally disabled.[93]

This lack of both capacity and antecedents may limit the rate at which mentally ill and disabled clients can be moved into managed-care arrangements, as may the greater political resources of both providers and client groups involved in these programs as compared to the AFDC population. The lack of any groups, either public or private, with experience with managing managed care for these populations may mandate a slower rate of growth simply because there are few organizations with claims to experience or expertise in these areas. Alternatively, particularly hard-pressed states may be tempted to assume a network and attempt to move these clients into managed care without any extended period of preparation.[94] Tennessee, which has been the only state to follow a version of this strategy by integrating mental health and MR services into its managed-care plans, is reported to have experienced the same types of confusion, service interruptions, enrollment declines, and conflicts with plans and interest groups as over other managed-care issues.[95]

Plan Monitoring and Quality Assurance

A final management problem likely to arise around large-scale expansions or extensions of managed care is the ability of states to monitor the performance of plans adequately. Since previous efforts have frequently been limited in their scale, ongoing responsibility for oversight of plan performance has frequently been added to the duties of existing units within state agencies, or assigned to relatively small, newly created offices of managed care. Responsibility for oversight of managed care has thus frequently been fragmented among a number of state agencies, many of whom have other responsibilities and limited experience with overseeing the operations of managed-care agencies.[96] Some state insurance agencies, for example, have experience in licensing and evaluating the financial solvency of some types of managed-care organizations, but may have little experience with other types of organizations or in working with health departments or Medicaid agencies on the particular problems associated with plans serving the Medicaid population. In many states Medicaid managed-care plans are not required to hold HMO licenses or meet associated capital or other financial requirements, and responsibility for regulating these nontraditional forms may rest with some other agency.

In similar fashion, state capacity to regulate the quality of care provided to Medicaid clients under managed care is uneven and, in general, not well developed. There is widely shared concern among state officials about the potential created by managed care for reduced access and underservice in caring for Medicaid clients—who are appreciably sicker than demographically similar groups in the general population and have been repeatedly found to underuse such preventive services as prenatal care and immunization—and widely shared agreement on the general need for states to develop the capacity to monitor the quality of care provided to Medicaid clients. Developing this capacity requires states to create standards for adequate care, develop data systems to demonstrate compliance with these standards, monitor plans for compliance with these standards, and make appropriate use of the results of these evaluations ranging from technical assistance to changes in rates or termination of contracts.

While there has been considerable improvement in the measurement of quality of care in the last five years, the state of the art in this area is still widely argued to be relatively primitive. The National Committee for Quality Assurance (NCQA), which has emerged as the leading agency in this area, has developed the Health Plan Employer Data and Information Set

(HEDIS), a set of quality standards for HMOs and a process to accredit plans for compliance with these standards,[97] but the current versions of these standards—it is widely agreed—focus on more readily measured structural or process characteristics, such as rates of immunization or mammography, rather than on the outcomes of care.[98] NCQA has recently issued a version of HEDIS that focuses explicitly on the Medicaid population,[99] and HCFA has issued broadly used guidelines for quality assessment, known as the Health Care Quality Improvement Systems (HCQIS). These standards, while considerable improvements over earlier efforts, are subject to the same caveats as other standards, as well as failing to completely address particular technical problems associated with the Medicaid population.[100] Quality measures for other Medicaid populations that are candidates for inclusion in large-scale expansions of managed care, such as the mentally ill, are even less well developed.[101]

State success in effectively overseeing the quality of care provided in Medicaid managed care has not been evaluated in any systematic way, but anecdotal evidence suggests that it is mixed and uneven. Some states have invested considerable time and resources in working with plans to develop performance measures and monitor plan performance on a regular basis,[102] while others have invested fewer resources and have made dramatically fewer demands on plans. It is far from clear to what extent plans providing care to Medicaid programs currently have the information system capabilities to comply with HEDIS or any other reasonable standards, but the available evidence suggests the proportion of plans able to provide such information on a timely or any other basis may be limited. While NCQA's HEDIS standards have been widely used by private employers and plans serving these employers, as well as by some Medicaid programs, only about 40 percent of the plans reviewed for accreditation by NCQA have been granted full accreditation, and the standards have come under attack from some national HMOs for being overly demanding and expensive.[103] Given this limited penetration in the private sector, where pressure from employers to demonstrate quality has been considerable, it seems unlikely that plans serving Medicaid clients have achieved even this level of capability.

The Balanced Budget Act imposes a variety of procedural requirements intended to ensure adequate quality of care for Medicaid clients and protect against the arbitrary denial of care.[104] States are required to develop strategies for quality assessment and improvement that specify standards for access to care and the collection of data from plans to monitor the care provided to recipients. States are also required to initiate an annual review of the operations of individual plans by an entity independent of the state and to establish sanctions short of contract termination, such as suspending payments or enrollment to apply to plans which fail to provide adequate care or discriminate among enrollees on the basis of health status.

The effects of these safeguards are difficult to predict. The requirements are substantial, but much discretion over what constitutes compliance with them is left to the states. If past history is an adequate guide, some states will invest considerable energy and resources in developing and implementing these procedures, while others will make considerably smaller investments. As in other areas, large-scale expansions of Medicaid managed care create a strong incentive for states to skimp on quality assurance and plan oversight. The available technology for monitoring plan performance is still relatively undeveloped, and the experience of more aggressive states suggests that applying the measurement tools that exist is time-consuming and expensive for both states and plans. Given the fiscal pressures that are likely to drive future large-scale enrollments in managed care, requiring that plans have elaborate data systems in place to be eligible for contracts or providing state agencies with the staff to oversee plan operations at the level of detail that past experience has suggested is necessary to improve the quality of care is likely to be seen as time-consuming luxuries that interfere with the primary goal of increasing enrollments as rapidly as possible.

Conclusions

These arguments suggest that managed care has largely lost its appeal as a silver bullet that can solve Medicaid's long-standing problems of access and quality at relatively low cost. As more states have acquired experience with managed care, and the consequences for providers, clients, and state agencies have become better defined, public debates over managed care have become more contentious, and the large-scale expansion or extension of managed care beyond its traditional clientele in the healthier and cheaper AFDC population into the more expensive elderly and disabled Medicaid populations is likely to progress at a slower rate than in recent years. There are sharply fewer organizational antecedents or private sector models to follow in instituting managed care for these populations, and the providers and interest groups associated with services to these populations are more powerful than those that have historically provided care to the

AFDC population, so that instituting managed care for these groups is likely to be slower and more politically difficult.

The effects of devolution on the continued growth of managed care are also problematic. Medicaid expenditure growth has tailed off sharply, the political appeal of large-scale health reform using Medicaid as a centerpiece has declined, and the political opportunity cost of managed care has increased significantly, so that there may be less pent-up demand among states for the flexibility to do large-scale managed care than previously. While it may be reasonably argued that more states would have tried more managed care on a larger scale if there had been no need to secure federal approval of these arrangements, changes in political and financial circumstances in many states suggest that local, rather than federal, politics may be more important to future managed-care efforts than in the immediate past. The argument here suggests that the primary circumstances likely to produce large-scale movement toward managed care in the future are sharp declines in state financial conditions or sharp increases in Medicaid spending as a result of recession or sharp increases in the rate of health care inflation.

While prediction is difficult, there is at least some evidence that Medicaid spending growth, at least in the short term, may remain modest. Recent CBO estimates of Medicaid baseline spending through 2002 have declined steadily, reducing both the size of the total projected deficit and the political visibility of Medicaid as a target for further efforts aimed at reducing the deficit. A second factor that might further depress Medicaid growth in the short term is the recently enacted federal welfare reform legislation, which potentially eliminates large numbers of AFDC recipients, who are automatically eligible for Medicaid, from the newly created temporary assistance to needy families (TANF) program. While states are required to continue Medicaid eligibility for recipients who would have been eligible under earlier rules even if they are no longer eligible for TANF, advocates have expressed concern that states will not establish new systems for re-establishing eligibility in a timely fashion, and many recipients who lose welfare eligibility may be without coverage for an extended period.[105] If this transition proves to be prolonged, Medicaid expenditures could be reduced further.

This moderate outlook for future Medicaid spending, the strong financial position of most state governments, and the financial flexibility provided by the repeal of the Boren amendment and other changes in the Balanced Budget Act suggest that most states may be under less immediate pressure to use managed care as a means of generating large short-term budget savings. Under these conditions, more states may likely have adequate time and resources to develop the neccessary managerial and information infrastructure to adequately manage managed care and phase in buildups in managed-care enrollment at a pace more appropriate to their ability to oversee plan operations adequately.

This potentially favorable outlook, however, has to be balanced against questions of how states will use the increased control over mandatory enrollment, contracting terms, and quality assurance provided in the Balanced Budget Act. By allowing states to institute mandatory managed care for most Medicaid recipients without waivers, limit recipient choice, contract with plans without commercial enrollees, and define compliance with requirements to ensure the quality of care, the Balanced Budget Act also creates the potential for states that are so inclined to configure managed-care programs primarily as a device for reducing Medicaid expenditures and generating budget savings. Past experience suggests that state reaction to this increased flexibility is likely to be extremely uneven. Some states will invest appreciable amounts of time and resources in developing an oversight infrastructure, while others may take advantage of lessened federal requirements and reduce their oversight efforts.

The argument here also suggests that, if presented with conditions that make large-scale expansion of managed care attractive, states are more likely, at least initially, to resort to expansion of managed care for the AFDC or TANF populations rather than extending managed care to the more expensive disabled or elderly populations. Because states and managed-care plans have more experience with operating managed-care programs for the AFDC population than for other groups, the "technology" required to manage such issues as rate setting and quality assurance is better developed than for other populations, and recipients and providers are less well organized and less powerful, making it politically easier to implement large-scale managed care in a relatively short period of time.

Under these circumstances, there are very real possibilities that states will underinvest in the management capacity required to realize the potential improvements in access and quality that managed care represents. While there is clear evidence that managed care, if done right, provides states with considerable opportunities to improve the health care provided to Medicaid clients, there is also considerable evidence that doing it right requires a sizable upfront investment in staff, systems, and time with regard to client education, enrollment, marketing oversight, capacity development, quality assurance, and a variety of other areas. States looking to managed care as a source of large-scale budget savings are likely to view these investments as unnecessary luxuries that prolong the process of enrolling large numbers of clients. Under these conditions, the political need to reduce expenditures is likely to take precedence over considerations of quality and access.

Notes

1. Jocelyn Guyer, "Trends in Medicaid Managed Care Enrollment and Plan Arrangements" (Center for Health Care Strategies Web Page [http://www.chcs.org/CHCS/jg_enrol.htm], 1996).

2. The eight states are Oregon, Pennsylvania, Tennessee, Washington, California, Michigan, Florida, and New York—which contained less than half of all Medicaid recipients in 1994. Guyer, "Trends in Medicaid Managed Care Enrollment," table 1.

3. For detailed descriptions of the range of PCCM programs, see Robert E. Hurley, Deborah A. Freund, and John E. Paul, *Managed Care in Medicaid: Lessons for Policy and Program Design* (Ann Arbor, Mich.: Health Administration Press, 1993).

4. The share of enrollees in health insuring organizations and prepaid health plans, the other two types of managed-care arrangements recognized by HCFA, declined from 25 percent of total enrollment in 1992 to 16 percent in 1995. Enrollment data are from Guyer, "Trends in Medicaid Managed Care Enrollment," fig. 3; and Hurley, Freund, and Paul, *Managed Care in Medicaid.*

5. Guyer, "Trends in Medicaid Managed Care Enrollment," fig. 5; and Lewin-VHI, "States as Payers: Managed Care for Medicaid Populations" (Washington, 1995).

6. Jocelyn Guyer, "States' Options for Using Medicaid Managed Care" (Princeton: Center for Health Care Strategies, not dated).

7. For a general description of mental health managed-care programs, see Bazelon Center for Mental Health Law, *Mental Health Managed Care: Survey of the States* (Washington, May 1996).

8. *Background Material and Data on Programs within the Jurisdiction of the Committee on Ways and Means, 1996 Green Book*, Committee Print, House Committee on Ways and Means, 104 Cong. 2 sess (Government Printing Office, 1996), p. 905, table 16-18.

9. As noted in the text, primary-care case-management programs generally pay a primary-care physician to act as a case manager responsible for providing or approving all care received by clients who select them as a case manager. Payment for approved care under these arrangements is made on a fee-for-service basis and cannot be separated from other vendor payments in the HCFA data from which these figures are taken. The health insurance organizations in Texas and California are private companies that manage portions of the Medicaid program under contract arrangements that do not put them at risk for overspending in the same fashion as conventional capitation arrange-

ments. The Texas program is large, amounting to more than $3 billion in 1995, while payments to the California program amount to approximately $650 million.

10. Lewin-VHI, "States as Payers," exhibit A-3, p. 26.

11. Fred Hellinger, "Selection Bias in HMOs and PPOs: A Review of the Evidence," *Inquiry*, vol. 32 (Summer 1995), pp.135–42.

12. See National Academy for State Health Policy, *Medicaid Managed Care: A Guide for States* (Portland, Maine, 1995) for an exhaustive description of enrollment requirements as of 1994; and Michael Sparer, "Managing the Managed Care Revolution: States and the New Medicaid," (1996).

13. National Academy for State Health Policy, *Medicaid Managed Care.*

14. Ibid.

15. Deborah A. Freund and Eugene M. Lewit, "Managed Care for Children and Pregnant Women: Promises and Pitfalls," *The Future of Children*, vol. 3 (Summer/Fall 1993); Mike Hanson in Nelson A. Rockefeller Institute of Government and the Brookings Center for Public Management, "Devolution and Medicaid: A View from the States" (Washington, unpublished transcript, May 23–24, 1996), pp. 320–21; Terence Driscoll, "The Interconnected Factors Which Lead to the Success of the Massachusetts Medicaid HMO Program," master's thesis, State University of New York (SUNY) at Albany, 1996.

16. Ron Winslow, "Welfare Recipients Are a Hot Commodity in Managed Care Now," *Wall Street Journal*, April 12, 1995, p. A1; Driscoll, "The Interconnected Factors"; Doug Cook in "Devolution and Medicaid," pp. 469–70; Karen Schimke, in "Devolution and Medicaid," p. 316; Mike Hanson in "Devolution and Medicaid," p. 321.

17. Historical data on Medicaid expenditures can be found on the HCFA website at http://www.hcfa.gov/medicaid/2082-1.htm.

18. See David Mirvis and others, "TennCare—Health System Reform in Tennessee," *Journal of the American Medical Association*, vol. 274 (October 18, 1994), pp. 1235–41; Lawrence D. Brown, "Commissions, Clubs, and Consensus: Florida Reorganizes for Health Reform," *Health Affairs*, vol. 12 (Summer 1993), pp. 7–26; Driscoll, "The Interconnected Factors"; Doug Cook in "Devolution and Medicaid," pp. 29–33.

19. For a detailed discussion of these debates, see James W. Fossett and James H. Wyckoff, "Has Medicaid Growth Crowded Out Education Spending?" *Journal of Health Politics, Policy and Law*, vol. 21 (Fall 1996), pp. 409–32.

20. For an account of this period, see David S. Broder and Haynes Johnson, "The Interests," in Haynes and Broder, *The System: The American Way of Politics at the Breaking Point* (Little, Brown, 1996), pp. 194–224.

21. See John Holahan and others, "Insuring the Poor through Section 1115 Medicaid Waivers," *Health Affairs*, vol. 14 (Spring 1995), pp. 199–216.

22. See the eight case studies in *Health Affairs*, vol. 12 (Summer 1993), pp. 27–88.

23. See, for example, James W. Fossett, "The Legislative Politics of Health Care Reform: Medicaid Managed Care in New York," working paper, SUNY at Albany, Department of Public Administration and Policy, 1994.

24. For a sampling of such stories, see David Hilzenrath, "Cutting Costs—or Quality?" *Washington Post Weekly Edition*, August 28–September 3, 1995, pp. 6–7; Milt Freudenheim, "Not Quite What Doctor Ordered: Drug Substitutions Add to Discord over Managed Care," *New York Times*, October 8, 1996, pp. D1, D6; Laura

Johannes,"More HMOs Order Outpatient Mastectomies," *Wall Street Journal*, November 6, 1996, pp. B1, B8.

25. Thomas Bodenheimer, "The HMO Backlash—Righteous or Reactionary?" *New England Journal of Medicine*, vol. 335 (November 21, 1996), pp. 1601–04.

26. Penelope Lemov, "The Strange Bedfellows of Managed Care," *Governing* (June 1996), pp. 21–24; and Bodenheimer, "The HMO Backlash."

27. Milt Freudenheim, "HMO's Cope with a Backlash on Cost Cutting," *New York Times*, May 19, 1996, pp. A1, A22.

28. Laura Johannes, "Managed Care Group Softens View on Hospital Stays after Mastectomies," *Wall Street Journal*, November 14, 1996, p. B6.

29. For surveys of recent activity, see Marc A. Rodwin, "Consumer Protection and Managed Care: The Need for Organized Consumers," *Health Affairs*, vol. 15 (Fall 1996), pp. 110–23; Lemov, "The Strange Bedfellows of Managed Care"; and Freudenheim, "HMO's Cope with a Backlash."

30. Milt Freudenheim, "Pioneering State for Managed Care Considers Change," *New York Times*, July 14, 1997, pp. A1, D8.

31. For accounts of these political alignments, see Lemov, "The Strange Bedfellows of Managed Care"; and George Anders and Laura Johannes, "Doctors Are Losing a Lobbying Battle to HMOs," *Wall Street Journal*, May 15, 1995, pp. B1, B2. For descriptions of the debate around the California and Oregon ballot propositions, see Robert Pear, "Stakes High as California Debates Ballot Issues to Rein in HMOs," *New York Times*, October 3, 1996, pp. A1, B9; Rhonda Rundle and Laurie McGinley, "California Voters Are Cool to 'Hot' HMO Issue," *Wall Street Journal*, October 31, 1996, pp. B1, B12; Bob Davis and G. Pascal Zachary, "Affirmative Action, Shareholder Lawsuits, and Tax Increases Are Rejected by Voters," *Wall Street Journal*, November 7, 1996, p. A17.

32. Lynn Etheredge, Stanley B. Jones, and Lawrence Lewin, "What Is Driving Health System Change?" *Health Affairs*, vol. 15 (Winter 1996), pp. 93–104.

33. Ron Winslow, "Managed Care Acts to Mollify Clients, Doctors," *Wall Street Journal*, December 17, 1996, pp. B1, B6.

34. For descriptions of this litigation, see William M. Sage, "'Health Law 2000': The Legal System and the Changing Health Care Market," *Health Affairs*, vol. 15 (Fall 1996), pp. 9–27; Edward Felsenthal, "When HMOs Say No to Health Coverage, More Patients Are Taking Them to Court," *Wall Street Journal*, May 17, 1996, pp. B1, B7; Edward Felsenthal, "Arcane State Laws Bedevil Managed Care," *Wall Street Journal*, September 6, 1996, p. B4; Robert Pear,"Medicare Patients in HMOs Win a Case," *New York Times*, October 31, 1996, p. B15; Linda Greenhouse, "Justices Refuse Case on Whether Health Care Networks Must Be Open to All Doctors," *New York Times*, November 5, 1996, p. A16.

35. For arguments along these lines, see Sage, "'Health Law 2000'"; Etheredge, Jones, and Lewin, "What Is Driving Health System Change?"; James F. Blumstein, "Rationalizing the Fraud and Abuse Statute," *Health Affairs*, vol. 15 (Winter 1996), pp. 118–28; Edward Hirshfeld, "Assuring the Solvency of Provider-Sponsored Organizations," *Health Affairs*, vol. 15 (Fall 1996), pp. 28–30.

36. Ann Murphy, "Formation of Networks, Corporate Affiliations, and Joint Ventures among Mental Health and Substance Abuse Treatment Organizations" (U.S. Department of Health and Human Services, Substance Abuse and Mental Health Services

Administration, 1995); Hirshfeld, "Assuring the Solvency of Provider-Sponsored Organizations," p. 29–30.

37. See, among others, General Accounting Office, *Medicaid: States Turn to Managed Care to Improve Access and Quality*, GAO/HRD-93-46; Marsha Gold, Michael Sparer, and Karyen Chu, "Medicaid Managed Care: Lessons from Five States," *Health Affairs*, vol. 15 (Fall 1996), pp. 153–66; and Marsha Gold and Michael Sparer, "Lessons in Medicaid Managed Care," *Health Affairs*, vol. 15 (Winter 1996), pp. 220–21; Ian Fisher with Esther B. Fein, "Forced Marriage of Medicaid and Managed Care Hits Snag," *New York Times*, August 28, 1995, pp. B1, B5; Martin Gottlieb, "A Free-for-All in Swapping Medicaid for Managed Care," *New York Times*, October 2, 1995, p. A1; United Hospital Fund, "New York City Returns to Direct Enrollment," *Medicaid Managed Care Currents,* vol. 1 (Summer 1996), pp. 1, 4; Geraldine Dallek, "A Consumer Advocate on Medicaid Managed Care," *Health Affairs*, vol. 15 (Fall 1996), pp. 174–77.

38. On enrollment declines in Tennessee, see Gordon Bonnyman,"Tenn-Care: Where It Stands Today—March 1996" (Center for Health Care Strategies Web Page [http://www.chcs.org/CHCS/gb.march.htm]) and "Policy and Coverage Changes—August 1996" (CHCS Web Page [http://www.chcs.org/CHCS/gb.aug.htm]); on New York, see United Hospital Fund, "Medicaid Managed Care in Transition," *Medicaid Managed Care Currents* (Spring 1996), pp. 1, 5.

39. Michael Hanson in "Devolution and Medicaid," pp. 393–99.

40. Donna Checkett, "A State Medicaid Director on Medicaid Managed Care," *Health Affairs*, vol. 15 (Fall 1996), pp. 172–73.

41. Karen Peed in "Devolution and Medicaid," pp. 313–14; Peggy Bartels in "Devolution and Medicaid," p. 315; Sparer, "Managing the Managed Care Revolution."

42. Michael Murphy in "Devolution and Medicaid," p. 317; Mike Hanson in "Devolution and Medicaid," p. 322; Peggy Bartels in "Devolution and Medicaid," p. 315.

43. For details on the various types of waivers, see Guyer, "States' Options for Using Medicaid Managed Care."

44. See Lawrence Brown, "The National Politics of Oregon's Rationing Plan," *Health Affairs*, vol. 10 (Summer 1991), pp. 28–51.

45. Doug Cook in "Devolution and Medicaid," pp. 342–44; Karen Peed in "Devolution and Medicaid," p. 344–45.

46. Joshua M. Wiener in "Devolution and Medicaid," pp. 69–71; James Tallon in "Devolution and Medicaid," pp. 346–47.

47. Wiener in "Devolution and Medicaid," p. 70.

48. Ibid., p. 339.

49. This description of these provisions is drawn from National Health Law Program, "Balanced Budget Act of 1997: Reshaping the Health Safety Net for America's Poor" (http://www.healthlaw.org/BBAtoc.html).

50. National Health Law Program, "Balanced Budget Act of 1997" (http://www.healthlaw.org/BBAsecIA.html#SecI).

51. See Michael Sparer and Lawrence D.Brown, "Nothing Exceeds Like Success?: Managed Care Comes to Medicaid in New York City" (Columbia University, Department of Health Policy and Management, June 1996); and James Tallon in "Devolution and Medicaid," pp. 346–47.

52. For an extended statement of this argument, see James W. Fossett and Janet

Perloff, "The 'New' Health Reform and Access to Care: The Problem of the Inner City," (Kaiser Commission on the Future of Medicaid, 1995).

53. New York State Office of Mental Health, *Statewide Comprehensive Plan for Mental Health Services 1994–1998* (Albany, 1993), appendix A, table 4.

54. See James W. Fossett and Janet Perloff, "The Politics of Medicaid Access: The Problem of the Inner City," working paper, SUNY at Albany, 1990.

55. Driscoll, "The Interconnected Factors"; Karen Peed in "Devolution and Medicaid," p. 296.

56. Karen Schimke in "Devolution and Medicaid", p. 265.

57. Driscoll, "The Interconnected Factors."

58. For evidence on Tennessee, see Gordon Bonnyman, "Policy and Coverage Changes," p. 1; on Florida, see Michael Hanson in "Devolution and Medicaid," p. 326.

59. United Hospital Fund, *Medicaid Managed Care Currents*, vol. 1 (Fall 1996).

60. Karen Peed in "Devolution and Medicaid," pp. 325–26.

61. Fossett, "The Legislative Politics of Health Reform."

62. For examples of the role of advocacy groups in waiver debates, see Sparer and Brown, "Nothing Exceeds Like Success?"

63. Steven Greenhouse, "The Odd Couple That Did the Heavy Lifting on Pataki's Managed-Care Medicaid Deal," *New York Times*, July 16, 1997, p. B4.

64. Alan Weil in "Devolution and Medicaid," pp. 157–58.

65. Donald Berwick, "Payment by Capitation and the Quality of Care," *New England Journal of Medicine*, vol. 335 (October 17, 1996), pp. 1227–31.

66. Peggy Bartels in "Devolution and Medicaid," pp. 280–82.

67. Ibid., pp. 283–85, 327.

68. Doug Cook in "Devolution and Medicaid," p. 329; Karen Peed in "Devolution and Medicaid," p. 301; Driscoll, "The Interconnected Factors."

69. Gold, Sparer, and Chu, "Medicaid Managed Care: Lessons from Five States."

70. See, among others, GAO, *Medicaid: States Turn to Managed Care*; Gold, Sparer, and Chu, "Medicaid Managed Care: Lessons from Five States"; Gold and Sparer, "Lessons in Medicaid Managed Care"; Fisher, "Forced Marriage"; Gottlieb, "A Free-for-All"; United Hospital Fund, "New York City Returns to Direct Enrollment"; Dallek, "A Consumer Advocate."

71. For one example of this dynamic, see Sparer and Brown, "Nothing Exceeds like Success?"

72. More precisely, Medicaid covers the cost of inpatient psychiatric hospitalization for all clients, but under the so-called IMD rule does not cover inpatient care for adults between ages twenty-one and sixty-five at institutes for mental disease or state psychiatric facilities and specialized psychiatric hospitals. It does, however, cover stays at IMDs for those under twenty-one and over sixty-five.

73. Joseph P. Newhouse, "Patients at Risk: Health Reform and Risk Adjustment," *Health Affairs*, vol. 13 (Spring I 1994), pp. 132–46.

74. For a sampling of this debate, see Newhouse, "Patients at Risk"; Richard Kronick, Zhiyuan Zhou, and Tony Dreyfus, "Making Risk Adjustment Work for Everyone," *Inquiry*, vol. 32 (Spring 1995), pp. 41–55; and Elizabeth J. Fowler and Gerard F. Anderson, "Capitation Adjustment for Pediatric Populations," *Pediatrics*, vol. 98 (July 1996), pp. 10–17.

75. See GAO, *Medicaid: States Turn to Managed Care*; and Dallek, "A Consumer Advocate on Medicaid Managed Care."

76. Gold, Sparer, and Chu, "Medicaid Managed Care: Lessons from Five States," pp. 156–57.

77. Marsha Gold and Michael Sparer, "Letter: Lessons in Medicaid Managed Care," *Health Affairs*, vol. 15 (Winter 1996), pp. 220–21.

78. James W. Fossett, Janet Perloff, John Petersen, and Phillip Kletke, "Medicaid in the Inner City: The Case of Maternity Care in Chicago," *Milbank Quarterly*, vol. 68 (1990), pp. 111–42.

79. James W. Fossett, Janet Perloff, Phillip Kletke, and John Petersen, "Medicaid and Access to Child Health Care in Chicago," *Journal of Health Politics, Policy and Law*, vol. 17 (Summer 1992), pp. 273–99.

80. Ibid.

81. Fossett and Perloff, "The 'New' Health Reform."

82. Sara Rosenbaum and others, *Negotiating the New Health System: A Nationwide Study of Medicaid Managed Care Contracts*, vol. 1 (George Washington University Medical Center, Center for Health Policy Research, February 1997).

83. Office of the Public Advocate for the City of New York, "Two Lists: Commercial and Medicaid Managed Care Providers" (New York, 1996).

84. Janet D. Perloff and James W. Fossett, "Staffing Medicaid Managed Care: Physician Supply and Network Capacity in New York City," unpublished paper, SUNY at Albany, School of Social Welfare, 1997.

85. Ibid.

86. For a detailed discussion of these questions, see ibid.

87. New York State Office of Mental Health, *Statewide Comprehensive Plan*.

88. James W. Fossett, Carol Ebdon, and Sheila Donahue, "Medicaid and Mental Health Reform: Financial Deinstitutionalization in New York," working paper, SUNY at Albany, Department of Public Administration, 1995.

89. John Iglehart, "Managed Care and Mental Health," *New England Journal of Medicine*, vol. 334 (January 11, 1996), pp. 131–35.

90. Medicaid inpatient hospital rates in New York are set by the state's Department of Health by a methodology resembling the Medicare Prospective Payment System in its reliance on prospective payment for a series of diagnosis related groups. For a detailed description of the current system, see New York State, Department of Health, Division of Health Care Financing, *Hospital Reimbursement in New York State (NYPHRM IV)* (Fall 1991).

91. See, for example, *Heard* v. *Cuomo*, 610 N.E.2d 348 (New York, 1993).

92. See Carol A. Boyer and David Mechanic, "Psychiatric Reimbursement Reform in New York State: Lessons in Implementing Change," *Milbank Quarterly*, vol. 72 (1994), pp. 621–51.

93. Gary Smith and John Ashbaugh, *Managed Care and People with Developmental Disabilities: A Guidebook* (Washington: National Association of State Directors of Developmental Disabilities Services, Inc., 1996).

94. The phrase is taken from Laurence E. Lynn Jr., "Assume a Network: Reforming Mental Health Services in Illinois," *Journal of Public Administration Research and Theory*, vol. 2 (1996), pp. 297–314.

95. Bonnyman, "Policy and Coverage Changes"; Bonnyman, "Access to Care" (CHCS Web Page [http://www.chcs.org/CHCS/gb.sept.htm] September 1996); and Bonnyman, "Rural Health Outreach and Conflicts of Interest Controversy" (CHCS Web Page [http://www.chcs.org/CHCS/gb.nov.htm] November 1996).

96. For examples of state oversight arrangements, see Marsha Gold, Hilary Frazer, and Cathy Schoen, "Managed Care and Low-Income Populations: A Case Study of Managed Care in Tennessee" (Washington: Mathematica Policy Research, 1995), and Sparer and Brown, "Nothing Exceeds like Success?"

97. For descriptions of these efforts, see John K. Iglehart, "The National Committee for Quality Assurance," *New England Journal of Medicine*, vol. 335 (September 26, 1996), pp. 995–99.

98. Robert H. Brook, Elizabeth A. McGlynn, and Paul D. Cleary, "Measuring Quality of Care," *New England Journal of Medicine*, vol. 335 (September 26, 1996), pp. 966–70; and Iglehart, "The National Committee for Quality Assurance."

99. National Committee for Quality Assurance, *Medicaid HEDIS (final)*, Washington, undated document.

100. Ibid.

101. For descriptions of the state of the art in these areas, see Harold Alan Pincus, Deborah A. Zarin, and Joyce C. West, "Peering into the 'Black Box': Measuring Outcomes of Managed Care," *Archives of General Psychiatry*, vol. 53 (October 1996), pp. 870–77; and Smith and Ashbaugh, *Managed Care and People with Developmental Disabilities*, pp. 225–29.

102. See Karen Peed in "Devolution and Medicaid"; Peggy Bartels in "Devolution and Medicaid"; and Driscoll, "The Interconnected Factors."

103. Iglehart, "The National Committee for Quality Assurance."

104. See National Health Law Program, "Reshaping the Health Safety Net for America's Poor" (http://www.healthlaw.org/BBAsecIE-G.html#SecIE).

105. Laura Summer, Sharon Parrott, and Cindy Mann, "Millions of Uninsured and Underinsured Children are Eligible for Medicaid" (Center on Budget and Policy Priorities Web Page [http://www.cbpp.org/mcaidprt.htm], April 1997); "The Medicaid Clearinghouse" (Families USA Web Page [http://www.familiesusa.org/medicaid/]).

5

Safety Net Providers and the New Medicaid

Choices and Challenges

Michael S. Sparer

DURING THE 1980s, federal officials required the states to increase the Medicaid reimbursement paid to many health care providers. These federal mandates enabled hospitals, community health centers, and other safety net providers to cope (more or less) with the rising number of uninsured. This pattern continues today: Medicaid revenue subsidizes much of the care rendered to the uninsured. Looking ahead, however, the Medicaid subsidy (and the fiscal health of the medical safety net) is at risk. The Balanced Budget Act of 1997 eliminated an important reimbursement mandate and required the phasing out of another. Federal regulators are already waiving some of the remaining mandates for some of the states. States are using their expanded flexibility to reduce Medicaid reimbursement. The new Medicaid federalism is increasing state authority and decreasing provider reimbursement.

Safety net providers are likely not only to receive less reimbursement for each Medicaid beneficiary, but also to have fewer of these publicly insured patients. The reason for the expected decline is that commercial managed-care companies, which until recently discouraged Medicaid beneficiaries from enrolling, are now competing for the Medicaid business. These companies recognize that Medicaid clients can be profitable, especially at a time when nearly every state is encouraging (or requiring) beneficiaries to enroll in managed care. As a result many beneficiaries who have long received health care in a public hospital, public health clinic, or community health center can today enroll in a commercial managed-care company.

To be sure, not all Medicaid beneficiaries will enroll in managed care. Moreover, some beneficiaries will enroll in "safety net" health plans (formed by safety net providers in an effort to maintain market share). Others will sign on with commercial plans but will continue to see their safety net provider (because the provider signs a contract with the plan). Some safety net providers may even prosper in the new health care marketplace. The transition to Medicaid managed care will be nonetheless turbulent for many safety net providers.

During this transition era, federalism issues loom large. With the safety net at risk, federal Medicaid officials could require states to enact safety net protection policies. For example, federal officials could require states to pay supplemental funds to safety net health plans. Such a policy would be a change, however, from the current trend toward loosened federal oversight. Alternatively, state governments could pursue more of a laissez-faire approach, removing themselves from the policy arena and letting the market alone determine the fate of the current safety net. Still another option is for local governments to dismantle the current safety net (by privatizing public hospitals and public health clinics) with the hope that other institutions take its place. Under any of these scenarios, however, the intergovernmental balance of power is important to the future of the medical safety net.

This chapter considers the politics of the medical safety net and the policy options available to the different levels of government. It recommends that federal officials reassert control over Medicaid policy and require states to enact explicit safety net protection policies. Before summarizing the policy options and recommending a policy path, however, the chapter summarizes the evolution of the medical safety net and examines the current status of five types of safety net institutions: public hospitals, academic medical centers, community health centers, public health clinics, and community-based specialty clinics. This history provides an important framework for the policy discussion that follows.

The Pre-Medicaid Era

For much of U.S. history, the federal government was only a minor player in the nation's health and welfare system. During the nineteenth century, for example, the only federal social welfare program was a pension program for Civil War veterans (and Confederate veterans were ineligible for such benefits).[1] The only federal health care program of note was a fairly small initiative to fund maternal and child health clinics, and that initiative was not enacted until 1921 (it was then repealed in 1929 and revived in 1935).[2] National health insurance was not seriously debated until 1912, and even then President Theodore Roosevelt's proposal for universal insurance was quickly labeled un-American and was easily defeated. Later initiatives by Presidents Franklin Roosevelt and Harry Truman fared no better.[3]

The bias against federal action was due in large part to the influence in America of the English poor-law tradition. Under this tradition social welfare was a local responsibility: neither the states nor the federal government had an important role to play. Moreover, only the so-called deserving poor (or those persons outside the labor force through no fault of their own) were entitled to assistance. Others were left to fend for themselves.

Lacking either federal leadership or federal funding, many local governments established a two-part medical safety net. First were institutions that focused on the acutely ill. These began as infirmaries connected to almshouses (which were residential institutions for the poor). Over time many of the infirmaries evolved into public hospitals. The second approach focused not on individuals but on the health of the community. Local health codes were enacted and public health departments established to enforce the codes. Initiatives were made to reduce infectious disease by improving sewage and garbage disposal. Public health clinics provided preventive health services to the community at large.

Before 1965 these municipal programs (supplemented by a few privately operated charity hospitals and the charity care component of the individual provider's practice) constituted the nation's medical safety net. Neither the states nor the federal government played much of a role. This changed in 1965 with the enactment of Medicaid, Medicare, and the community health center initiative (then called the neighborhood health center program).

Medicaid and the Bias against Primary Care: 1966–85

Medicaid and Medicare were efforts to provide the aged and the poor with access to the existing mainstream health care system. These were publicly funded health insurance programs. These were not efforts to alter or expand the existing health care system. The community health center program, in contrast, was an effort to create community-run primary care clinics in low-income communities. The policy assumption was that locally controlled but federally funded clinics could provide coordinated, comprehensive, and cost-effective health care to otherwise underserved poor persons. The five-year plan was to establish more than 1,000 clinics, serve 25 million poor persons, and receive direct federal subsidies of more than $3 billion annually.[4]

By the early 1970s, however, it was clear that most Medicaid beneficiaries and the uninsured would continue to have inadequate access to primary and preventive health care. The problem was threefold: (1) federal Medicaid law favored inpatient specialty care and disfavored community-based primary care, (2) the community health center program grew more slowly than expected, and (3) the nation continued to suffer from a geographic maldistribution of health care providers; nearly 43 million Americans currently live in medically underserved communities.

Between 1965 and the late 1980s, for example, Congress required state Medicaid programs to pay hospitals for their reasonable costs but provided states with nearly unfettered discretion in setting reimbursement for outpatient primary care.[5] As a result, Medicaid payments to hospitals were relatively generous, covering almost 95 percent of costs, while payments to office-based primary-care providers were extraordinarily low (less than 40 percent of the average private insurance rate).[6] In some states the disparity between inpatient and outpatient rates was even more marked. In New York, for example, a hospital that treated a Medicaid beneficiary received approximately 101 percent of the cost of the care.[7] A primary-care physician, in contrast, received only 16 percent of the rate paid by private insurers.[8]

The low rates dissuaded most office-based physicians from treating Medicaid clients. In New York, for example, only 44 percent of the state's doctors participated in Medicaid, and only 20 percent of those that did billed the program more than $10,000 per year.[9] During this era most Medicaid beneficiaries received health care, if at all, in hospital emergency rooms and hospital clinics.

To be sure, there was (and is) a small cadre of office-based physicians with a medical practice composed primarily of Medicaid beneficiaries. These doctors, who generally practice in inner-city low-income communities, are referred to as traditional Medicaid providers. The providers compensate for low Medicaid rates by treating a high volume of Medicaid patients. Nonetheless, the number of traditional Medicaid providers is too few to provide health care access to most Medicaid beneficiaries.

The federal bias against community-based care also slowed the growth of the community health center program. The Medicaid reimbursement received by community health centers was generally inadequate to cover the cost of their Medicaid patients. The rates for covered services were too low, too many services were not covered at all (such as those, like social work counseling, that straddled the boundary between medical and social services), and the nonphysician providers relied on by many centers were too often ineligible for Medicaid reimbursement. Along with lower-than-expected Medicaid reimbursement, community health centers received smaller-than-expected federal grants. The nation's rising Medicaid bill left fewer dollars for health center grants.

By the mid-1980s community health centers also were coping with a growing shortage of health care providers. The shortage resulted from a dramatic reduction in the funding allocated to the National Health Service Corps (NHSC). This program, enacted in 1970, provides loans and grants to health profession students who agree to practice for at least two years in a medically underserved community.[10] By the late 1980s the program had awarded thousands of scholarships.[11] More than half of the physicians then working in community health centers were NHSC graduates.[12] In the early 1980s, however, President Ronald Reagan encouraged Congress to eliminate funding for new NHSC positions. While the program was never fully defunded, it was significantly curtailed—so much so that by 1985 only thirty-four physicians received new scholarships (compared with more than 2,500 scholarship awards in 1978).[13] By the mid-1980s the health center community was feeling the pinch: not only were federal Medicaid dollars continually scarce, but centers were increasingly short-staffed.

The health center work force shortages reflect a more generic problem in the U.S. health care system: there are too few physicians willing to practice in low-income or rural communities and too many anxious to practice in upscale neighborhoods and wealthy suburbs. In Bedford-Stuyvesant, New York, for example, there are less than seventy-five office-based physicians per 100,000 population; in the city's fashionable Upper East Side, in contrast, the number is 1,136 per 100,000 population.[14] The best explanation for the maldistribution of medical resources is money. Physicians who treat the privately insured earn much more than do those working with the poor. There are lifestyle issues as well: many health care professionals are reluctant to live in isolated rural communities (especially as they raise families) or to practice in crime-filled inner cities; a suburban office and a middle-class clientele seem safer and easier.

Federal Efforts to Improve Access to Care (1985–96)

Beginning in the late 1980s federal Medicaid officials adopted two strategies to increase the access to care available to the poor and uninsured.[15] First was an effort to increase Medicaid reimbursement for the medical safety net. For example, Congress required the states to increase the reimbursement paid to community health centers. At the same time Congress (and the states) developed more expansive definitions of covered services and covered providers, all of which provided additional reimbursement as well. Congress also provided supplemental funds to hospitals that served a disproportionate share of the poor and the uninsured. Congress even required increased reimbursement for obstetricians and gynecologists.[16]

The second strategy was to encourage managed-care organizations that had previously covered the middle class and the privately insured to enter the Medicaid market. The hope was that managed-care companies would encourage (or require) their affiliated physicians to treat Medicaid beneficiaries. The goal was to shift—from the statehouse to the marketplace—responsibility for the geographic maldistribution problem. Managed-care plans would be required, for example, to develop provider networks that were adequate to serve the newly enrolled Medicaid beneficiaries. Government's role would be to monitor and regulate health plan performance.

The impact of the beneficiary access programs is hard to judge. The good news is that the increased Medicaid reimbursement enabled public hospitals to survive, encouraged community health centers to expand, and convinced some ob/gyns to accept new Medicaid patients. At the same time, however, the number of medically underserved communities is increasing. In 1992, for example, the federal government classified 2,271 communities as health profession shortage areas; by 1995 the number had grown to 2,677.[17] Meanwhile, the impact of Medicaid managed care on beneficiary access is hard to gauge. Without doubt, commercial managed-care companies are now competing fiercely for the Medicaid business. There is nonetheless little evidence that the companies are persuading large numbers of physicians to move their practices into medically underserved communities.[18] Moreover, as the commercial health care industry continues to evolve, there is a risk that current safety net providers could be forced out of business. The result could be an even greater geographic maldistribution of providers.

Managed Care

The U.S. health care system is in the midst of a rapid and remarkable transition. The change began in the 1980s, when health care economists persuaded the private sector that soaring health care premiums were due largely to a system in which doctors delivered unnecessary care (because they were paid a separate fee for every service) and consumers did not care (since the bill was paid by a third-party insurer). The recommended alternative was prepaid managed care: in exchange for a fixed fee, managed-care organizations would assume responsibility for all (or most) of an employee's health care needs. The policy assumption was that managed-care plans would lower health care costs and that the dramatic rise in employer health insurance premiums would thus taper off.

By the early 1990s most employers were persuaded: by 1993, 51 percent of those with employer-sponsored insurance were enrolled in managed care; two years later the number was up to 73 percent.[19] At the same time the movement to managed care helped to reduce health care costs.[20] Between 1994 and 1995, for example, employer health insurance premiums increased only 2.3 percent, the lowest rate in almost a decade.[21]

To be sure, researchers disagree on whether the cost savings are short term or long term. For example, many health plans use their market leverage to negotiate discounts with hospitals and other providers. Large savings of this sort are not likely to be replicated over time. Similarly, many managed-care advocates tout the cost-containment potential of so-called practice guidelines (which tell health care providers how to treat particular symptoms). The practice guideline movement, however, is both controversial and in its infancy.

Managed-care advocates also point to savings generated by actually managing client care. The primary-care provider, for example, should be a case manager, supervising and controlling client access to specialty and hospital services. But case managers often do little case management. The trend toward looser forms of managed care, such as point-of-service plans, reduces even further the amount of case management.[22] Finally, the trend toward capitation should encourage providers to provide less care. The long-term savings from this trend are nonetheless still unclear (as is the long-term impact on quality of care).[23]

Despite these uncertainties, public officials have jumped on the managed-care bandwagon. President Clinton argued in 1993 that (managed) competition between managed-care plans could produce enough savings to finance health insurance for the nation's 37 million uninsured.[24] More recently, the Balanced Budget Act of 1997 amended the Medicare program in an effort to encourage Medicare beneficiaries to enroll in managed care. The goals of the new initiative are to increase beneficiary choice and to reduce and control program expenditures.[25] Meanwhile, nearly every state now encourages (or requires) Medicaid beneficiaries to enroll in managed care.[26]

The growth in managed care has prompted a second fundamental change in the U.S. health care system: the trend toward mergers and consolidations. The trend began with those who pay the health care bill: the business and insurance communities. Large corporations, for example, formed purchasing alliances in an effort to increase their leverage when negotiating with insurance companies.[27] Similarly, insurance companies began to consolidate in an effort to increase their leverage with the health care provider community.[28] The increasingly powerful insurance industry (especially the large managed-care companies) used their leverage to negotiate discounts from the fragmented provider community.

In response to the consolidating payer community, health care providers are now consolidating as well. Physicians are forming group practices, hospitals are buying group practices (and merging with other hospitals), and physicians and hospitals are together forming integrated delivery systems (thereby competing with the traditional managed care companies). In Minneapolis, for example, three integrated delivery systems now control more than 75 percent of the health care market.[29] The lines between insurer and provider are growing increasingly thin.

The changing health care system has a profound impact on the nation's medical safety net. The movement toward managed care requires safety net providers either to form their own managed-care organizations or to enter into contracts with managed-care companies already in place. The movement toward mergers and consolidations requires safety net providers to consolidate themselves, either joining with other providers or aligning with a more mainstream health care system. At the same time, however, the capacity of the safety net to survive the transition varies significantly. Community health centers, for example, seem well positioned (though hardly secure). Public hospitals and public health clinics, especially those in rural communities, face a more daunting task. The following section examines these three types of safety net providers along with academic medical centers and community-based specialty clinics. The goal is to compare and contrast the future prospects of the current safety net.

Public Hospitals

There are over 1,300 government-owned acute-care hospitals scattered throughout the United States.[30] Most are owned by cities and counties.[31] Nearly two-thirds are small (fewer than 200 beds), are located in rural communities, and have relatively low occupancy rates (generally well below 50 percent). Many of the urban institutions, in contrast, are quite large and have relatively high occupancy rates. For example, the 100 biggest public hospitals average 581 beds each[32] and have an average occupancy rate of 79 percent.[33]

The Urban Public Hospital. Most urban public hospitals, unlike their rural counterparts, were established as safety net facilities. These institutions, many of which date back to the eighteenth century, were part of the nation's original safety net. Two hundred years later the mission of the urban public hospital is the same. These institutions provide care to the poor, the aged, and the uninsured. In 1991, for example, nearly 50 percent of the patient population was on Medicaid and another 25 percent was uninsured.[34] Only 12 percent had private health insurance.[35]

High levels of uncompensated care are not, however, the only obstacle facing the urban public hospital. These institutions treat a sicker and more difficult population than do most of their commercial or nonprofit counterparts, provide communities with necessary but unprofitable services (such as trauma care), struggle with an aging and inadequate physical infrastructure, employ a surplus of health care workers, suffer from significant cutbacks in local government funding, and face the unenviable organizational task of converting struggling acute care facilities into thriving managed-care entities. They must do all this in a political environment that favors privatization and in a bureaucratic environment that sharply limits decisionmaking authority.

For example, public hospitals undoubtedly treat the sickest and most difficult cases of the poor. These are the providers of last resort, caring for the homeless mentally ill, the noncompliant tuberculosis patient, and the babies addicted to cocaine. In addition, at a time when private hospitals are closing emergency rooms and trauma centers, public hospitals are increasingly providing the only trauma services in town. Victims of violence are therefore disproportionately treated in public facilities.

At the same time, most urban public hospitals are located in aged and inadequate physical plants. For example, while the average private hospital is in a seven-year-old building, the average urban public hospital is in a twenty-six-year-old plant—and some public hospitals (in Chicago, Los Angeles, and New York) are more than fifty years old.[36] Moreover, few public hospitals can afford significant modernization efforts. Indeed, the average per bed capital expenditure for public hospitals is just over half of the national average for all hospitals.[37] As one study noted:

> The aging infrastructure not only increases operating expenses as maintenance costs rise, it also reduces the ability to provide high-quality care and to attract paying patients. Indeed, in many public hospitals, medical equipment is often outdated, elevators are often out-of-order, and visitor waiting rooms are old and depressing. To be sure, some public hospitals are engaged in significant modernization efforts, but financing the large amount of necessary debt is a task few public hospitals can now undertake.[38]

Urban public hospitals also cope with a surplus of health care workers. According to one study, for example, the average hospital spends 53 percent of its budget on labor; in the typical public hospital, in contrast, the figure is more like 70 to 75 percent.[39] For this reason many public hospitals are trying hard to reduce the size of their work force. In the early 1990s, for example, New York City's public hospital system reduced its work force from 48,000 to 38,000; over the next couple of years the city hopes to eliminate 8,000 additional jobs.[40] Similarly, the Los Angeles public hospital system eliminated nearly 3,000 positions in 1995.[41]

The work force reductions have the potential to harm quality of care. To avoid adverse outcomes, hospital managers need to make the remaining work force more productive. One task is to require more from staff physicians. This is particularly important in systems in which doctors work both for the public hospital and for an affiliated academic medical center. These doctors need to spend more time treating public hospital patients and less time teaching and training. New York City is demanding this sort of change in its current negotiations with affiliated academic medical centers.[42] At the same time, staff physicians need more support, especially from nonprofessional hospital staff. This requires hospital managers and union leaders to compromise on work rules, seniority systems, and job descriptions.

Improving the productivity of the public hospital work force is not an easy task. Indeed, the former head of New York City's hospital system suggests that "[w]orkforce re-engineering is the hardest operational issue facing public hospitals."[43] One problem is the political strength of both the physicians and the unions that represent nonprofessional health care workers. Even more problematic, however, are the bureaucratic and political constraints that limit management discretion. In most cities, for example, public hospital officials are appointed by the mayor and serve at his or her pleasure. The line between politics and management is often blurred. In New York, for example, the city's Office of Collective Bargaining conducts all public hospital labor negotiations. City officials must also approve all capital projects.[44] These rules clearly limit management's autonomy. The bureaucratic politics are especially problematic where, as in New York, political leaders hope to privatize the public system. Bureaucratic maneuvering lessens the likelihood of innovative leadership.

Even with this rather staggering set of obstacles, however, the financial position of many public hospitals improved during the late 1980s and early 1990s. One reason was the new reimbursement mandates: increased Medicaid funding subsidized the cost of the uninsured. The Medicaid disproportionate share hospital (DSH) program was particularly helpful. Under this initiative, states are required to provide supplemental Medicaid funding to those hospitals that serve large numbers of the poor and the uninsured. This program initially was rather small ($500 million in 1988), but by 1995 it distributed more than $19 billion in supplemental funds.[45] Public hospitals were primary beneficiaries: in 1992, for example, DSH funds accounted for 12 percent of the revenue received by ninety-five of the nation's largest public hospitals.[46]

A second factor was the new eligibility mandates: Congress in the late 1980s required the states to provide expanded coverage to pregnant women and young children. These mandates, along with expanded coverage for certain low-income elderly persons, increased total program enrollment from around 22 million in 1988 to nearly 35 million in 1995.[47] As a result, the number of paying customers was significantly increased.

Finally, many public hospital systems actually were becoming more efficient. The size of the hospital work force was reduced, third-party collection efforts were improved, there was some increased worker productivity, and there was even an effort to reduce some of the bureaucratic obstacles to good performance.

By the mid-1990s, however, the outlook for the urban public hospital seems far bleaker. The problems are well known. First, the Medicaid subsidy is at risk. Hospitals are likely to receive less reimbursement for each Medicaid patient (as states cut Medicaid rates and Congress scales back the DSH program), and they are likely to have fewer Medicaid patients as well (as commercial managed-care companies persuade healthy Medicaid enrollees to leave the public hospital system). Second, other sources of public hospital revenue are also at risk. For example, Congress is poised to reduce Medicare funding for graduate medical education. At the same time, local governments are reducing their public hospital subsidy. Third, the demands on the public system are increasing. The number of uninsured is growing, as is the number of high-risk, high-cost Medicaid clients that are unattractive to the typical commercial managed-care company. Put simply, the fear is that the public systems will need to treat more patients for less money.

Even with these obstacles, however, there is still some room for optimism. Urban public hospitals often own and operate the largest primary-care infrastructure in their community. This infrastructure enables some public institutions to become effective competitors in a managed-care world. For example, the public hospital HMO in Minneapolis is doing quite well in the competition for both Medicaid beneficiaries and county employees.[48] Only by following this model are most urban public hospitals likely to survive.

The Rural Public Hospital. Most rural public hospitals were built during the 1950s, an era when federal policy explicitly encouraged an expanded hospital supply. For example, the federal Hill-Burton program enacted in 1946 provided federal dollars to build (or modernize) hospitals (mainly in rural and poor communities). The policy assumption was that every community needed its own state-of-the-art hospital. The program worked (perhaps too well). By the mid-1970s there was an oversupply of hospital beds. Hospital costs grew rapidly, aided by generous third-party payers (such as Medicare, Medicaid, and most private insurers) that generally paid whatever the hospital charged.

By the 1980s the oversupply of hospital beds had caused occupancy rates to dip quite low (below 50 percent) in many rural hospitals. At the same time, third-party payers (now with growing leverage) reduced the reimbursement they paid. The result was a fiscal crisis in many small institutions. More than 340 rural public hospitals closed during the 1980s and early 1990s, and hundreds more are struggling to survive.[49]

It will be especially difficult for these rural institutions to adjust to the new managed-care environment. The first problem is that rural public hospitals generally do not own or operate a primary-care infrastructure. As a result, these institutions are unlikely to form their own managed-care organization. Nor are they likely to become a primary-care provider for some other managed-care entity. At the same time, however, most rural public hospitals do not offer the latest high-tech medicine. For this reason, few managed-care organizations are likely to refer patients in need of specialty care.

As managed care moves to rural America, more and more rural public hospitals will close. The rationale for these institutions is no longer apparent. The rural public hospitals that survive will be those that emphasize and expand outpatient and primary-care services. In effect, the rural public hospital needs to be restructured into a rural health clinic. This is the best prescription for survival.

Academic Medical Centers

The managed-care revolution is forcing the nation's medical education system to reconsider its mission and task. At the same time, medical educators, long accustomed to generous Medicaid and Medicare reimbursement, are battling with federal and state officials anxious to reduce medical education payment levels. Like their public hospital counterparts, academic medical centers are having to do more with less.

Consider first the changes prompted by the movement toward managed care. The most obvious is the specialty mix of the nation's medical work force. The market is demanding more primary-care physicians and fewer medical specialists. Physicians are responding to the changing market. As recently as 1992 only 19 percent of graduating medical students entered generalist residency programs; by 1996 the number was greater than 50 percent.[50] Medical schools and teaching hospitals need to adjust. For example, medical schools have traditionally recruited students with a strong background in science (and an interest in specialized research), hired faculty members who are themselves specialists (who become student role models), and offered a curriculum that emphasized the specialties. At the same time, teaching hospitals (which train young physicians following their graduation from medical school) have long preferred specialist residents: such residents not only generate more income for hospitals than do generalists (especially from Medicare); they also provide faculty members with time to pursue their own research. As the medical marketplace changes, however, these patterns are changing as well.

A second challenge for the academic medical center is to become more cost-efficient. These are high-cost institutions. One study suggests that costs incurred by teaching facilities are 25 percent higher than those incurred by their nonteaching counterparts.[51] Teaching hospital staffs treat the most complicated cases, order more tests, and use the latest (and most expensive) technology. Teaching hospitals employ a higher-than-average number of specialists. Teaching hospitals treat large numbers of the poor and uninsured. In short, teaching hospitals teach as well as treat, and performing both functions simultaneously is generally expensive and often inefficient.

Until recently, both public and private payers have subsidized the high cost of the academic medical center. Consider Medicare. Between 1965 and 1983 Medicare reimbursed hospitals (including teaching hospitals) for their actual costs. In 1983, in an effort to control costs, Congress enacted a new payment system under which a hospital's reimbursement depends largely on the patient's diagnosis: the more complicated the case, the more generous the reimbursement. At the same time, however, Congress also provided teaching hospitals with a significant bonus to compensate for the higher costs incurred in educating doctors. The direct medical education adjustment reimburses hospitals for a portion of residents' and faculty salaries, and the indirect medical adjustment compensates for the sicker patients and more rigorous care that are generally associated with teaching facilities. By 1992 these medical education supplements provided teaching hospitals with approximately $5.2 billion a year.[52]

In most states Medicaid also provides teaching hospitals with a supplemental payment to cover the costs of graduate medical education. According to one study, Medicaid in 1992 spent more than $1.8 billion on graduate medical education.[53] Most states also provide direct subsidies to academic medical centers. This is particularly true where, as in California, the majority of academic medical centers are owned and administered by the state. Finally, even private insurers have historically shared the cost of graduate medical education, paying inflated hospital bills that included subsidies for the teaching program.

Today, however, both public and private subsidies are at risk. The Republicans in Congress have proposed cutting Medicare funding for graduate medical education. So too have Medicaid policymakers. And managed-care companies often bypass teaching facilities (as too expensive), use them only as a high-tech referral source, or negotiate low-cost deals (that eliminate the graduate medical education subsidies).

The risks to the academic medical center community are illustrated by recent events in Tennessee. In early 1994 Tennessee implemented the TennCare program, under which roughly 800,000 Medicaid beneficiaries and 400,000 of the uninsured were enrolled in one of twelve managed-care organizations. The program was funded, in part, by reducing payments for clinical care, eliminating funding for graduate medical education and capital expenditures, and redirecting Medicaid DSH payments from safety net hospitals to managed-care companies. To compensate for these cutbacks, the state established an essential provider fund, which provided transitional funding for both hospitals and community-based providers (such as community health centers). The transition funds targeted to hospitals were, however, far less than the expected loss of revenue. Moreover, the fund itself was raided to cover unexpected budget shortfalls and therefore provided even lower-than-expected assistance.[54]

TennCare has had a devastating effect on at least some of Tennessee's academic medical centers. First, patient volume in the teaching hospitals is down 10 to 15 percent.[55] The decline in the number of routine births is especially dramatic. At the University of Tennessee's teaching hospital, for example, the number of deliveries has dropped by 50 percent.[56] Second, the remaining patient population is sicker. The University of Tennessee maternity ward again illustrates the point: nearly 90 percent of the remaining births are from high-risk pregnancies.[57] Third, Medicaid payments for particular services have declined significantly. One hospital reported that its Medicaid revenue has declined from 65 cents on the dollar to 38 cents.[58] The loss of revenue makes it more difficult for the hospitals to provide charity care to the state's 400,000 or so remaining uninsured. At the same time, academic medical institutions are also reducing their teaching programs.[59]

As the Tennessee experience illustrates, academic health centers face a formidable challenge. These institutions must restructure their teaching programs toward primary care while at the same time lowering costs and becoming more competitive. One strategy is to consolidate with other teaching facilities. In New York City, for example, Columbia Presbyterian Medical Center is joining forces with New York Hospital. The merger is part of a broader effort to become an integrated service network. It is quite possible, however, that newly created networks of this sort will be unable to compete with the lower-cost commercial competition. If that is the case, teaching hospitals will survive only as high-tech referral sources, making it nearly impossible for these institutions to fulfill their primary-care education mission. It also would leave the poor and the uninsured who rely on these institutions with one less safety net provider.

Community Health Centers

There are over 600 federally funded community health centers, delivering care at more than 1,600 sites and treating more than 7 million persons.[60] Nearly 75 percent of health center patients are children or young women.[61] Most are poor or uninsured: 40 percent are on Medicaid, 38 percent are uninsured, 10 percent are on Medicare; 12 percent have private insurance.[62] As a result, health center revenue is generated primarily from Medicaid (34 percent) and federal grants (35 percent).[63] Most health centers generate additional revenue from state and local governments and from a variety of private foundations. The centers also bill the uninsured, though on a sliding-fee scale. The patchwork funding enables most centers to survive, but barely: a recent case study of ten health centers found each with inadequate cash reserves.[64]

Despite their fiscal troubles, most community health centers provide coordinated, comprehensive, and cost-effective health care. The evidence suggests, for example, that Medicaid beneficiaries who use community health centers spend less time in the hospital, cost less, and generally receive better health care than does the typical Medicaid client. According to one study of six health centers in New York, Medicaid beneficiaries who used the centers were nearly 30 percent less expensive than other beneficiaries.[65] Another study reported that health centers in Maryland ranked quite high on quality-of-care measures, despite ranking quite low on cost.[66]

Health centers are especially good at providing social services that enable beneficiaries to have access to medical care. They provide case managers (to guide clients through the maze of available services), interpreters (for non-English-speaking clients), and transportation services (to enable

patients to travel to the center). They have health educators and social workers and outreach workers. They also offer job training programs, substance
abuse counselors, nutrition initiatives, pregnancy prevention programs,
school-based health services, child care programs, violence prevention initiatives, GED workshops, and HIV testing and counseling programs.[67] While
no health center provides every service, every center provides more than
just medical care.

Health centers are able to finance these services primarily because of
the 1989 federal law that required states to pay cost-based reimbursement
for covered Medicaid services and expanded the definition of covered services (to include such enabling services as transportation, translation, and
case management). This requirement significantly increased health center
revenue. One study of ten health centers reported that total revenues increased between 35 and 142 percent between 1989 and 1993.[68] The same
study reported that all ten centers used the increased revenue to pay for the
uninsured and to cover additional enabling services.[69] While health centers
were hardly awash in excess cash, this was indeed an era of optimism and
expansion.

More recently, however, an era of caution has replaced the era of optimism. One problem is that Congress is phasing out the cost-based reimbursement mandate. A second problem is that federal regulators have already
waived the reimbursement mandate for nine states with mandatory managed-care initiatives. In these states health center reimbursement is negotiated between health plan and health center and is usually less than cost-based.

In this changing environment, community health centers have two options. The first is to become a participating provider in a managed-care
network. This requires entering into a contract with a managed-care organization. The contract details the services covered, rates paid, and administrative procedures to be followed. The second option is to form health
center–based managed-care organizations. This route also requires a contract, although the agreement here is made directly with the Medicaid agency
rather than with a managed-care network.

Either approach can be perilous. The rates paid could be less than cost-
based,[70] the services covered could be fewer than the center generally provides, and the information systems required could be beyond the center's
capacity. At the same time, the contract could require a health center with
little experience in managing risk to accept capitation, and it could impose
such risk on a center with minimal cash reserves.

Nonetheless, those health centers that survive the transition to managed care should do very well. Health centers are experienced safety net providers with an expertise in primary health care for low-income populations. Commercial managed-care organizations are often anxious to hire health centers as primary-care providers. Health centers could find themselves with unexpected bargaining leverage. As part of the contract, the center could receive improved management information systems, expanded quality improvement programs, and better-than-expected rates. At the same time, those health centers that form their own managed-care organizations could do quite well in the competition for the Medicaid business. This is especially so if the center affiliates with other safety net providers and achieves some efficiencies of scale.

Public Health Clinics

Local health departments, unlike other safety net providers, do not qualify automatically for Medicaid reimbursement. The problem is that Medicaid does not reimburse services provided free to the public (and most health departments provide their services free to the public). In response, many health departments have established third-party billing systems, if for no other reason than to qualify for Medicaid funding. (These departments rarely seek to collect from other third-party payers.) Even with this expanded Medicaid reimbursement, however, health departments rely more on direct local (and state) appropriations than do any other component of the medical safety net. In 1992, for example, local governments provided approximately $13.7 billion to support local public-health activities.[71]

Despite this historic pattern, health department funding is generally a low priority for most local politicians. This pattern is worsening: antigovernment politicians often are anxious to defund or to scale back public health funding. The policy assumption is that managed-care organizations will care for the Medicaid population and that other safety net providers will service the uninsured.

To be sure, local health departments do far more than provide primary care to the poor and uninsured. Indeed, the historic mission of the local health department was to assess the public health needs of the local community and develop programs to meet those needs. Public health departments collected data on disease epidemics, regulated the quality of the water supply, enforced local health codes, conducted health education campaigns, and generally tended to the needs of the public rather than the individual.

Only rarely would health department doctors themselves deliver health care, and when they did it was usually to supplement a broader public health campaign (immunizing children, for example, as part of an immunization campaign).

In recent years, however, health departments have shifted resources away from infectious disease control (and other public health initiatives) and increased their efforts to become direct providers of care. Health departments have become the provider of last resort for large numbers of the poor and uninsured. Health departments have become an increasingly important part of the medical safety net. By the late 1980s, for example, 92 percent of all health departments were immunizing children, 84 percent provided other child health services, and more than half delivered prenatal care services.[72] At the same time, many health departments provide large amounts of specialty-care services, especially to populations underserved by the traditional medical community. For example, most county health departments provide mental health services. Others treat sexually transmitted diseases. Still others care for persons with AIDS.

The increased attention to direct-care provision has limited the resources available for traditional public health activities. Some observers believe the trend is inappropriate.[73] For this reason, some states (such as Washington) now seek to shift the health department emphasis back to traditional public health functions.[74] For these states the changing health care marketplace is an opportunity to encourage that shift. In other states, however, the public health department is too large a part of the medical safety net for any such shift to occur. This is especially common in rural southern states like Alabama.[75] In these states the health departments need to survive the transition to managed care, the cutbacks in public funding, and the tension inherent in an effort to simultaneously care for the individual and plan for the public—a task that is quite difficult.

Community-Based Specialty Clinics

There are literally thousands of small community-based clinics that provide specialty-care services. Some of the clinics are affiliated with a hospital, community health center, or local health department. Others are freestanding institutions. There are mental health clinics, substance abuse treatment centers, and AIDS care facilities. There are women's health clinics and clinics that serve the homeless.

On their own, the freestanding specialty clinics are not likely to survive the changing health care marketplace. As the market moves to managed care, the clinics need either to affiliate with a larger provider (most likely a larger safety net institution) or to diversify their services. One strategy is to add a primary-care practice to the package of services provided. Planned Parenthood, for example, is converting many of its women's health clinics into full-service primary-care clinics. This approach makes the clinics more attractive to potential managed-care partners.

Not all specialty clinics have the resources to follow the Planned Parenthood model. In fact, most do not. Without such a shift, however, many of the clinics are unattractive managed-care partners. They are high-cost, have little experience in managing risk, and generally have inadequate management information services. But the services they provide are important, as is their experience in serving hard-to-treat populations. These are the providers most in need of government protection. State and federal officials need to decide whether providing such protection is good policy.

Options and Obstacles

Nearly all safety net providers rely on Medicaid funding to subsidize care rendered to the uninsured. There is little choice: aside from the bad debt and charity programs in place in a few states and the few dollars the uninsured themselves pay directly, care provided to the uninsured is unreimbursed. Until recently, however, Medicaid funding was too low to provide a useful subsidy: rates barely covered the cost of the Medicaid clients, much less the cost of others. This changed during the late 1980s. Community health centers were suddenly entitled to cost-based reimbursement. Hospitals that treated large numbers of poor people were guaranteed supplemental Medicaid funding. Even local health departments were able to dramatically increase their Medicaid funding. As a result, most safety net providers could cope with the rapid rise in the number of uninsured (and the increased care demands placed on the safety net as a result).

The fragile system of Medicaid mandates and implicit cross-subsidies is about to end. Some changes are already taking place. For example, several Medicaid managed-care demonstration programs permit managed-care companies to pay community health centers less-than-reasonable cost reimbursement. Medicaid managed-care initiatives are also likely to reduce (or eliminate) reimbursement for services that are more social than medical (such as transportation to and from clinics). At the same time, both Congress and the states are looking to cut Medicaid reimbursement in the traditional fee-for-service program. The Balanced Budget Act of 1997 eliminated the Boren amendment (which guaranteed hospitals reasonable and adequate reimbursement), established a schedule for phasing out the requirement that Medicaid pay cost-based reimbursement to federally qualified community health centers, and reduced Medicaid DSH payments by $10.4 billion over the next five years.

Safety net providers also expect less revenue from other government programs. Congress is likely to cut Medicare reimbursement, reducing both the per-procedure fees and the funding for graduate medical education. Local governments will also cut back, reducing their appropriations to public health departments and public hospitals. And governments at all levels are cutting back on funding for programs designed to remedy the geographic maldistribution of providers.

Safety net providers need to respond to this changing policy environment. One strategy is to find new funding sources. There are two possibilities: First, safety net providers can expand their patient base and serve more of the privately insured. For example, academic medical centers are well positioned to become referral centers for commercial managed-care companies. Some academic medical centers will even become the primary-care hub of successfully integrated service networks—as will some prestigious nonprofit hospitals.

Most safety net providers, especially those that are publicly owned, are nonetheless unlikely to attract a significant commercial enrollment. The stigma of public ownership is too much of an obstacle. As a result, even the most successful public institutions hesitate to try. For example, the Minneapolis public hospital system recently created a managed-care entity in an effort to compete in the changing health care marketplace. The managed-care entity, called Metropolitan Health Plan, successfully competes for Medicaid beneficiaries and county employees. It has done so well that it is now considering moving into the Medicare market as well. Metropolitan officials insist, however, that they have no plans to compete for privately insured enrollees. The competition is too fierce and the effort would divert attention from the organization's core constituency and primary market.[76]

A second source of additional funding is private foundations. The target foundations are those established during the conversion of nonprofit insurers or providers into for-profit entities. Many nonprofits hope to raise significant capital by converting to for-profit status and then selling stock.

State law, however, generally requires these organizations to use their current cash value to continue the nonprofit mission. The theory is that the nonprofit has received a significant public benefit through the use of its nonprofit status (tax benefits, regulatory benefits, rate benefits, and the like) that should now be returned to the public. The most common approach so far is for companies to create an independent nonprofit foundation to distribute these funds. These foundations may well distribute funds to safety net providers.

The for-profit conversion of Blue Cross of California (BCC) illustrates the potential sums available for distribution. In 1992 BCC proposed the creation of a for-profit subsidiary called Well-Point Health Networks. The California Department of Corporations and BCC then began a long process to determine how the conversion should proceed. The final agreement, reached in May 1996, required BCC to spend $3 billion to endow two independent foundations—the California Health Care Foundation and the California Endowment.[77] These newly created foundations are working now to determine their funding priorities. So far the emphasis seems to be on programs targeting the uninsured and medically underserved populations.[78] Two caveats are nevertheless important. First, in many states (such as New York) the conversion battles are just beginning. Second, even in California, the foundations are newly formed and the funding priorities just established. Most of the nation's safety net providers will not receive grants anytime soon.

Since safety net providers cannot expect major infusions of new funding in the short term, the more immediate challenge is twofold: to preserve as much of the current funding streams as possible and to become cost-efficient in the use of such funds. The tasks are connected. Consider the effort to preserve current funding streams. One strategy is for safety net providers to affiliate with a Medicaid managed-care health plan. The terms of the affiliation will vary. The provider might deliver primary care or specialty services or both. The provider may have control over the beneficiaries it serves, or it may be required to accept any and all referrals. The provider may need to follow the plan's practice guidelines or it may retain significant care autonomy.

Under any of these scenarios, however, the provider is likely to be reimbursed on a capitated basis. Fewer and fewer health plans are willing to reimburse on a fee-for-service basis. The shift toward capitation requires providers to become more cost-effective. Only by keeping costs low will providers prosper under managed care. Only by becoming more efficient can providers simultaneously provide good-quality care.

This need for efficiency is even more pronounced when safety net institutions form their own managed-care health plans. The transition is hard. One or more safety net providers create a new managed-care entity. The new organization then relies on the member institution(s) to deliver most of the care, though contracts with other providers are often needed as well. The new entity has a board of directors (with each member institution represented) and a small administrative staff. The obstacles to success are apparent. The health plan needs capital to get started, and most safety net providers have little extra capital to invest. The new plan needs to meet state licensing requirements, which can be quite rigorous. The plan needs to determine its target population, develop a marketing and enrollment program, and educate enrollees in the workings of managed care. It also needs to establish a provider reimbursement system, a quality-assurance program, and a provider education initiative. This all needs to happen at a time when the member institutions (usually community health centers and hospitals) are struggling to remain viable and to contract with as many other managed-care plans as possible. The process is complicated and time consuming, and it is not always successful.

In this environment, government needs to decide whether it should help safety net providers survive the transition to the managed-care marketplace. There is no consensus on this issue, however. Consider the federal role. Until the Balanced Budget Act of 1997, states could not require Medicaid beneficiaries to enroll in managed care unless federal regulators waived various federal laws (such as the law that guarantees beneficiaries the freedom to select any willing provider). As states jumped on the managed-care bandwagon and pressed for mandatory managed care, federal regulators used the waiver process to impose a variety of regulatory mandates. Clearly, however, the mandates focused on beneficiary protection and not provider protection. Indeed, most waivers permit states to end the requirement that community health centers receive cost-based reimbursement. Federal regulators also concluded that managed-care companies were not bound by the Boren amendment.

The movement to delegate more authority to the states makes it unlikely that federal regulators will impose safety net protection plans anytime soon. Indeed, the trend is moving in the opposite direction.

With increased discretion states are likely to adopt very different approaches to the safety net protection issue. At one extreme is California. Under California's mandatory managed-care initiative Medicaid beneficiaries in twelve of the state's largest counties will choose between one of two managed-care health plans: a commercial plan and a government-run safety net plan (that would feature the county-run public hospital system). Clients who do not choose will be assigned to the government-run plan (at least until that plan achieves its minimum enrollment targets). This will not only ensure the survival of the public plan, but also enable county hospitals to maintain most of their federal DSH income. In addition, the government plan must offer contracts to all qualified safety net providers; the commercial plan is encouraged to do so as well.[79]

At the other extreme are states that let the market alone determine the fate of the current safety net. Florida illustrates this point. According to one observer, the Florida legislature is likely to "just say no" to safety net protection programs.[80] The opposition is both political and pragmatic. There is little political gain from programs that protect safety net providers. At the same time, government efforts to favor certain providers over others are at odds with the nation's antigovernment mood. After all, lots of providers think they are essential to the medical safety net, and government (arguably) should not pick and choose which providers to protect.[81]

The Need for a Safety Net Protection Plan

The laissez-faire approach would be more persuasive if the country had a program of national health insurance. This is not about to happen anytime soon. Instead, the number of uninsured persons is likely to grow, as are the demands on the medical safety net. The safety net is the provider of last resort, and the uninsured often have nowhere else to go. Health plans and providers do not compete for the business of the uninsured: on the contrary, the fiscal pressures on both plans and providers make the uninsured even less attractive than in years past.

Even with national health insurance, however, there would still be a need for a safety net protection plan. An insurance card does not guarantee access to care. There must be an adequate supply of health care providers in each community, and the providers must be willing to treat the covered populations. The United States falls short on both tests. First, nearly 45 million Americans live in medically underserved communities;[82] the medical safety net in these communities needs to be protected and expanded. Second, the nation's experience with Medicaid illustrates that health care providers will not always care for the insured.

To be sure, there is no single formula for the content of a safety net protection plan. There are, however, four safety net protection strategies that states should be encouraged to adopt.

Licensure Requirements

In most states the department of insurance regulates the HMO industry. HMO applicants are required to demonstrate financial soundness, which requires high levels of financial reserves; the goal is to minimize the possibility of bankruptcy. Unfortunately, however, many fledgling safety net health plans cannot meet the reserve requirements. One alternative is to impose lower reserve requirements on safety net plans, at least during a transition period. California, for example, temporarily exempts safety net health plans from the stringent cash reserve and capitalization requirements imposed on traditional managed-care plans.[83] A second strategy is to create a new form of Medicaid managed-care company (usually regulated by the state's Medicaid agency) that has lower reserve requirements. New York follows this model. A third approach is to permit publicly sponsored health plans to waive reserve requirements as long as government officials provide a written guarantee of financial backing. Arizona has adopted this strategy.[84]

The advantage of special licensing rules is that safety net health plans are more likely to form. The disadvantage is that underfinanced organizations could be created. Perhaps the best approach is illustrated by an Illinois law that requires community-based health plans to have a net worth of $1 million, as opposed to the $2 million requirement imposed on HMOs.[85] The requirement is low enough to encourage safety net participation but high enough to protect against insolvency.

Supplemental Funding

Several states provide supplemental funding to safety net health plans. The goal is to enable the plans to compete with the commercial managed-care organizations. One strategy is to provide special start-up grants. In California, for example, state officials established a $500,000 fund to help safety net clinics make the transition to managed care.[86] New York also provides start-up funding for some safety net health plans.[87] A second approach is to adjust capitation rates for patient case mix. The goal here is to pay higher rates to those plans that have a more costly patient population. Unfortunately, however, case mix risk adjustment efforts are still in their infancy. For this reason, the better strategy is simply to pay enhanced rates to safety net health plans. Massachusetts, for example, plans to pay an enhanced rate to the managed-care organization formed by two public hospitals (Boston City and Cambridge).[88] Rhode Island has a similar program for community health centers that form managed-care plans.

Guaranteed Enrollment

In mandatory managed-care initiatives, beneficiaries who do not choose a health plan are assigned to one. Most states develop a formula for making assignment decisions. The usual goal is to assign beneficiaries to a primary-care provider that is geographically accessible. States can also use the assignment process to encourage greater participation in safety net health plans. Under California's two-plan initiative, for example, beneficiaries will be assigned to the publicly sponsored plan until and unless that plan reaches a specified enrollment goal.[89] New York has a more complicated formula, under which provider-based plans are given a slight preference.[90]

Essential Community Provider Contracts

The most common safety net protection strategy is to encourage or require health plans to contract with safety net health plans. In Minnesota, for example, managed-care plans are required to offer contracts to all so-called essential community providers. The contract must offer community health centers cost-based reimbursement (for at least three years) and must offer other safety net providers a competitive rate as well. In addition, once a contract is signed, the health plan must include the safety net provider on the list of providers offered to privately insured enrollees (as well as to those on Medicaid).[91]

To be sure, essential community provider contracts generally do not require actual referrals. Moreover, not all referrals are desirable: if a health plan assigned only the most difficult-to-treat patients, or only high-cost patients, the safety net provider could be worse off, not better. Nonetheless, required contracts of this sort, if regulated carefully, may well ease the transition to managed care.

Some Final Thoughts

The content of the new Medicaid will determine the future of the medical safety net. The movement toward Medicaid managed care, for example, places the medical safety net at risk. Some safety net providers (such as community health centers) are better positioned than others (such as small specialty clinics), but all must fundamentally transform. Some will survive; others will not. At the same time, the trend toward Medicaid devolution makes the transition even more difficult. Some states will adopt aggressive safety net protection plans. Most will not. The nation's geographic maldistribution of providers will worsen. The poor and the uninsured will have a harder time obtaining care.

These trends suggest the need for a more forceful federal role. Congress should require states to enact a safety net protection plan. Federal regulators should approve such plans and oversee their implementation. The new Medicaid needs to accommodate (or at least acknowledge) the existing safety net. The plans need not be identical. There is surely room for state diversity and discretion. Some states could enact essential community provider requirements. Others could ease licensure requirements for safety net health plans. Still others could provide supplemental funding (or guaranteed enrollment) to safety net health plans. But federal officials should not allow a laissez-faire Medicaid.

Had the nation enacted national health insurance, the troubles of the safety net would be less pressing. There would presumably be some competition for the 40 million or so who are now uninsured (though the Medicaid experience suggests caution about this assumption). Without national health insurance, however, and with the number of uninsured persons rising, there is a greater need for a federally guaranteed safety net protection plan. This is one policy arena in which a nationally managed federalism is a better policy approach than the state-centered federalism toward which we are moving.

Notes

1. Ann Shola Orloff, "The Political Origins of America's Belated Welfare System," in Margaret Weir, Ann Shola Orloff, and Theda Skocpol, eds., *The Politics of Social Policy in the United States* (Princeton University Press, 1988), pp. 37–80.

2. Karen Davis and Cathy Schoen, *Health and the War on Poverty: A Ten-Year Appraisal* (Brookings, 1978), p. 122.

3. Paul Starr, *The Social Transformation of American Medicine* (Basic Books, 1982).

4. Davis and Schoen, *Health and the War on Poverty*, p. 163.

5. Michael S. Sparer, *Medicaid and the Limits of State Health Reform* (Temple University Press, 1996), pp. 38–39.

6. Prospective Payment Assessment Commission, *Medicare and the American Health Care System* (Washington, June 1995), p. 133; and Sparer, *Medicaid and the Limits of State Health Reform*, pp. 39–41.

7. Prospective Payment Assessment Commission, *Medicare and the American Health Care System*, p. 133.

8. Sparer, *Medicaid and the Limits of State Health Reform*, p. 41.

9. Thomas Fanning and Martin de Alteriis, "The Limits of Marginal Economic Incentives in the Medicaid Program: Concerns and Cautions," *Journal of Health Politics, Policy and Law*, vol. 18, no. 1 (Spring 1993), pp. 29–30.

10. *The Emergency Health Personnel Act of 1970.*

11. General Accounting Office, *National Health Service Corps: Program Unable to Meet Need for Physicians in Underserved Areas*, GAO/HRD-90-128 (August 1990).

12. Michael S. Sparer, "Reform and the Medical Work Force: Choices and Challenges," in John J. DiIulio Jr. and Richard P. Nathan, eds., *Making Health Reform Work: The View from the States* (Brookings, 1994), p. 119.

13. Ibid. The NHSC survived the Reagan challenge and is now receiving increased funding. In 1991, for example, 287 physicians received awards. Nonetheless, NHSC funding remains well below peak levels.

14. Lucetter Lagnado, "Inner-City Hospital Begs for Life Support," *Wall Street Journal*, February 12, 1997, p. B-1.

15. A third strategy, unrelated to the Medicaid program, was to expeditiously process immigration visas for foreign physicians who agreed to practice in medically underserved communities.

16. This effort coincided with new Medicaid eligibility requirements that increased the number of covered pregnant women: the eligibility expansions would be irrelevant unless there were physicians willing and able to provide prenatal and postnatal care.

17. Tim Henderson, "State Health Notes," Intergovernmental Health Policy Project, National Conference on State Legislatures, November 1996.

18. Marsha Gold, Michael Sparer, and Karyen Chu, "Medicaid Managed Care: Lessons from Five States," *Health Affairs*, vol. 15, no. 3 (Fall 1996), p. 163.

19. Gail A. Jensen and others, "The New Dominance of Managed Care: Insurance Trends in the 1990s," *Health Affairs*, vol. 16, no. 1 (January/February 1997), p. 126.

20. Jack Zwanziger and Glenn A. Melnick, "Can Managed Care Plans Control Health Care Costs?" *Health Affairs*, vol. 15, no. 2 (Summer 1996), p. 196.

21. Jensen and others, "The New Dominance of Managed Care," p. 129.

22. Under a point-of-service plan, consumers have a fiscal incentive to use in-network providers but can, for a higher fee, see other providers as well. The flexibility of this approach is attractive to many consumers, and this is the fastest-growing managed-care model (Jensen and others, "The New Dominance of Managed Care, pp. 126–27). Nonetheless, the increased consumer choice leads to decreased health plan management.

23. Zwanziger and Melnick,"Can Managed Care Plans Control Health Care Costs?" pp.196–97.

24. Commerce Clearing House, Inc., "President Clinton's Health Care Reform Proposal and Health Security Act," as presented to Congress, October 27, 1993 (Chicago, November 1, 1993).

25. Ironically, however, Medicare so far has lost money on its managed-care program. This is because Medicare payments are based on the average beneficiary in a particular community, while managed-care companies have enrolled primarily healthy and low-cost beneficiaries. John D. Wilkerson, "Messing with Medicare: Markets and Politics in the 104th Congress," in John D. Wilkerson, Kelly J. Devers, and Ruth S. Given, eds., *Competitive Managed Care: The Emerging Health Care System* (San Francisco: Jossey-Bass, 1997), pp. 297, 313.

26. Michael S. Sparer, "Managing the Managed Care Revolution: States and the New Medicaid," in Wilkerson, Devers, and Given, eds., *Competitive Managed Care*, pp. 231–58.

27. Linda A. Bergthold and others, "Group Purchasing in the Managed Care Marketplace," in Wilkerson, Devers, and Given, eds., *Competitive Managed Care*, pp. 59–82.

28. Recently, for example, Aetna purchased U.S. Healthcare for $8.8 billion. Indeed, four managed-care companies now control over 50 percent of the nation's HMO enrollment. Kenneth E. Thorpe, "The Health System in Transition," *Journal of Health Politics, Policy and Law*, vol. 22, no. 2 (April 1997), pp. 339–61.

29. Allan Baumgarten, *Minnesota Managed Care Review: 1994* (Minneapolis: Allan Baumgarten), p. 7.

30. Bruce Siegel, "Public Hospitals—A Prescription for Survival" (New York: Commonwealth Fund, October 1996), p. 1.

31. As of late 1992 there were about 340 federal veterans' hospitals; the rest were owned by cities and counties. National Commission on the State and Local Public Service, "Frustrated Federalism: Rx for State and Local Health Care Reform" (Albany, N.Y.: Nelson A. Rockefeller Institute of Government, 1993), p. 36.

32. Siegel, "Public Hospitals," p. 1.

33. National Association of Public Hospitals, "America's Urban Health Safety Net" (Washington, January 1994), p. 32.

34. Ibid., p. 41.

35. Ibid.

36. Ibid., p. 65.

37. Ibid., p. 64.

38. National Commission on the State and Local Public Service, "Frustrated Federalism," p. 37.

39. Siegel, "Public Hospitals," p. 17.

40. Peter Klemperer in Nelson A. Rockefeller Institute of Government and the Brookings Center for Public Management, "Devolution and Medicaid: A View from the States" (Washington, unpublished transcript, May 23–24, 1996), pp. 372–73.

41. Siegel, "Public Hospitals," p. 17.

42. Esther B. Fein, "In Columbia Pact, New York City Ties Pay to Hospital Productivity," *New York Times*, January 8, 1997, p. A1.

43. Siegel, "Public Hospitals," p. 18.

44. Ibid., p. 13.

45. Diane Rowland, "Medicaid's Role," testimony at Hearing on Medicaid Reform before the Subcommittee on Health and Environment of the House Committee on Commerce, 105 Cong., 1 sess. (Government Printing Office, 1997), p. 4.

46. See National Association of Public Hospitals, "America's Urban Health Safety Net," p. 136.

47. Kaiser Commission on the Future of Medicaid, *Medicaid Facts: Medicaid Enrollment and Spending Growth* (1996).

48. Michael S. Sparer, Marilyn R. Ellwood, and Cathy Schoen, "Managed Care and Low-Income Populations: A Case Study of Managed Care in Minnesota," report prepared for the Henry J. Kaiser Family Foundation and the Commonwealth Fund (Washington: Mathematica Policy Research, Inc., May 1996), pp. 18–20.

49. Siegel, "Public Hospitals," p. 1.

50. Spencer Foreman, "Market Forces and Physicians: The Author Responds," *Health Affairs*, vol. 15, no. 4 (Winter 1996), p. 222; Association of American Medical Colleges, *AAMC Data Book* (Washington, December 1992), table B13; and Henry A. Waxman, "Health Care Workforce Reforms: Meeting Primary Care Needs," *Academic Medicine*, vol. 68 (December 1993), pp. 898–99.

51. Thorpe, "The Health System in Transition," p. 20.

52. General Accounting Office, *Graduate Medical Education Payment Policy Needs to Be Reexamined*, GAO/HEHS-94-33 (May 1994), p. 1.

53. James R. Boex and Mohan L. Garg, "State Medicaid Payments in Support of Graduate Medical Education and Teaching Hospital Infrastructure," report to the Kellogg Foundation (1993), p. 6.

54. Gregg S. Meyer and David Blumenthal, "The Initial Effects of TennCare on Academic Health Center," report submitted to the Task Force on Academic Health Centers, established by the Commonwealth Fund (November 1996).

55. Ibid., p. 13.

56. Ibid.

57. Ibid.

58. Ibid.

59. Gregg S. Meyer and David Blumenthal, "TennCare and Academic Medical Centers: The Lessons from Tennessee," *Journal of the American Medical Association*, vol. 276, no. 9 (September 4, 1996), p. 674.

60. General Accounting Office, *Community Health Centers: Challenges in Transitioning to Prepaid Managed Care*, GAO/HEHS-95-138 (May 1995), pp. 1, 4.

61. Ibid.

62. Julie Rovner, "The Safety Net: What's Happening to Health Care of Last Resort," special supplement to *Advances*, issue 1 (Robert Wood Johnson Foundation, 1996), p. 4.

63. GAO, *Community Health Centers*, p. 5.

64. Ibid., p. 3.

65. Center for Health Policy Studies, "Utilization and Costs to Medicaid of AFDC Recipients in New York Served and Not Served by Community Health Centers" (Columbia, Md.: June 1994), cited in National Association of Community Health Centers, Inc., "America's Health Centers: Value in Health Care: A Report on the Cost-Effectiveness of Health Centers" (Washington: May 1995), p. 2.

66. Barbara Starfield, "Costs vs. Quality in Different Types of Primary Care Settings," *Journal of the American Medical Association*, vol. 272, no. 24 (December 28, 1994).

67. GAO, *Community Health Centers*, p. 14. See also Robert Cunningham, ed., "CHC's Loss of Medicaid Stealth Subsidy Jeopardizes Uninsured," *Medicine and Health: Perspectives* (New York: Faulkner and Gray, July 29, 1996).

68. GAO, *Community Health Centers*, p. 24.

69. Ibid., p. 19.

70. Under TennCare, for example, community health centers suffered a 20 to 25 percent decline in Medicaid reimbursement. Note "The Impact of Medicaid Managed Care on the Uninsured," *Harvard Law Review*, vol. 110 (January 1997), p. 764.

71. Rovner, "The Safety Net," p. 2.

72. National Commission on the State and Local Public Service, "Frustrated Federalism," p. 41.

73. Ibid., p. 42.

74. Ken Cameron in "Devolution and Medicaid," p. 430.

75. Michael Murphy in "Devolution and Medicaid," p. 439.

76. Sparer, Ellwood, and Schoen, "Managed Care and Low Income Populations: A Case Study of Managed Care in Minnesota," p. 19.

77. Leonard D. Schaeffer, "Health Plan Conversions: The View from Blue Cross of California," *Health Affairs*, vol. 15, no. 4 (Winter 1996), pp. 183-87.

78. See, for example, the announcement of the California Endowment's funding priorities set forth in *Health Affairs*, vol. 15, no. 4 (Winter 1996), p. 197.

79. Michael Sparer, Marsha Gold, and Lois Simon, "Managed Care and Low-Income Populations: A Case Study of Managed Care in California," report prepared for the Henry J. Kaiser Family Foundation and the Commonwealth Fund (Washington: Mathematica Policy Research, Inc., May 1996), pp. 9–10, 43.

80. Michael Hanson in "Devolution and Medicaid," p. 397.

81. Ibid., p. 391.

82. National Commission on the State and Local Public Service, "Frustrated Federalism," p. 7.

83. Sparer, Gold, and Simon, "Managed Care and Low Income Populations: A Case Study of Managed Care in California," p. 47.

84. Larry S. Gage and others, "The Safety Net in Transition: Increasing Your Role in State Design of Medicaid Managed Care Programs" (National Association of Public Hospitals, June 1996), p. 10–11.

85. Ibid., p. 10.

86. Sparer, Gold, and Simon, "Managed Care and Low-Income Populations: A Case Study of Managed Care in California," p. 37.

87. Michael Sparer and Karyen Chu, "Managed Care and Low-Income Populations: A Case Study of Managed Care in New York," report prepared for the Henry J. Kaiser Family Foundation and the Commonwealth Fund (Washington: Mathematica Policy Research, Inc., 1996), p. 4.

88. Gage and others, "The Safety Net in Transition," p. 12.

89. Sparer, Gold, and Simon, "Managed Care and Low Income Populations: A Case Study of Managed Care in California," p. 40.

90. United Hospital Fund, "Medicaid Managed Care Legislation Passes," *Currents: Medicaid Managed Care*, vol. 1, no. 3 (Fall 1996), p. 6.

91. Karen Peed in "Devolution and Medicaid," pp. 410, 412, 422. See also Sparer, Ellwood, and Schoen, "Managed Care and Low Income Populations: A Case Study of Managed Care in Minnesota," p. 31.

6

Long-Term Care and Devolution

Joshua M. Wiener

MEDICAID AND long-term care are very deeply intertwined.[1] Older people and persons with disabilities account for two-thirds of Medicaid expenditures, about half of which is for long-term care.[2] In 1994 long-term care accounted for 45 percent or more of Medicaid program expenditures in eleven states.[3] Indeed, Medicaid is the dominant source of public funding for long-term care, accounting for almost two-thirds of government spending for nursing homes, intermediate-care facilities for the mentally retarded (ICF/MRs), and home-care services in 1993.[4] Largely because of the aging of the population, real, inflation-adjusted Medicaid spending on long-term care for the elderly is projected to double between 1993 and 2018.[5]

Many policymakers and analysts disparage the large role that long-term care plays in the Medicaid budget, claiming that it was unintended. That role, however, is consistent with the program's historical antecedents and legislative intent. Federal support for nursing-home care for the elderly poor substantially predates Medicaid, going back to the Social Security amendments of 1950. The immediate antecedent for Medicaid was the Kerr-Mills medical assistance program, which was developed in 1960 specifically to provide medical care to the "deserving elderly."[6] In fact, the House-Senate conference report for the 1965 Social Security amendments establishing Medicaid refers to the program as a means to provide a more effective Kerr-Mills medical assistance program for the aged and to extend its provisions to additional needy persons.[7]

If long-term care is important to Medicaid, it is nearly impossible to overstate the importance of Medicaid to the long-term care industry. In 1994, 69 percent of nursing home residents and virtually all ICF/MR residents depended on Medicaid to help pay for their care.[8] Indeed, in many parts of the country nursing homes have their historical antecedents in county poorhouses.

In grappling with how reform of the Medicaid program will affect long-term care, state and federal policymakers must address four key questions: First, how should responsibility for long-term care be apportioned between the federal and state governments? Closely related to this question is the issue of what national standards related to long-term care should be imposed on the states in their operation of the Medicaid program. Second, should the legal entitlement to long-term care services be retained? Like the rest of the Medicaid program, states have considerable flexibility in what long-term care services they cover, but they must provide them to all persons who meet the financial and need criteria. Third, especially if federal Medicaid reform is linked to deficit reduction, is it possible to substantially reduce the rate of increase in long-term care expenditures without adversely affecting beneficiaries? In long-term care, the options are much more varied than they are for acute care, where there is a single-minded focus on increasing managed-care enrollment. Finally, how should federal Medicaid funds be allocated to the states, and what are the implications of this distribution system for dividing resources at the state level between acute and long-term care, institutional and noninstitutional services, and among the elderly, disabled, children, and nondisabled adults?

The Medigrant proposal passed by Congress in 1995 and President Clinton's Medicaid plan (proposed in 1995 and again, with minor changes, in 1997) provided starkly different answers to these questions. The Medigrant plan would have radically changed the Medicaid program; President Clinton's proposal was much more modest. The Medigrant plan would have given vast new authority to the states, eliminated most federal long-term care requirements, terminated the entitlement to services, required deep cuts in spending, and allocated federal money to the states in substantially different ways. President Clinton's plan would have given states some additional freedom to organize long-term care services, but otherwise would have retained the current structure of the program. States would have faced some spending constraints under the president's plan, but they would not have been severe and the current system of allocation would not change radically.

While Congress and the president disagreed on policy directions, the issues raised by their proposals did not go away. This chapter focuses on how the four major policy questions mentioned previously play out for Medicaid policy for long-term care, primarily highlighting policy issues affecting the elderly population.

Background

Although states have substantial flexibility in how they run their Medicaid programs, they must meet numerous minimum federal requirements in terms of service coverage, reimbursement, quality of care, and eligibility in order to obtain federal matching funds. Over the last seven years Medicaid long-term care expenditures have increased rapidly, but far less quickly than acute care spending. As with the rest of the Medicaid program, states vary enormously in terms of service coverage, provider reimbursement, and expenditures. While eligibility does vary, the range is not as extreme for long-term care as it is for acute care.

Service Coverage

States are required to provide a basic package of acute and long-term care services to federally determined populations. The mandatory services include nursing home care and home health care (for those who require nursing home-level care). Even where states all cover the same service, utilization can vary tremendously. For example, in 1992, 2 percent of the elderly population of Nevada was in nursing homes, while 7.6 percent of the elderly in Minnesota were institutionalized.[9]

At their option, states can cover a broader range of services, and there is considerable variation across states in the kinds of optional long-term care services that are available. For example, while all states cover ICF/MRs, only thirty-one states cover personal care services.[10] States may apply for waivers of federal rules in order to provide a wide range of home- and community-based services to persons at high risk of institutionalization. Under these waivers, the Health Care Financing Administration (HCFA) must find that the average per capita cost of serving this population with the waiver is not greater than the average per capita cost without the waiver. As of 1997 there were a total of two hundred home- and community-based waiver programs in effect, serving about 250,000 people.[11] Thus many waiver programs are quite small, and the bulk of the funds is for persons with mental retardation or developmental disabilities (MR/DD).

Provider Reimbursement

Until the requirements were repealed by the Balanced Budget Act of 1997, states had to pay nursing homes and hospitals (including mental hospitals) according to rates that were adequate to cover the costs of an economically and efficiently operated facility (the so-called Boren amendment requirements). States now have almost complete freedom in how they set nursing home reimbursement rates. As of the end of 1993, forty-two states reimbursed nursing homes using a prospective payment methodology, mostly based on facility-specific historical costs.[12] In 1993 the average Medicaid nursing home rate was $85.05, and ranged from a low of $50 in Tennessee to a high of $315 in Alaska.[13] There are no federal requirements regarding reimbursement of home- and community-based providers or ICF/MRs. In general, Medicaid beneficiaries have less access to services than do private-pay clients, because Medicaid payment rates are lower.

Eligibility

The striking fact about long-term care financing is that only a small portion of the bill is paid by Medicare or private insurance. Instead, the disabled elderly and younger population who use long-term care pay for it out of their own or their family's income and assets until they are impoverished, and then they turn to Medicaid.

Long-term care is very expensive, with a year in a nursing home costing an average of $37,000 in 1993.[14] As a result, many Medicaid nursing home residents were not poor when they entered the nursing home but became poor by depleting their income and assets paying for care, a process known as spending down.[15]

Medicaid eligibility requirements for long-term care are complex and differ depending on whether the applicant resides in an institution or in the community. Whether they need services at home or in an institution, unmarried people are not eligible for Medicaid if they have more than $2,000 in assets, generally not counting the value of the home. The asset limits for married couples, one of whom still lives at home, were liberalized under the Medicare Catastrophic Coverage Act of 1988; a spouse of a nursing home resident now may keep substantially more of the couple's income and assets than was previously permitted.[16] Meeting the asset limits by transferring assets to other parties at less than fair market value is strictly prohibited. States are required to recover the cost of Medicaid institutional and home care from the estates of deceased Medicaid beneficiaries.

Nursing home and other institutional residents who meet the asset test must contribute all of their income toward the cost of their care, after deducting a small allowance (usually $30 a month) to pay for personal items. Only then will Medicaid help pay the bills. Most states permit people with incomes of any level to qualify for Medicaid institutional care if they meet the asset test and if their medical expenses exceed their income. In some states, however, individuals with income above a set amount—usually 300 percent of the Supplemental Security Income (SSI) level ($5,808 per year in 1997)—are ineligible regardless of how high their medical expenses may be.[17] (SSI is the cash welfare program for the aged, blind, and disabled.) Some people find that they have too much income to qualify for Medicaid but not enough to pay for nursing home care.

Older people and persons with disabilities living in the community become eligible for Medicaid in two ways. First and most common, people whose income and assets are low enough to qualify for the SSI program also qualify for Medicaid, although the so-called 209(b) states may apply stricter eligibility requirements. Second, most states have medically needy programs that allow people with higher levels of income to qualify for Medicaid if, after deducting their medical expenses, their incomes are below the medically needy income level. Although many institutional residents qualify for Medicaid under this provision, relatively few community-based elderly people or persons with disabilities do.

Medicaid Long-Term Care Expenditures

As shown in tables 6-1 and 6-2, total (federal and state) Medicaid long-term care expenditures increased from approximately $25 billion in 1988 to $52 billion in 1995, increasing at an average annual rate of 10.8 percent, which, while substantial, is much less than for the acute care portion of Medicaid.[18] The rate of increase has fallen in recent years, averaging 6.8 percent between 1992 and 1995. Holahan and Liska project that Medicaid long-term care expenditures will increase by 8.9 percent per year between 1996 and 2002.[19]

Table 6-1. *Medicaid Expenditures, by Type of Service, 1988–95*

Millions of dollars

Service	1988	1989	1990	1991	1992	1993	1994	1995
Total	54,100	60,777	72,063	94,154	119,597	130,748	143,729	156,994
Acute care	26,627	30,674	36,741	46,809	55,065	65,041	71,178	80,152
DSH[a]	449	667	1,378	5,316	17,526	17,016	16,890	18,988
Other	1,546	1,211	1,553	5,080	4,432	3,354	6,616	5,644
Long-term care	25,478	28,226	32,391	36,949	42,575	45,338	49,044	52,209
Nursing facilities	15,103	16,230	18,396	21,102	24,577	26,297	28,253	30,318
ICF-MR[b]	5,978	6,633	7,679	8,357	8,907	9,502	9,417	9,602
Mental health	1,753	1,906	2,192	2,525	3,078	2,556	2,869	2,688
Home care	2,644	3,457	4,125	4,965	6,013	6,984	8,506	9,601
Frail elderly	—	—	—	—	21	6	25	35
Home- and community-based waiver	735	1,044	1,337	1,702	2,256	2,880	3,754	4,631
Home health	519	652	820	1,048	1,266	1,457	1,657	1,923
MR-DD[c]	—	—	—	—	11	56	86	124
Personal care	1,390	1,761	1,968	2,215	2,459	2,585	2,984	2,888

Source: Urban Institute analysis of data from HCFA Forms 64 and 2082.

a. Disproportionate share hospital payments.

b. Intermediate-care facilities for the mentally retarded.

c. Mental retardation/developmental disabilities.

Table 6-2. *Rates of Increase in Medicaid Expenditures, by Type of Service, 1988–95*

Percent

Service	1988–89	1989–90	1990–91	1991–92	1992–93	1993–94	1994–95	1988–92	1992–95
Total	12.3	18.6	30.7	27.0	9.3	9.9	9.2	21.9	9.5
Acute care	15.2	19.8	27.4	17.6	18.1	9.4	12.6	19.9	13.3
DSH[a]	48.6	106.5	285.7	229.7	(2.9)	(0.7)	12.4	149.9	2.7
Other	(21.7)	28.2	227.2	(12.8)	(24.3)	97.3	(14.7)	30.1	8.4
Long-term care	10.8	14.8	14.1	15.2	6.5	8.2	6.5	13.7	7.0
Nursing facilities	7.5	13.3	14.7	16.5	7.0	7.4	7.3	12.9	7.2
ICF-MR[b]	11.0	15.8	8.8	6.6	6.7	(0.9)	2.0	10.5	2.5
Mental health	8.7	15.0	15.2	21.9	(17.0)	12.3	(6.3)	15.1	(4.4)
Home care	30.8	19.3	20.4	21.1	16.1	21.8	12.9	22.8	16.9
Frail elderly	—	—	—	—	(71.0)	316.7	40.2	—	19.3
Home- and community-based waiver	42.1	28.1	27.3	32.6	27.7	30.3	23.4	32.4	27.1
Home health	25.7	25.7	27.9	20.8	15.0	13.7	16.1	25.0	14.9
MR-DD[c]	—	—	—	—	396.9	53.9	44.9	—	122.9
Personal care	26.7	11.7	12.5	11.0	5.1	15.5	(3.2)	15.3	5.5

Source: Urban Institute analysis of data from HCFA Forms 64 and 2082.

a. Disproportionate share hospital payments.

b. Intermediate-care facilities for the mentally retarded.

c. Mental retardation/developmental disabilities.

Table 6-3. *Medicaid Long-Term Care Expenditures, per Capita,*
Ages 85 and Older, 1994

	Expenditures (millions)	Population (thousands)	Spending per capita
Total United States	$27,674	3,519	$7,866
New England	$2,443	216	$11,313
Connecticut	651	53	12,325
Maine	235	20	11,691
Massachusetts	1,145	102	11,261
New Hampshire	159	15	10,447
Rhode Island	184	18	10,372
Vermont	69	8	8,200
Middle Atlantic	$8,487	575	$14,762
New Jersey	969	110	8,838
New York	5,648	270	20,899
Pennsylvania	1,870	195	9,575
South Atlantic	$3,656	619	$5,915
Delaware	63	8	7,720
District of Columbia	194	9	22,659
Florida	981	258	3,797
Georgia	422	69	6,120
Maryland	404	55	7,363
North Carolina	668	84	7,987
South Carolina	270	38	7,154
Virginia	435	70	6,227
West Virginia	219	28	7,836
East South Central	$1,322	211	$6,249
Alabama	334	56	5,963
Kentucky	325	51	6,335
Mississippi	212	36	5,865
Tennessee	451	68	6,623
West South Central	$2,219	336	$6,592
Arkansas	253	40	6,378
Louisiana	443	49	9,016
Oklahoma	239	51	4,650
Texas	1,284	196	6,536

Given the range in coverage and payment rates, it is not surprising that
there is substantial variation in Medicaid long-term care spending per beneficiary and per capita. Table 6-3 shows that for the elderly population age
eighty-five and older, per capita long-term care expenditures averaged $7,866
in 1994, ranging from a low of $2,027 in Arizona to a high of $20,899 in
New York.

Table 6-3. (*continued*)

	Expenditures (millions)	Population (thousands)	Spending per capita
East North Central	$4,236	597	$7,091
Illinois	770	163	4,711
Indiana	638	79	8,086
Michigan	880	120	7,351
Ohio	1,293	153	8,431
Wisconsin	655	82	7,992
West North Central	$2,030	327	$6,201
Iowa	212	58	3,631
Kansas	186	46	4,018
Minnesota	798	75	10,697
Missouri	481	90	5,351
Nebraska	174	31	5,539
North Dakota	95	13	7,543
South Dakota	84	14	5,936
Mountain	$727	164	$4,423
Arizona	99	49	2,027
Colorado	214	39	5,497
Idaho	66	14	4,821
Montana	81	12	6,576
Nevada	66	11	6,154
New Mexico	94	17	5,424
Utah	68	17	3,990
Wyoming	39	5	7,196
Pacific	$2,553	472	$5,412
Alaska	39	2	22,906
California	1,757	347	5,066
Hawaii	99	13	7,842
Oregon	197	45	4,343
Washington	461	65	7,074

Source: Urban Institute calculations based on HCFA Form 64 data and current population reports.

Although institutional services (nursing home, mental hospitals, and ICF/MRs) account for the bulk of Medicaid long-term care expenditures (83 percent in 1994), spending for home- and community-based services (personal care, home- and community-based waivers, home health, and the frail elderly program) are growing at a much faster rate. As shown in table 6-4, home- and community-based services constitute a substantial portion of long-term care spending in a few states, such as Oregon (41.7 percent),

Table 6-4. *Distribution of Medicaid Long-Term Care Expenditures by State, 1994*[a]

Percent

State	SNF/ICF-Other[b]	ICF/MR[c]	Mental health	Home health
Total United States	57.6	19.2	5.9	17.3
New England	63.7	13.7	2.5	20.1
Connecticut	63.8	14.9	2.6	18.7
Maine	65.5	15.1	4.2	15.2
Massachusetts	63.6	15.0	2.0	19.3
New Hampshire	66.6	2.2	3.8	27.5
Rhode Island	61.2	12.7	3.3	22.8
Vermont	59.2	4.7	0.1	36.0
Middle Atlantic	50.0	19.9	6.7	23.3
New Jersey	57.7	19.6	3.5	19.1
New York	44.5	21.0	6.0	28.5
Pennsylvania	63.0	16.9	10.9	9.2
South Atlantic	60.5	18.6	5.1	15.8
Delaware	50.1	22.6	4.9	22.4
District of Columbia	49.5	20.4	24.5	5.6
Florida	70.4	14.0	0.9	14.7
Georgia	70.8	14.8	1.9	12.4
Maryland	62.3	8.8	1.6	27.3
North Carolina	54.1	28.1	2.6	15.2
South Carolina	45.5	33.6	9.4	11.5
Virginia	53.4	21..6	12.3	12.7
West Virginia	62.4	3.9	6.7	27.1
East South Central	68.3	16.4	6.2	9.1
Alabama	70.3	14.5	3.5	11.7
Kentucky	63.5	12.3	5.6	18.6
Mississippi	68.2	23.7	5.5	2.6
Tennessee[d]	70.6	17.3	8.8	3.3
West South Central	55.1	26.2	4.4	14.3
Arkansas	54.9	19.0	10.4	15.8
Louisiana	53.1	31.0	9.8	6.2
Oklahoma	55.1	19.9	5.9	19.1
Texas	56.1	27.2	0.0	16.7

Table 6-4. (*continued*)

State	SNF/ICF-Other[b]	ICF/MR[c]	Mental health	Home health
East North Central	64.2	20.0	5.1	10.6
Illinois	62.5	26.7	2.4	8.5
Indiana	67.1	28.2	1.7	3.1
Michigan	61.7	10.2	9.2	18.9
Ohio	67.2	19.0	6.9	6.8
Wisconsin	61.4	16.8	3.6	18.2
West North Central	59.4	20.6	3.0	17.0
Iowa	53.2	35.6	5.0	6.1
Kansas	49.3	25.8	6.0	18.9
Minnesota	64.9	16.0	2.0	17.2
Missouri	56.9	19.2	2.2	21.7
Nebraska	67.0	12.2	2.7	18.1
North Dakota	57.5	23.5	2.0	17.0
South Dakota	57.4	21.0	3.7	17.9
Mountain	53.4	16.2	11.1	19.3
Arizona[d]	46.7	19.3	28.9	5.1
Colorado	56.3	9.2	4.8	29.8
Idaho	53.5	30.0	0.0	16.5
Montana	59.8	9.0	9.8	21.5
Nevada	59.4	16.6	13.9	10.1
New Mexico	52.8	18.9	9.1	19.1
Utah	50.8	23.3	3.8	22.1
Wyoming	52.5	9.0	0.2	38.3
Pacific	57.3	16.8	9.7	16.2
Alaska	66.0	15.1	13.2	5.7
California	59.6	16.7	11.9	11.8
Hawaii	80.2	6.8	0.0	13.0
Oregon	35.4	17.8	5.1	41.7
Washington	55.2	18.7	5.3	20.8

Source: Urban Institute calculations based on HCFA Form 64 data.

a. Does not include DSH payments, administrative costs, accounting adjustments, or the U.S. territories. Totals may not add due to rounding.

b. SNF/ICF: skilled nursing facilities/other intermediate care facilities.

c. ICF/MR: intermediate care facilities for the mentally retarded.

d. For Arizona and Tennessee expenditure and beneficiary data are based on figures reported directly by the state; adjustments were made to categorize these numbers in the same manner as other states reporting to the HCFA.

while in states such as Tennessee (3.3 percent) and Mississippi (2.6 percent) virtually all expenditures are for institutional care.

The Medicaid Reform Proposals and Long-Term Care

During 1995, 1996, and 1997 Congress, the president, and the National Governors' Association (NGA) developed proposals to restructure Medicaid. In each case long-term care under the Medicaid program would have been substantially altered.

The Medigrant Proposal

In keeping with the rest of the Medigrant proposal, the long-term care components of the plan would have eliminated the open-ended entitlement to services, terminated most federal standards and their enforcement, and held federal matching payments to a level substantially below projected spending under current law. Among the provisions to be repealed or substantially weakened were the requirements that (1) states provide nursing home and home health care, (2) states pay nursing homes enough to cover the costs of an efficient provider that met the quality standards, (3) states may not hold adult relatives financially responsible for the cost of nursing home care, (4) the federal government ensure that states enforce the nursing home quality standards, (5) states obtain a budget-neutral waiver in order to cover nonmedical services targeted to the population at risk of institutionalization, and (6) services be provided to all eligible population groups with comparability in terms of "amount, duration, and scope." States would have been allowed to cover a very broad range of long-term care services.[20] Earlier versions of the plan would also have repealed almost all nursing home quality standards, allowed unlimited imposition of family responsibility requirements, and dropped provisions that protect the community-based spouses of married nursing home residents from impoverishment; however, these were dropped from the final plan because of political opposition.

To ensure that each group of low-income people that received coverage under the current Medicaid program received some services, the bill established spending minimums for certain groups of people. The proposal required states to sustain or set aside a share of the block grant spending to use on any services they might choose for three groups: low-income mothers and children, people with disabilities, and low-income elderly. The set-asides were determined by states' historical spending on coverage of these groups for the mandatory services plus nursing home care for the optional population. These maintenance-of-effort requirements were very weak and amounted to only 85 percent of their 1992–94 expenditures (which were not indexed for inflation) for the mandatory services for the mandatory eligibility groups plus nursing home care; most expenditures for home- and community-based services were excluded from the base. Within these very modest constraints, states could spend Medigrant money as they chose.

President Clinton's Proposal

President Clinton's Medicaid reform plan was much more modest, both in terms of the level of savings proposed and the amount of additional flexibility granted the states. His 1995 and 1997 proposals were virtually the same in structure. His plan would have retained the entitlement to services but established a limit on year-to-year growth in average federal payments per enrollee (commonly referred to as a per capita cap). Different per capita caps would have been established for the aged, disabled, adults, and children. Thus, unlike under the congressional plan, federal funds would automatically rise if enrollment increased. For long-term care, states would have been allowed greater flexibility to provide a broad range of home- and community-based services, the nursing home reimbursement standards would have been eliminated, and a few minor nursing home quality requirements would have been repealed. Under current law states must obtain a waiver from HCFA in order to provide certain nonmedical home- and community-based services; under the president's proposal waiver approval would no longer be required. All other federal requirements would be retained.

The NGA Resolution

Following the collapse of budget talks in 1996, the NGA developed a broad outline of a proposal that attempted to marry the block grant approach of Medigrant with the average per beneficiary limits on the growth of expenditures proposed by the Clinton administration. Because it was only a six-page outline and not a full-fledged proposal, many issues were not addressed. In general it sought to provide states with very broad flexibility but guarantee coverage for certain mandatory groups and services. However, because most nursing home residents are not eligible through mandatory-coverage provisions, they would not be protected under the NGA plan; nor would the use of home- and community-based services be allowed to increase automatically. States would be given flexibility to provide home- and community-based services, to enforce nursing home quality standards with only weak federal oversight, and to set nursing home payment rates as they saw fit.

Responsibility for Long-Term Care

At the heart of the issue of devolution and Medicaid is the question of how responsibility for long-term care should be allocated between the federal and state governments; and, relatedly, what national standards should be imposed on the states as a condition of receipt of federal funds? Currently the financing of acute and long-term care services for young and older persons with disabilities is splintered among many payers. Acute care for elderly persons and some younger persons with disabilities is paid largely by the federally run and financed Medicare program; however, Medicaid also plays a role, primarily by paying the Medicare cost sharing and premiums and covering additional services such as prescription drugs. At the same time, long-term care is financed primarily by Medicaid and state-financed programs, but Medicare spending for nursing home and home care has increased dramatically in recent years. Within Medicaid, although both federal and state governments are involved in the financing and policymaking, operational responsibility for managing the system is primarily the responsibility of the states.

What Level of Government Should Have Primary Responsibility for Long-Term Care?

Over the past fifteen years there have been numerous proposals to consolidate financing and responsibility for long-term care at either the federal or state level. In various swap proposals put forth by President Reagan, the NGA, and former senator Nancy Kassebaum, long-term care has alternately been proposed as a fundamentally federal or fundamentally state responsibility. During the late 1980s a variety of social insurance proposals drafted by former senator George Mitchell, Senator Edward Kennedy, Representative Henry Waxman, Representative Pete Stark, and the Pepper commission would have made long-term care predominately a federal responsibility. As part of health reform in 1993, President Clinton's long-term care proposal for a new non-means-tested home care program would have been very heavily federally financed, but would have relied on states almost entirely to design and administer the new program. Recent long-term care reforms in a variety of countries have struggled with the question of what level of government should be responsible for long-term care.[21]

There are three main arguments in favor of consolidating responsibility at the national level or for maintaining extensive national standards. First, national programs provide equity across geographic areas to all citizens of the country. Uniform national programs eliminate the undesirable variation in coverage, access, and quality of services that exist with more decentralized programs. For proponents of national programs, it is unfair that a severely disabled elderly person in New York should be able to obtain extensive personal care services, while a person with a similar level of disability in Mississippi should not. Moreover, given variations in fiscal capacity and political cultures, some states may choose not to provide certain services or cover certain groups for which there is otherwise a national consensus.

Second, since Washington provides the lion's share of Medicaid's funds, it is only reasonable to expect federal legislators and administrators to retain a major voice in how the money is spent.[22] The notion is that the person who pays the piper gets to call the tune. If federal oversight were scaled back, Congress and the president may see less reason to financially support Medicaid adequately. If they have little say in how that money is used, it will be politically more difficult for federal lawmakers to raise taxes, cut other programs, or increase public borrowing to appropriate more money for Medicaid.

Third, consolidation of long-term care at the national level would make the federal government responsible for virtually all important programs for the elderly population (that is, Medicare, Social Security, SSI, and veterans' programs), allowing for better coordination and integration of services and programs. For health care, a fundamental problem facing policymakers and providers is that older and younger persons with disabilities do not come with just acute care needs or just long-term care needs; rather they have both, and the current system fragments responsibility. Because of the bifurcation of financial responsibility for acute (Medicare) and long-term (Medicaid) care, there is a strong incentive for the federal government to shift costs to the states and vice versa. Or, at the very least, there is a relative indifference about initiatives that would save money for the other level of government. Thus the largely state-run Medicaid program has little incentive to reduce hospital use by elderly persons who are jointly Medicare and Medicaid beneficiaries, because these savings will accrue mostly to the federal government. By the same token, Medicare has little interest in controlling unskilled nursing home and home care use, because these savings will be captured mostly by state governments.

On the other side, there are three arguments in favor of decentralization. First, far more than the federal government, states are already heavily involved in the day-to-day operation and management of long-term care services. States assess client need, regulate the supply and quality of care, set reimbursement rates, write contracts with providers, process claims, and coordinate the care of clients. In most other countries subnational governmental units have the predominant role in long-term care.[23] Thus a configuration where states have a strong role would capitalize on their creativity and experience in developing long-term care delivery systems.

Second, long-term care is an intensely personal service involving a variety of quality-of-life issues. Therefore the planning and delivery of services should be influenced by local circumstances, norms, and values, and by the local preferences of the population with disabilities, their caregivers, and providers. For example, a thoughtfully designed care plan in rural Alabama might not make sense in New York City because the resources, service delivery patterns, and lifestyles vary so greatly between these two locations.

Third, because they are less driven than the federal government to routinize their decisionmaking process and because individual cases loom larger in the policy process, state and locally administered programs are arguably less rigid and bureaucratic then centrally run programs. For example, Wisconsin's community options program is far more flexible and individually tailored than is the Medicare home health benefit.

While state and local officials often support the programmatic reasons for designing and administering long-term care programs at the subnational level, they are usually less enthusiastic about having to pay for services. Long-run demographics guarantee large increases in need for long-term care, and some officials worry that efforts at decentralization may be thinly disguised efforts to dump the fiscal burden on another level of government.

Should Existing Medicaid Long-Term Care Standards Be Eliminated?

During 1995 and 1996 the debate over what level of government should be responsible for long-term care focused mostly on the federal standards that would be repealed by the Medigrant plan. At its core, the issue is what should be allowed to vary across the states and what should be the same (or at least meet minimum standards) throughout the country? Within long-term care, all of the major Medicaid reform proposals would have given states substantial additional flexibility in the provision of home- and community-based services. However, the debate over the Medigrant proposal raised questions about at least three areas of current federal law and regulation: prohibitions against the imposition of so-called family responsibility requirements, standards on nursing home (and hospital) reimbursement, and nursing home quality standards.

FAMILY CONTRIBUTIONS TO NURSING-HOME COSTS. Since the beginning of the Medicaid program, federal law explicitly has prohibited states from requiring adult children to contribute to the cost of nursing home care of their parents as a condition of Medicaid eligibility (Section 1902(a)(17)(D) of the Social Security Act)—commonly referred to as family responsibility requirements. The Medigrant proposal passed by Congress would have allowed states to impose these requirements on adult children who have more than the state's median income.

Advocates of family responsibility programs see them as a way to promote equity, reduce costs, and encourage family care.[24] Some policymakers argue that it is unfair to tax lower- or moderate-income people to pay for care of the parent of an affluent adult child, as sometimes happens in the current system. A family responsibility program could also encourage informal caregiving by delaying the point at which families seek institutional placement for their elderly kin. Advocates also contend that family members who know that they would be held financially responsible for part of the cost of institutional care of their parents might be more inclined to seek noninstitutional alternatives or to purchase private long-term care insurance for them. Elderly nursing home candidates themselves also might be more resistant to placement that could lead to a financial burden on their children.

Opponents of family responsibility initiatives take issue with the implicit assumption that family members of many disabled elderly do not do enough to help these relatives. A substantial volume of research finds that relatives provide enormous amounts of informal home care to disabled elderly relatives.[25] Fully 84 percent of disabled elderly people who were admitted to nursing homes between 1982 and 1984 received assistance from relatives and friends.[26] Other studies suggest that caring for disabled elderly relatives imposes large emotional and physical strains on families.[27] Opponents of family responsibility argue that adult children should not be punished because they have a parent who needs expensive nursing home care, and they question the wisdom of discouraging people who need institutional care from seeking it.

Because family financial responsibility is prohibited by current law, there is little direct evidence on potential savings; but the available data suggest that it would generate few savings. Administrative costs, in particular, could be high and could largely offset savings.[28] In the early 1980s Idaho took advantage of a Reagan administration reinterpretation of the law that allowed family responsibility requirements when contributions are enforced under a law of general applicability and not imposed solely on Medicaid beneficiaries. The Idaho family responsibility initiative had a goal of $1.5 million in annual collections, but succeeded in collecting less than $32,000 in its six months of operation.[29]

NURSING HOME REIMBURSEMENT RATE STANDARDS. Under current law states may set Medicaid payment rates at whatever level they choose for home- and community-based services, but until recently they were required to meet a federal minimum standard for nursing home and hospital reimbursement.[30] This standard was prescribed by the Boren amendment, which required that providers be reimbursed under rates that the state "finds and makes assurances satisfactory to the Secretary [of the Department of Health and Human Services] are reasonable and adequate to meet the costs which must be incurred by efficiently and economically operated facilities in order to provide care and services in conformity with applicable State and Federal laws, regulations and quality and safety standards" (Section 1902(a)(13) of the Social Security Act). Within this standard, states could use a wide variety of reimbursement methodologies. Although this law was designed to relax previous requirements, many states had difficulty meeting the standard; as of 1993 at least forty-three nursing home reimbursement lawsuits were filed for violation of the Boren amendment's substantive or procedural standards.[31] Repeal of the Boren amendment has been long sought by state governors, who contend that it unnecessarily limits their flexibility in setting reimbursement rates. All of the major proposals for Medicaid reform would have repealed the Boren amendment and given states complete freedom to set payment rates. The Balanced Budget Act of 1997 eliminated virtually all federal standards on nursing home reimbursement.

Although the Boren standards appeared very minimal, states contended that they have been nearly impossible to operationalize and that the courts were unreasonable in their interpretation of them. Moreover, Boren's procedural requirements compounded the difficulty of defending the state's methodology in court. Medicaid officials believed that the lawyers representing the state are inadequate when compared to the high-priced lawyers that nursing home providers hire. Because of their poor prospects of winning in court, states saw the threat of a lawsuit as being nearly as important as actually having a lawsuit when it comes to affecting state payment policy. Furthermore, many state officials felt it was unfair that they were forced to give rate increases to nursing homes and not to home- and community-based care and other providers. The net result was that states believed that they were forced into reimbursement systems that went far beyond the minimalist standard embodied in the plain language of the statute. As a result, they spent more money on nursing homes than they would otherwise choose.

The problem with repealing the reimbursement standards is that Medicaid nursing home payment rates are already fairly low, especially in comparison with Medicare and private-pay rates. In 1993 average Medicaid nursing home payment rates were $82 a day, while average Medicare payment rates were $170 a day.[32] In addition, although there is great variation across facilities and states, private-pay charges generally tend to be substantially higher than Medicaid rates.[33] Indeed, some states have an implicit policy of having private-pay residents subsidize Medicaid beneficiaries. Not surprisingly, then, nursing homes prefer private-pay to Medicaid patients.[34] As a result, Medicaid beneficiaries often have difficulty gaining access to nursing homes. To the extent that states cut reimbursement rates and the payment differential between private-pay and Medicaid patients widens, access problems may worsen.

In addition, while there is little evidence of a simple relationship between cost and quality, there is probably some threshold level of reimbursement below which it is impossible to provide adequate quality of care. Repeal of the Boren amendment without any substitute eliminates the safeguard that Medicaid payment levels not go below that threshold. While the quality of care in nursing homes has improved over the last twenty years, nursing home resident advocates remain extremely concerned about the quality of care provided in many nursing homes.[35]

FEDERAL QUALITY STANDARDS FOR NURSING HOMES. Largely in response to concerns about inadequate care in nursing homes, the Omnibus Budget Reconciliation Act of 1987 (OBRA87) dramatically revised and strengthened the Medicaid and Medicare quality standards and the survey and certification process for nursing homes. This federal law spells out in tremendous detail what facilities and states must and must not do and when; in contrast, federal standards for most home care services are nonexistent.[36] Facilities that do not meet the standards are not eligible for Medicaid and Medicare reimbursement.

Some states chafe under these very specific requirements and would like to see them changed. The House of Representatives passed a version of the Medigrant program that would have eliminated most of these national standards. While the final Medigrant legislation would have retained the current requirements, it also would have given states much more flexibility in the implementation of the survey and certification process, with federal enforcement of the standards being almost entirely eliminated. The NGA proposal was close to the Medigrant plan. In contrast, the Clinton proposal would make only small changes in the survey and certification process.

Advocates for greater state flexibility in quality enforcement argue that the existing system is unduly bureaucratic and inflexible, with many standards that do not really relate to quality of care.[37] Moreover, they contend that state government is concerned about ensuring adequate quality of care in nursing homes because it is their citizens who are in the nursing homes. From a financial perspective, different quality standards might make reimbursement cuts more feasible.

Consumer advocates strongly oppose the proposed changes in the Medigrant proposal. They note that quality standards and their enforcement were weak in many states before OBRA87.[38] Advocates moreover argue that it is the threat of the loss of federal funds that motivates states to make the quality improvements. In addition, if accompanied by repeal of the Boren amendment, they worry that state reimbursement rates will be inadequate to provide quality care. Thus there will be a strong incentive for state surveyors to "look the other way" because they know that it is unfair to require facilities to meet certain staffing and other standards if the state will not pay enough to satisfy those standards.

There is substantial evidence that the quality standards imposed by OBRA87, while not perfect, have improved quality of care and may have saved money. An evaluation led by Research Triangle Institute, Inc., found that the OBRA87 standards reduced the use of physical and chemical restraints, lowered hospitalizations, lessened use of indwelling catheters, and decreased the number of dehydrated patients.[39] The standards also increased the percentage of residents who participated in activities and the proportion of residents who used hearing aids if they needed them.

Medicaid Entitlement to Long-Term Care

A key issue in Medicaid reform, especially as it relates to long-term care, is whether individuals should have an entitlement—a legal obligation on the part of government to provide services to individuals who meet preestablished criteria regardless of the cost to the government. For example, within Medicaid long-term care this means that if a state chooses to cover personal care services, it must pay for services for all individuals who meet the medical and disability criteria and who use services; it cannot say that it will spend $100 million and that is all.[40] As with the rest of the Medicaid program, the Medigrant plan would have eliminated the entitlement to long-term care services; President Clinton's proposal retained it. While complicated, the NGA proposal would have eliminated, for the most part, the entitlement for most persons and services.

Those who would retain individual entitlements argue that, combined with national minimum standards, they provide the population with an important sense of security that adequate resources will be available.[41] Individuals know that if they become destitute and need long-term care services they can obtain certain benefits. Entitlement is the mechanism that links expenditures to need, that is, to the number of beneficiaries and the cost of care. This linkage is lacking with block grants or other appropriated programs; fixed budget programs simply do not have the automatic engine of spending increases inherent in entitlement programs. Once the entitlement is eliminated, funding can be set at any desired level and Congress could easily reduce federal spending without deliberating on how cuts would actually be implemented at the state, local, facility, or individual level. The end result may be that some needy people will be denied assistance.

On the question of whether resources would be adequate, the Medigrant proposal clearly sounded alarms. While there were some efforts to distribute funds among the states based on the size of their elderly population (which is a proxy for need for long-term care services), aggregate levels of spending into the future were not explicitly adjusted for growth in the disabled population (elderly or nonelderly) or inflation in long-term care services, and the growth factor adopted was far below historical levels. (This issue is discussed in greater detail later in this chapter.)

In addition, it would be an overstatement to contend that Medicaid long-term care expenditures are rampaging out of control. As noted, Medicaid long-term care expenditures have increased much more slowly than acute care spending and have not been subject to the level of manipulation that has characterized Medicaid acute care expenditures. In addition, through certificate-of-need programs and moratoriums on new construction, states have substantial control over the utilization of nursing homes and ICF/MRs, which account for the bulk of Medicaid long-term care expenditures. Moreover, eligibility and expenditures for long-term care are probably less sensitive to recession and other general macroeconomic factors, because the population in need is outside of the labor force. Thus Medicaid long-term care expenditures are relatively predictable and less likely to fluctuate wildly.

People who favor ending the individual entitlement to benefits argue that spending for public programs should be decided as part of a deliberative process in which all programs compete for resources within an overall spending limit. Advocates of this position contend, first and foremost, that eliminating entitlements is the only sure way to control spending and provide needed budget predictability at both the federal and state levels. Neither the federal nor state governments can permanently afford to have Medicaid expenditures increase faster than revenues without squeezing out other desirable spending. If Medicaid funds are depleted, federal and state legislators can always appropriate additional money if that is a priority. In this view, entitlement programs have a blank check that inevitably leads to spending levels that are higher than policymakers or the public would deliberately choose.

Advocates of ending the entitlement also argue that changing Medicaid to a program with a fixed annual budget could change the nature of the program in beneficial ways. States would no longer have an incentive to manipulate the Medicaid financing system in order to maximize federal reimbursement. Over the last twenty years states have refinanced many state-funded long-term care programs to be Medicaid-covered services. In some cases the net result was an increase in federal spending without an increase in the number of persons receiving services. In addition, a capped program would put states in a much stronger bargaining position with providers over reimbursement rates and the provision of services, because all parties would know that only a limited amount of money would be available.

Block grant proponents contend that states are not heartless and will not turn their backs on the poor and people with long-term care needs.[42] But without federal requirements for states to provide specified services to particular groups, it is not obvious what they will do if the federal and state money runs out before the end of the year. For example, would states deny Medicaid eligibility to a severely disabled elderly person who needed nursing home care and had no place else to go? Or would they find that they had to spend additional funds, even though Medicaid was no longer an entitlement?

Finally, and most important for long-term care, without the constraint of having to provide services on an entitlement basis states would have freedom to tailor services to local and individual needs. Disabled persons, especially the non-elderly, need a very wide range of services. The philosophy of the disability movement holds that services should be tailored to the individual disabled person. Inevitably each individual has different needs and wants. As a result, the range of services provided should be much broader than institutions and homemaker and personal care services, and arguably should include anything that maximizes the independence of the individual.[43] Many advocates go so far as to urge provision of cash benefits instead of services, thus giving disabled persons complete freedom to choose whatever services they like from whatever provider they want.

The basic dilemma is that the more flexible the set of services provided, the more difficult it is to provide services on an entitlement basis and still keep expenditures within the desired amount. The broader the range of available services, the more likely persons will use them even if they do not need them, thus raising the level of overall expenditures. Bluntly put, people cannot be entitled to everything they might possibly want. Some states are reluctant to cover certain home- and community-based services in an entitlement program because the definition of need is hard to establish and the number of people who meet the criteria is large. However, they might be willing to offer at least some of these services if they can fix the level of expenditures. In addition, from a federal perspective, the broader the possible services the greater the incentive for states to refinance state-funded programs, such as vocational rehabilitation, through the Medicaid program without expanding services. The conflict between coverage of a broad range of long-term care services and an open-ended entitlement led even the Clinton administration to propose a major expansion of home care without an entitlement to services as part of its health reform plan in 1993.[44]

Although there is little doubt that a block grant would give states additional long-term care flexibility, current Medicaid law gives states the opportunity to cover a range of home- and community-based services. In terms of flexibility, the home- and community-based waivers are probably the most important mechanism for doing so. Under these programs, federal rules relating to statewideness, comparability of services, income and resource rules, and requirements for states to provide services to all persons in the state on an equal basis may be waived. Federal legislation specifically allows provision of case management, home health aide services, personal care services, adult day health, habilitation, and respite care as specifically allowable services; other services may be covered if approved by the secretary of the Department of Health and Human Services (HHS) (Section 1915 (c) of the Social Security Act). Although conflict between the federal government and the states was substantial during the Reagan and Bush administrations over whether waiver services were cost-effective, regulatory changes implemented by the Clinton administration have made obtaining waivers fairly easy. President Clinton's Medicaid reform proposal would have allowed states to implement these programs without having to obtain a waiver.

As a practical matter, however, it may be extremely hard for states to run a program as large as Medicaid long-term care (let alone Medicaid as a whole), in which services are tailored to the needs of individuals. While states have a lot of experience administering nonentitlement long-term care programs, these programs tend to be fairly small, whereas 9.6 million elderly and disabled persons received Medicaid benefits in 1995.[45] The administrative complexities of implementing an individually tailored program for such large numbers of people could be overwhelming. Furthermore, basic legal standards prohibit states from being arbitrary and capricious in their determinations of who will and will not receive services and how much. The Americans with Disabilities Act (ADA) may also deter states from limiting the enrollment of persons with disabilities. States establishing large programs that give government officials broad discretion may face an avalanche of litigation, especially in the early years of the program. It is probable, although not certain, that states would establish standard administrative rules about who will be eligible and what services they will cover. In other words, they may run their new programs as *de facto* state entitlements or quasi-entitlements.

Controlling Long-Term Care Expenditures

A key issue in evaluating Medicaid reform plans is how states will live within the budget levels established by these proposals.[46] The Medigrant proposal in particular envisioned a much lower rate of increase in Medicaid expenditures than has occurred historically. Unlike proposed welfare and Medicare reforms, advocates of greater state flexibility and substantially reduced federal Medicaid spending have not put forth a blueprint or even a theory of how states could stay within their budgets. The policy debate begins and ends with the notion that if states are given enough flexibility, they will figure out how to reduce the rate of growth in expenditures without hurting beneficiaries. Indeed, block grant advocates explicitly reject the argument that reduced federal funding and requirements will adversely affect the poor.

Overall there are three broad strategies that states might use to control long-term care spending: (1) bring more private resources into the long-term care system to offset Medicaid's expenditures, (2) reform the delivery system so that care can be provided more cheaply, and (3) reduce Medicaid eligibility, reimbursement, service coverage, and quality standards. Based on the available research, there is little evidence to suggest that large savings are possible without adversely affecting beneficiaries' eligibility, access to services, and quality of care received. As a result, claims that large Medicaid long-term care savings can be obtained easily should be viewed with caution.

Increase Private Resources

The first general strategy to control spending is to bring additional private resources into the long-term care system. This could be done in three ways: (1) by encouraging private long-term care insurance, (2) by more strictly enforcing prohibitions against transfer of assets before receiving Medicaid, and (3) by aggressively recovering money from the estates of deceased Medicaid nursing home residents. This strategy builds on the observation that a substantial proportion of Medicaid nursing home residents were not poor before they entered the nursing home.[47] Thus those nursing home residents may have private resources that can be more effectively drawn on to offset their Medicaid expenditures.

ENCOURAGE PURCHASE OF PRIVATE LONG-TERM CARE INSURANCE. One way to reduce Medicaid long-term care expenditures might be to encourage the purchase of private long-term care insurance. For initially nonpoor Medicaid nursing home residents, private long-term care insurance might prevent both their impoverishment and subsequent Medicaid expenditures. Only about 4 to 5 percent of the elderly currently have any type of long-term care insurance, much of which is deficient in terms of coverage.[48]

While there are several reasons why so few people have private long-term care insurance, the most important is that such insurance is unaffordable for most of the elderly. The average annual premium for high-quality insurance policies sold by the leading insurers in 1993 was $2,137 if bought at age sixty-five and $6,811 if bought at age seventy-nine.[49] Most studies have found that only 10 to 20 percent of the elderly can afford private long-term care insurance.[50]

One way to increase purchase of private long-term care insurance that has been of interest to many states is the so-called Robert Wood Johnson Foundation Public-Private Partnership, in which easier access to Medicaid is provided to purchasers of state-approved private long-term care insurance policies. In these public-private partnerships—which are being tried in California, Connecticut, Indiana, and New York—policyholders are allowed to keep far more of their financial assets than usually permitted and still receive long-term care benefits under Medicaid.[51] This strategy allows the insured to obtain lifetime asset protection without having to buy an insurance policy that pays lifetime benefits. Moreover, supporters argue that the scheme will be roughly budget neutral, with Medicaid savings offsetting the additional benefits. Participation in this initiative was disappointing, with only 11,399 policies in force as of December 1995, over half of which were in New York State.[52] At the May 1996 conference on Medicaid it was suggested that the possibility of transferring assets to obtain Medicaid eligibility had dampened participation in New York.

To estimate the potential impact of various private long-term care insurance options on Medicaid expenditures, Wiener, Illston, and Hanley simulated several different private long-term care insurance options using the

Brookings-ICF Long-Term Care Financing Model.[53] The simulations suggest that private long-term care insurance is unlikely to substantially affect Medicaid nursing home expenditures. With generous assumptions about the willingness of the elderly to purchase insurance, Medicaid nursing home expenditures might be 1 to 4 percent less than what they would be without private long-term care insurance in 2018—basically rounding error for long-range projections. Private long-term care insurance has little impact on expenditures, because it is too expensive for the elderly who depend on Medicaid to pay for their nursing home care.

Only where large numbers of younger persons purchase private long-term care insurance through their employers is there potential for significant reductions in Medicaid nursing home expenditures and the number of Medicaid nursing home beneficiaries. Premiums are much lower if bought at younger ages and through group rather than individual policies. If employers sponsor but do not help pay for private long-term care insurance, Medicaid expenditures could decline as much as 31 percent, and the number of Medicaid nursing home residents could fall by as much as 17 percent by the year 2018. This option would require an extraordinary increase in the employer-sponsored market, however, since less than 0.1 percent of the nonelderly population currently has private long-term care insurance.[54] Moreover, most middle-aged workers are not interested in buying private long-term care insurance, because they have more pressing expenses, such as child care, mortgage payments, and college education for their children. The risk of needing long-term care is too distant to galvanize many younger people into buying insurance. Nonetheless, according to one official at the May 1996 conference, in order to increase the number of younger people with insurance, Washington State enacted legislation to offer private long-term care insurance to state employees.

PREVENT TRANSFER OF ASSETS. Over the past few years policymakers and the media have focused attention on so-called Medicaid estate planning, where middle- and upper-class elderly persons transfer, shelter, and underreport assets in order to artificially appear poor so that they can qualify for Medicaid-financed nursing home care.[55] Despite the fact that Congress has legislated against this practice, some observers argue that the legislative prohibitions are easy to circumvent and that the prevalence of Medicaid estate planning has increased dramatically in recent years, substantially increasing Medicaid spending.[56]

At the May 1996 conference there was substantial disagreement over how prevalent transfer of assets actually was. One official from Washington State questioned whether stopping it would produce enough "juice to be worth the squeeze." On the other hand, noting that Medicaid estate planning seminars are common in their state, New York officials contended that it was a major problem. Even in New York, however, there was not unanimous agreement with one observer unable to reconcile the enormous number of anecdotes with survey data on the low level of assets held by disabled elderly widows.

While it seems likely that an increasing number of persons are transferring assets, the very limited available evidence suggests that the current numbers are much smaller than commonly thought, and thus savings are likely to be small. The only direct evidence is from a 1993 U.S. General Accounting Office (GAO) study of applicants for Medicaid nursing home care in Massachusetts, a state chosen in part because asset transfer was believed to be common there.[57] Of the 403 Massachusetts Medicaid applicants reviewed, 49 had transferred assets, three-quarters of whom had shifted less than $50,000 in resources. Furthermore, twenty-six of the forty-nine applicants were either denied eligibility or withdrew their application. Six of the seven applicants who transferred more than $100,000 were denied eligibility. Thus, although some clients did transfer assets, existing rules kept most off the Medicaid rolls.

Beyond this direct evidence, there are more indirect data to suggest that asset transfer is not as common as often assumed. First, logically, older persons cannot transfer large amounts of assets they do not have. Existing data suggest that very elderly, disabled widows, who account for the vast bulk of nursing home patients, have quite low incomes and assets.[58] For example, using a synthetic estimate based on data on the noninstitutionalized elderly population from the Survey of Income and Program Participation, Wiener, Hanley, and Harris calculated that only about 12 percent had the level of assets ($100,000 or more) considered typical of estate planners' clients. Of this more wealthy population, about half had enough annual income to pay for nursing home care without recourse to any assets. Thus this group has little incentive to engage in Medicaid estate planning.

Second, if a large and rapidly increasing number of the elderly are transferring their assets, then the number of Medicaid nursing home beneficiaries should be rising rapidly. But the number of Medicaid nursing home beneficiaries is increasing slowly and only slightly faster than the number of nursing home beds. Between 1990 and 1994 the average annual compound rate of increase in Medicaid nursing home beneficiaries was 2.9

percent a year, while the increase in the number of nursing home beds was 1.6 percent a year.[59] All of the excess increase in Medicaid beneficiaries is due to a relatively large increase in Medicaid nursing home residents in one year—1991–92—which probably reflects implementation of the spousal impoverishment provisions of the Medicare Catastrophic Coverage Act of 1988.

Expand Estate Recovery. In general, the home is an excluded asset in determining financial eligibility for Medicaid. However, states have long had the option of recovering Medicaid expenditures for nursing home care from the estates of deceased Medicaid beneficiaries, principally from the sale of their houses. The Omnibus Budget Reconciliation Act of 1993 mandated that all states operate such programs, but some states have refused to do so because these efforts are politically unpopular. As of 1995 only five states (Alaska, Georgia, Michigan, Tennessee, and Texas) did not have some type of program in place.[60]

It is likely that a significant proportion of elderly persons discharged from nursing homes own their homes, but not as many as commonly assumed.[61] In an analysis of eight states in 1985, the GAO found that only 14 percent of nursing home applicants for Medicaid owned a home, with an average value of about $31,000.[62]

Experience with currently operating estate-recovery programs suggests that they are likely to recoup only a small proportion of nursing home expenditures. The amount recovered from the estates of deceased Medicaid beneficiaries averaged only 1.4 percent of Medicaid nursing home expenditures in 1994 for the top ten states, falling rapidly from a high of 3.8 percent in Oregon to a low of 0.4 percent in Montana.[63] Because of the efforts already under way in many states, additional savings are likely to be limited largely to those states not currently operating estate-recovery programs.

System Reform

Another general strategy for saving money is to reorganize the delivery system in ways that make care more efficient and effective. This can be done by adding long-term care to the acute care services provided by managed-care organizations, or by expanding home care and nonmedical residential long-term care services.

INTEGRATE ACUTE AND LONG-TERM CARE SERVICES THROUGH MANAGED CARE.
Persons with disabilities currently receive care through a fragmented and
uncoordinated financing and delivery system.[64] A major consequence of
this fragmentation may be that total costs are higher than they would be in
an integrated system.[65] Because of the growing awareness of the inadequa-
cies of the current system, there is increasing interest among policymakers
in finding ways to integrate the acute and long-term care sectors, primarily
by expanding managed care to include long-term care services. Under these
models, managed-care organizations receive a fixed payment per enrollee
to provide a range of acute and long-term care services, creating financial
incentives to avoid both the functional decline that can result from unmet
health care needs and the unnecessary costs associated with providing services in needlessly expensive settings.

Although the integration of acute and long-term care services offers
the opportunity for improved quality of care, some long-term care advocates have doubts about this model. One concern is that HMOs and other
managed-care providers have little experience with the low-income elderly
and disabled persons, and virtually none with long-term care. Another concern is that fiscal pressures within integrated systems will end up shifting
resources to acute care, thereby shortchanging long-term care.[66] Finally,
there is a fear that long-term care services will become overmedicalized
and less consumer-directed as the balance of power shifts from the individual client and his or her chosen provider to HMOs, insurance companies, or other administrative entities.

From the state perspective, projects that truly integrate acute and long-
term care services are extremely difficult to establish under current law
because they require waiver of both Medicare and Medicaid rules. Almost
all elderly and some disabled Medicaid beneficiaries receive most of their
acute care services through the Medicare program. For dually eligible Medicaid beneficiaries, Medicaid pays the Medicare Part B premium, deductibles
and coinsurance, uncovered services (mostly prescription drugs), and long-
term care. While the Balanced Budget Act of 1997 gives states greater freedom to fashion their Medicaid managed-care programs, states are not gaining
any control over the Medicare program. Thus they may not have much
leverage over the provision of acute care services to dual eligibles.

DEMONSTRATION PROJECTS AND OTHER INITIATIVES. Despite the difficulties in
establishing integrated financing and delivery systems, a substantial number of demonstration projects and other initiatives are under way to test

various approaches. The best known of these demonstrations are the Social Health Maintenance Organizations (Social HMOs), On Lok and its Program of All-Inclusive Care for the Elderly (PACE) replications, and the Arizona Long-Term Care System (ALTCS).[67] Although not directly involved in long-term care, conventional HMOs participating in the Medicare program are required to provide the full range of benefits, including home health and skilled nursing facility services. State-initiated efforts are also under way or under development in Wisconsin, Colorado, Texas, Minnesota, New York, Maine, and Florida. The six New England states have worked together to develop proposals within a common framework.

Social HMOs extend the traditional HMO concept by adding a modest amount of long-term care benefits.[68] Social HMOs are intended to serve a cross-section of the elderly population, including both functionally impaired and unimpaired persons. In fact, the overwhelming majority of enrollees are not disabled. While all enrollees are Medicare eligible, relatively few Medicaid beneficiaries are members. Enrollees generally pay premiums to cover the extra benefits. Although Social HMOs were originally a four-site initiative, Congress has authorized a second generation of demonstrations.

In 1983 On Lok Senior Health Services obtained federal waivers allowing it to receive monthly capitation payments from Medicare, Medicaid, and (in a few cases) individuals to provide a comprehensive range of acute and long-term care services.[69] In a broad test of this approach, PACE is replicating the On Lok model at eight sites throughout the country.[70] Enrollment is limited to persons who are so disabled that they meet nursing home admission criteria. Because expenditures per person are so high, very few persons can afford to pay an actuarially fair insurance premium out-of-pocket. As a result, almost all enrollees are Medicaid eligible, with the program financing the long-term care benefits. PACE sites operate as geriatrics-oriented, staff-model HMOs, that is, the primary-care physicians are employees of the organization. Finally, the approach makes heavy use of adult day health care, which is integrated with the provision of primary care. Some states, such as Wisconsin, are experimenting with variants of the PACE model.[71]

The Arizona Health Care Cost Containment system (AHCCCS) is a statewide demonstration project that finances medical services for the Medicaid-eligible population through prepaid, capitated contracts with providers. Beginning in 1989 the ALTCS program incorporated Medicaid long-term care services into the AHCCCS demonstration.[72] Participation in the program is limited to individuals who are certified to be at high risk of institutionalization. ALTCS covers acute care services as well as care in nursing facilities, ICF/MRs, and home- and community-based services. Under the ALTCS model, the state contracts with one entity in each county to assume responsibility for covered services to elderly and physically disabled eligibles. In the overwhelming majority of cases, the contractor for elderly people and persons with physical disabilities is the county government.

POTENTIAL FOR COST SAVINGS. As with more traditional acute care services, it appears that capitation can reduce expenditures. Evidence concerning Social HMOs and On Lok/PACE show that acute care utilization can be lowered in capitated care settings, but it is less clear that integrating acute and long-term care services generates additional savings.[73] Social HMOs did not appear to do substantially better than conventional HMOs in reducing acute care expenditures. The early evidence from On Lok/PACE is more encouraging, but the data are very preliminary, do not adjust for case mix, and involve a relatively small sample. A limitation of the PACE model is that demonstration sites tend to be very small, enrolling an average of only about 200 persons per site.

In an evaluation of the ALTCS, Laguna Research Associates compared the total costs of ALTCS with an estimate of what a traditional Medicaid program in Arizona would cost.[74] Evaluating the cost-effectiveness of the Arizona program was extremely difficult because the state has never had a conventional Medicaid program. As a result, evaluators were forced to develop a synthetic estimate of what the costs of a traditional Medicaid program in Arizona would have been had it had one. Unfortunately, the states used to develop the synthetic estimate were largely determined by data availability rather than whether states were comparable to Arizona in ethnicity, style of care, and other factors.

According to the evaluation, the ALTCS program appears to save money, largely because of how it provides services to the MR/DD population.[75] For fiscal year 1993 Laguna Research Associates estimated that service costs for the elderly population were 18 percent less for ALTCS than they would be under a conventional Medicaid program. Unlike many other Medicaid programs, the program appears to successfully limit services to persons at high risk of institutionalization.[76] However, because of the weakness of the research design, these results must be viewed with caution. In addition, ALTCS's higher administrative costs offset a significant portion of the overall savings.

EXPAND HOME- AND COMMUNITY-BASED SERVICES. The most persistent dream in long-term care is that the expansion of home- and community-based services could reduce overall long-term care expenditures. The fundamental hope has been that lower-cost home care could replace more expensive nursing home care. However, there is a substantial body of rigorous research to suggest that expanding home care is more likely to increase rather than decrease total long-term care costs.[77] This occurs because large increases in home care usage more than offset relatively small reductions in nursing home usage. To improve cost-effectiveness, many states, including Washington and Wisconsin, have tried to better target resources to persons at a higher risk of institutionalization.

A problem with expanding home- and community-based care as a savings strategy is that noninstitutional services may not be cost-effective for this population. Home care for persons who require nursing home–level care and who do not have extensive family support is expensive. In an analysis of Connecticut's Medicaid home- and community-based waiver program, Liu and his co-authors found that a substantial number of persons who met the eligibility criteria of being at high risk of institutionalization were prevented from receiving home care services because their care plan was too expensive.[78] These persons tended to be substantially more disabled and to have far less informal support—strong indicators of being at high risk of institutionalization—than persons who were allowed to participate in the program.

To some extent, ending the entitlement to home care and nursing home care as envisioned under the Medigrant plan could solve this cost problem by allowing states to predetermine how much money they will spend for institutional and noninstitutional services. To the extent that home care has been funded through nonentitlement programs rather than Medicaid, this limitation already exists for noninstitutional services (but not for institutional care). At the May 1996 conference, one official noted that in Wisconsin there is a substantial waiting list for home- and community-based services, but not for nursing home care. Some states, such as Wisconsin and Washington, have a conscious policy of limiting growth in nursing home supply while increasing home care services.[79] Indeed, according to one official at the May 1996 conference, Washington has incentives for nursing homes to close beds, a process that has been dubbed bed banking. Despite a growing elderly population, Washington is planning to reduce its supply of nursing home beds in nominal terms.

Recognizing that there are certain economies of scale in residential settings that are lacking in traditional home care, where services must be provided to one person at a time, Oregon (and, to a lesser extent, some other states, such as Washington) has developed nonmedical residential alternatives to nursing homes.[80] By aggressively expanding assisted living and adult foster care, Oregon hopes to promote residential settings that are more homelike, provide greater personal autonomy, and cost less.[81] In particular, the state has concentrated on older persons with Alzheimer's disease, who need a lot of supervision but not a great deal of medical care.

Although highly innovative, this approach has been very controversial. For example, the nursing home industry has charged that these alternative residential settings are just substandard nursing homes, and there have been some recent reports of quality-of-care problems.[82] For some residents, Stark and her coauthors found, going to an adult foster home in Oregon was associated with less improvement and more decline in physical functioning than going to a nursing home.[83]

Not much systematic research has been done on the effectiveness of these newer state strategies. Table 6-5 presents the percent increase in Medicaid long-term care expenditures for the elderly from 1988 to 1994 for the United States as a whole and for Oregon, Washington, and Wisconsin— states that have been active in reorganizing the long-term care delivery system.[84] Over that time period, both Oregon and Washington had rates of increase in Medicaid long-term care expenditures that were substantially greater than for the United States as a whole. Wisconsin had a far lower rate of increase, but much of its home- and community-based services is financed outside of the Medicaid program. Rather than reducing total long-term care spending, these states have used more dollars to serve more people.

Table 6-5. *Percent Increase in Medicaid Long-Term Expenditures, United States, Oregon, Washington, and Wisconsin, 1988–94*

Location	Total increase
United States	92
Oregon	116
Washington	110
Wisconsin	76

Source: Author's calculations based on: David Liska and others, *Medicaid Expenditures and Beneficiaries: National and State Profiles and Trends, 1988–1994,* 2d ed. (Washington, D.C.: Kaiser Commission on the Future of Medicaid, 1996), p. 112.

For persons with mental illness and MR/DD, there is some reason to believe that moving residents out of mental hospitals and ICF/MRs and into community-based services might save money. According to one New York official, "If you looked at the MR/DD population, well over 30,000 people were in large developmental centers. That's down to date to only 4,000. So this has been very successful in moving these people out of these large facilities, closing these large facilities, and moving them into the community. . .just a few years ago, we were anticipating that we were going to be setting up small residential settings of four, five, and six people. Now what's happened is that more and more people that are coming under the rules are living at home."[85] ICF/MRs are extremely expensive because of extensive regulatory requirements, antiquated physical plants, relatively highly paid staff (many of whom are state employees), and preferential reimbursement rates for state-run facilities. Average per person costs of home- and community-based waivers for this population are about half that for ICF/MRs.[86] However, the persons remaining in institutions are more severely disabled and may be very costly to serve in the community.[87] Moreover, to the extent that institutions lose residents but do not close, their fixed costs must be spread over a smaller number of residents.

Traditional Cuts in Eligibility, Reimbursement, Services, and Quality

If states do not succeed in substantially reducing the rate of increase in long-term care expenditures through increasing private resources or through delivery system reform, there are still a large number of more conventional mechanisms that can be used—especially if states are given more flexibility. More specifically, possible cuts include imposing family responsibility, reducing the amount of income and assets that the community-based spouses of institutionalized residents may retain, raising the level of disability needed for nursing home care, cutting nursing home and home care reimbursement rates, imposing moratoriums on new construction of nursing homes, curtailing coverage of home care services, and reducing nursing home quality standards. States already have considerable flexibility in several of these areas, and all of the major Medicaid reform proposals further increase their freedom of action. While these changes would almost certainly reduce Medicaid expenditures, they are not reforms of the system and would be painful to both beneficiaries and providers.

Distribution of Funds

Medicaid reform proposals are ultimately about money—how much does each state and each eligibility group and service within each state receive? All of the Medicaid proposals under consideration during 1995, 1996, and 1997 would have significantly changed the current dynamics of allocation across the states and within the program.

Allocation across States

Conflicts over allocations among states are inevitable when an open-ended matching grant program such as Medicaid is proposed to be converted into a block grant or per capita caps instituted.[88] Under an open-ended matching formula, the federal government simply pays a fixed percentage of the allowable costs incurred by states. The amount each state receives is determined by its own actions and is unaffected by the amounts received by other states or by any federal budget limit. As with the Medicaid program as a whole, states with high average incomes tend to have far more generous benefits and higher use than lower-income states and, therefore, higher expenditures. For example, in 1994 average annual long-term care expenditures for the elderly per resident age sixty-five and older was $2,412 in New York and $1,595 in Connecticut, but only $620 in Alabama and $623 in Mississippi.[89] Even after adjusting for differing match rates, federal Medicaid expenditures per elderly resident in Alabama and Mississippi were about three-fifths that of Connecticut and about one-third that of New York.[90] Low-income states could increase the size of their federal grants by spending more of their own money, but most choose not to. In fact, because of high federal matching rates, low-income states have to spend far less of their own funds per poor resident than rich states do to obtain the same amount of federal money.

Reformed allocation systems, be they block grants or per capita caps, could create significant inequities if they are based on historical spending patterns. They could lock in place much lower levels of spending in low-benefit states, while leaving high-benefit states with comparatively generous spending. Under block grants or per capita caps, funding levels and allocations that are not adjusted to reflect state differentials in the growth of the population in need and disparities in spending per recipient will disproportionately hurt states with low benefits and rapidly expanding populations in need.

The Medigrant proposal attempted to address this problem somewhat by adopting an allocation formula that included the number of state residents in poverty, an enrollment mix factor that included the state's caseload distribution (that its, proportion of children, elderly, persons with disabilities, and so forth), the state's expected spending on each group relative to the national average, and an index of input costs. States with high expenditures relative to need were given low growth rates. Political and policy considerations dictated that limits be placed on the amount of money that any state could gain or lose relative to its previous year's allocation. As a result, the amount of leveling that would have occurred across the states under the Medigrant program would have been modest.

Unfortunately, many of these adjustment factors are not particularly sensitive to long-term care needs. For example, nursing home use is very low until age seventy-five or eighty-five; thus allocations based on the population age sixty-five and older are not likely to mirror long-term care needs very closely. Moreover, although the institutionalized population tends to have lower incomes, the Current Population Survey and other surveys that measure poverty exclude this population from their sample. This is most important for the eighty-five and older population, nearly a quarter of whom are in nursing homes.[91] In addition, many persons receiving Medicaid long-term care services, especially in institutions, did not start off as poor but were impoverished by the high cost of care. Thus needs-based calculations using the poverty population in each state are likely to be inaccurate in regard to long-term care. Finally, even in generous states there is reason to question whether current funding is adequate to meet the long-term care needs of the elderly and disabled populations. Thus a high level of spending is not a sign of inefficiency or excessively generous benefits.

The indirect effect of this failure to make adequate adjustment for long-term care in the Medigrant plan was to disproportionately give low growth rates to states with high long-term care spending per capita. Eight of the top ten states in long-term care spending per elderly person would have received the lowest possible growth rate under the congressional formula of 2 percent a year.[92] Since a state would have received a low growth rate if its base is high, states spending high amounts on long-term care were likely to be worse off under the formula.

These adjustments only addressed how each year's funds would be allocated and did not affect the aggregate amount that would be distributed in any year. Under the plan, federal expenditures would have to increase by only an average of 4.8 percent a year.[93] This level was chosen largely to meet deficit reduction targets; the expected rate of increase in demand for long-term care and the projected cost increases in nursing home and home care did not appear to figure explicitly into the calculations. Given demographic changes and the underlying rate of increase in prices, this is a very low rate of increase. For example, the demand for nursing home care is projected to increase by about 1.9 percent a year between 1993 and 2018; the average cost of nursing home care increased approximately 7.6 percent a year between 1983 and 1993.[94]

President Clinton's proposal for limits on the growth in average per beneficiary expenditures was more favorable to long-term care but had its own problems. Under his plan, a state's allocation would be automatically adjusted for enrollment changes, whether caused by demographic trends, changed economic circumstances, or decisions by the state to expand or shrink eligibility. The per capita cap, however, locked into place the existing level of benefits and spending. If a state with a limited package of benefits decided to expand its package or reimburse its providers more generously, it would have had to pay for all of the marginal costs from state resources. In addition, the caps were calculated based on the average expenditures for the elderly and for the younger disabled populations. Since the per capita limit did not distinguish long-term care users, states' limits might be insufficient if they experience an increase in the proportion of long-term care users within the aged or disabled groups.[95] This approach may also give states an incentive to reduce the number of long-term care users, since they could substitute several lower-cost aged beneficiaries without long-term care use for one with long-term care needs and receive the same federal spending limit. States may also be discouraged from targeting home care services to persons at a high risk of institutionalization, since that would increase the average cost per person.

Allocation within Medicaid

The greater the cost pressures placed on the states and the greater the freedom the states have to design their own Medicaid programs, the more states will have to consciously choose how to allocate resources between acute and long-term care, institutional and noninstitutional services, public and private providers, and across eligibility groups (that is, families and children, people with disabilities, and the elderly). Under current law, many of these decisions have already been made by federal law and regulation. Governors and state legislators have little choice but to implement federal rules.

There are several reasons to expect that long-term care would do well in the competition for resources. Indeed, a persistent fear of advocates for children is that, in a zero-sum game, which is inevitable in a block grant, the elderly (and perhaps younger persons with disabilities) will succeed in protecting their services at the expense of younger people without disabilities. First, especially compared with unmarried women with children, the elderly are a politically favored group. It was media stories about the impact of the Medigrant proposal on long-term care, not on young welfare families, that made the congressional proposals politically unpopular. Indeed, given that programs that provide assistance to the poor are rarely favored, the role of Medicaid in financing long-term care for the middle class as well as for the low-income population should improve its ability to compete.[96]

Second, nursing homes and other long-term care providers have historically been extremely dependent on the Medicaid program, much more so than hospitals and physicians. As a result, long-term care providers have focused on Medicaid in a way that other providers have not. Nursing homes in particular are well situated to press their case to maintain their funds: they are well organized, contribute to the campaigns of state legislators, and are familiar to state bureaucrats.[97] In addition, in some states many long-term care providers are county-run. Thus a cut in reimbursement or coverage would be a cost shift to local government that would be strongly resisted.

Third, over the short to medium run, Medicaid long-term care expenditures, especially nursing home and other institutional spending, are relatively fixed by the number of beds in use. For obvious reasons it is practically and politically impossible to "kick little old ladies out of nursing homes." In contrast, eliminating eligibility for nondisabled adults only adds to the uninsured, who will probably continue to get some charity care from public hospitals and other providers. As one official at the May 1996 conference argued:

> What you're competing over is very different for the elders and disabled. My view is, we are mostly competing over services, whereas kids and young adults with children, you're competing over coverage. In other words, the dollar struggle is to offer more services to elderly and disabled, or to offer coverage to low-income families who wouldn't otherwise have coverage at

all. The consequences of that tradeoff are very different. You don't offer services to elderly or disabled. They die, or they end up on the streets, or they become county wards. You do not offer insurance to young families with children. They just get added to this amorphous 40 million Americans without health insurance that's now 40 million-and-one. Don't get me wrong. I care terribly much about those [people]. But our society seems perfectly comfortable allowing that 40 million number to increase every year.

Conclusions

While much of the debate over Medicaid reform has focused on low-income children and nondisabled adults, long-term care is a critical component of the Medicaid program, accounting for about one-third of expenditures. It is hard to change Medicaid without at least indirectly affecting older people and younger persons with disabilities. Moreover, long-term care providers are heavily dependent on Medicaid revenues.

In long-term care, as well as the rest of the Medicaid program, various reform proposals debated between 1995 and 1997 would have provided states with greater flexibility, ended the entitlement to services, reduced federal funding, and changed the system of allocation of federal funds. A strong argument can be made that states should have greater flexibility in organizing their long-term care delivery systems in order to provide more and more varied home- and community-based services. It is really the states and not the federal government that are deeply involved in the day-to-day running of long-term care programs. Moreover, to paraphrase Tip O'Neill, "all long-term care is local" and should reflect local values, needs, and lifestyles.

Nonetheless, the federal government clearly has a role to play, both in providing funding and in guaranteeing minimum standards. Despite protestations by the states that they have nothing but good in their hearts, it is hard to justify the repeal of national minimums regarding family responsibility, nursing home quality standards and enforcement, and spousal impoverishment, as was embodied in various versions of the Medigrant plan. There is little reason why these should vary across states. National standards regarding nursing home reimbursement were clearly not working as intended, but their repeal may open the way for inadequate reimbursement and quality problems in an industry that has been plagued by more than its share of substandard providers.

Given the desire to broaden the range of long-term care services and the potential for nearly unlimited demand for this aid, eliminating the entitlement to services makes much more sense in long-term care than it does in acute care. The key issue, however, is the level of funding. Almost by definition, spending in entitlement programs increases when the need for services rises. No such guarantee applies to block grants. The great fear of long-term care advocates is that, once the entitlement is eliminated, long-term care expenditures would not increase with need and the cost of services. Especially given the lack of attention to those issues in the construction of the Medigrant plan, this seems to be a valid concern—particularly in a political environment focused on deficit reduction and reducing government expenditures.

Because of the substantial flexibility that states already have in terms of coverage, reimbursement, and eligibility, there is little doubt that they could substantially lower long-term care spending if they were determined to do so—even under current law. However, while there are promising developments in the integration of acute and long-term care services and in creative home- and community-based services, there is little research at this time to support the claim that massive savings are possible. While it is conceivable that major changes in the structure of the Medicaid program could dramatically alter the Medicaid-provider dynamics so as to generate significant savings, the burden of proof rests on the shoulders of advocates of greater state flexibility and reduced funding to demonstrate why this would be true.

The hard reality is that the current method of Medicaid long-term care financing is actually a pretty economical system. Payment rates are much lower than Medicare and the private sector. Individuals receive government help only after using up almost all of their assets, and they must contribute virtually all of their income toward the cost of care. Medicaid pays only the costs that the institutionalized population cannot. Finally, the institutional bias of the delivery system limits services largely to persons with the most severe disabilities who do not have family supports. Within this system, it is hard to obtain large additional savings.

Finally, converting the open-ended financing system of Medicaid to a block grant or imposing per capita caps creates substantial problems of equity across states. Under the current system, states that want to spend more can do so without adversely affecting other states. This is reflected in the current wide variation across the states in Medicaid long-term care spending per capita. With either a block grant or per capita caps, there is a substantial danger that historical patterns of spending will be permanently in-stitutionalized. In such a situation, the low-benefit states will never be able to improve their long-term care systems. Formulas to mitigate these prob-lems for Medicaid as a whole have used general measures of poverty and population growth that are largely irrelevant to long-term care. Moreover, even in the most generous states, current Medicaid spending may not be adequate to meet the long-term care needs of the current elderly and younger population with disabilities. Thus efforts to move generous states more to-ward the average is probably inappropriate.

Notes

1. Definitions of long-term care vary. For this paper, long-term care includes nursing facilities, intermediate care facilities for the mentally retarded (ICF/MRs), mental hos-pitals, and home- and community-based services.

2. John Holahan and David Liska, "Where Is Medicaid Spending Headed?" (Wash-ington: Kaiser Commission on the Future of Medicaid, December 1996), p. 2.

3. David Liska, Karen Obermaier Marlo, Anuj Shah, and Alina Salganicoff, *Med-icaid Expenditures and Beneficiaries: National and State Profiles and Trends, 1988–1994*, 2d ed. (Washington: Kaiser Commission on the Future of Medicaid, November 1996), p. 49.

4. Office of the Assistant Secretary for Planning and Evaluation, Office of Dis-ability, Aging and Long-Term Care Policy, *Cost Estimates for the Long-Term Care Pro-visions of the Health Security Act* (U.S. Department of Health and Human Services, March 1994), pp. 5–6, tables 2–4.

5. Joshua M. Wiener, Laurel Hixon Illston, and Raymond J. Hanley, *Sharing the Burden: Strategies for Public and Private Long-Term Care Insurance* (Brookings, 1994), p. 10.

6. Robert Stevens and Rosemary Stevens, *Welfare Medicine in America: A Case Study of Medicaid* (Free Press, 1974), pp. 23–24, 28–32.

7. House Committee on Ways and Means, *Social Security Amendments of 1965*, Committee Print, 89 Cong. 1 sess. (Government Printing Office, March 29, 1965), p. 73.

8. American Health Care Association, *Facts and Trends: The Nursing Facility Sourcebook, 1996* (Washington, D.C., 1996), pp. 34–35.

9. Richard C. Ladd and others, *State LTC Profiles Report* (Minneapolis: Univer-sity of Minnesota, November 1995), p. 21.

10. Health Care Financing Administration, *Medicaid Services State by State* (Wash-ington: HCFA pub. no. 02155-96).

11. Except for Arizona, every state has at least one home- and community-based waiver program. Arizona's entire long-term care program is covered by a section 1115 research and demonstration waiver that has many of the same goals. See Health Care Financing Administration, "Medicaid Waivers," section B, no. 8 (http://www.hcfa.gov/medicaid/obs7.htm).

12. Health Care Financing Administration, *Medicaid: spDATA System, Characteristics of Medicaid State Programs, Part 1* (Washington: HCFA pub. no. 10130, 1993), pp. 322–28.

13. American Health Care Association, *Facts and Trends: The Nursing Facility Sourcebook, 1997* (Washington, D.C., 1997), p. 59.

14. Wiener, Illston, and Hanley, *Sharing the Burden*, p. 1.

15. Just over one-quarter of discharged and current residents who were eligible for Medicaid at some point began their nursing home stays as private-pay residents. Joshua M. Wiener, Catherine M. Sullivan, and Jason Skaggs, "Spending Down to Medicaid: New Data on the Role of Medicaid in Paying for Nursing Home Care," #9607 (Washington: American Association of Retired Persons, June 1996).

16. Under these so-called spousal impoverishment rules, in 1996 a spouse who remains in the community is allowed to keep income from his or her spouse of at least $1,254 (150 percent of the federal poverty level for an elderly couple) but no more than $1,919 a month (which may be increased if the spouse has excess shelter expenses for housing and utilities). States must also allow the noninstitutionalized spouse to keep half of the couple's combined assets totaling not more than $76,740 in 1996. Both income and assets figures are indexed to the consumer price index. See Brian Burwell and William H. Crown, "Medicaid Eligibility Policy and Asset Transfers: Does Any of This Make Sense?" *Generations*, vol. 20, no. 3 (Fall 1996), pp. 78–83.

17. Social Security Administration, "SSI Payment Amounts" (http//:www.ssa.gov/OACT/COLA/SSIamts.html/#Table, October 16, 1997).

18. Much of the very high rate of increase in the Medicaid program, especially during 1991 and 1992, was due to state manipulation of the disproportionate share hospital (DSH) provisions to maximize federal reimbursement. General Accounting Office, *Medicaid: Spending Pressures Drive States toward Program Reinvention*, GAO/HEHS-95-122 (April 1995).

19. Holahan and Liska, "Where Is Medicaid Spending Headed?" p. 11.

20. Allowable services would have included nursing facility services, ICF/MR services, mental hospital services, home- and community-based services (such as home health, nursing services, home health aide services, personal care, assistance with activities of daily living, chore services, day care services, respite care services, and training for family members), hospice, and case management.

21. Joshua M. Wiener, "Long-Term Care Reform: An International Perspective," in *Health Care Reform: The Will to Change*, Health Policy Studies, no. 8 (Paris: Organization for Economic Cooperation and Development, 1996), pp. 67–79.

22. Gary Burtless, R. Kent Weaver, and Joshua M. Wiener, "The Future of the Social Safety Net," in Robert D. Reischauer, ed., *Setting National Priorities: Budget Choices for the Next Century* (Brookings, 1997), p. 86.

23. Wiener, "Long-Term Care Reform," pp. 67–79.

24. Brian O. Burwell, "Shared Obligations: Public Policy Influences on Family Care for the Elderly," Medicaid Program Evaluation Working Paper 2.1 (Baltimore, Md.: HCFA, Office of Research and Demonstrations, May 1986), p. 99.

25. One study estimated that more than 27 million unpaid days of informal care are provided each week. See Korbin Liu and Kenneth G. Manton, "Disability and Long-Term Care," paper presented at the Methodologies of Forecasting Life and Active Life

Expectancy Workshop, sponsored by the National Institute on Aging, the American Council of Life Insurance, and the Health Insurance Association of America, Bethesda, Md., June 25–26, 1985, p. 14.

26. Raymond J. Hanley and others, "Predicting Elderly Nursing Home Admissions: Results from the 1982–1984 National Long-Term Care Survey," *Research on Aging,* vol. 12, no. 2 (June 1990), pp. 199–228.

27. Leonard I. Pearlin and others, "Caregiving and the Stress Process: An Overview of Concepts and Their Measures," *Gerontologist,* vol. 30 (October 1990), pp. 583–94; Bob G. Knight, Stephen M. Lutzky, and Felice Macofsky-Urban, "A Meta-Analytic Review of Interventions for Caregiver Distress: Recommendations for Further Research," *Gerontologist,* vol. 33 (April 1993), pp. 240–48; Ada C. Mui, "Caregiver Strain among Black and White Daughter Caregivers: A Role Theory Perspective," *Gerontologist,* vol. 32 (April 1992), pp. 203–12; Shirley J. Semple, "Conflict in Alzheimer's Caregiving Families: Its Dimensions and Consequences," *Gerontologist,* vol. 32 (October 1992), pp. 648–55; and Marilyn M. Skaff and Leonard I. Pearlin, "Caregiving: Role Engulfment and the Loss of Self," *Gerontologist,* vol. 32 (October 1992), pp. 656–64.

28. In 1983 HCFA estimated net savings of only $25 million per year for a national family responsibility initiative, projecting that 75 percent of the reductions in Medicaid expenditures would be offset by increased administrative costs. See Subcommittee on Human Services of the House Select Committee on Aging, *Medicaid and Family Responsibility: Who Pays?,* Committee Print, 98 Cong. 1 sess. (GPO, 1983), p. 4. These costs involve identification of responsible relatives, evaluation of their incomes, distribution of assessments to relatives, and enforcement of collections. Furthermore, compliance with a state's assessment cannot be assumed, especially if the relative lives in another state. Conceivably, states could lower their administrative costs by shifting the burden of collecting the funds to the nursing homes. However, if facilities were unsuccessful in obtaining the funds, then the Medicaid reimbursement level might be inadequate to provide reasonable quality care.

29. Burwell, "Shared Obligations," pp. 131–32.

30. The Boren amendment does not govern the contracting relationship between managed-care organizations and nursing homes and hospitals.

31. Charlene Harrington and others, "Nursing Home Litigation under the Boren Amendment: Case Studies" (San Francisco: University of California, Institute for Health and Aging, November 1993).

32. American Health Care Association, *Facts and Trends: The Nursing Facility, 1995* (Washington, 1995), p. 55. Since not all Medicaid providers participate in Medicare, and vice versa, these two figures are not the average of exactly the same facilities. In addition, more expensive hospital-based nursing facilities participate more actively in the Medicare program. Case mix differences between Medicare and Medicaid nursing home residents also account for some of the rate disparity. See Avi Dor, "The Costs of Medicare Patients in Nursing Homes in the United States," *Journal of Health Economics,* vol. 8 (1989), pp. 253–70.

33. In the 1980s private reimbursement rates tended to be 18 to 30 percent higher than Medicaid reimbursement rates. Author's estimates are based on the 1985 National Nursing Home Survey; Congressional Research Service, *Medicaid Source Book: Background Data and Analysis (A 1993 Update),* Committee Print, Subcommittee on Health

and Environment of the House Committee on Energy and Commerce, 103 Cong. 1 sess. (January 1993); Robert J. Buchanan, R. Peter Madel, and Dan Persons, "Medicaid Payment Policies for Nursing Home Care: A National Survey," *Health Care Financing Review*, vol. 13, no. 1 (Fall 1991); and Institute of Medicine, *Improving the Quality of Care in Nursing Homes* (Washington: National Academy Press, 1986).

34. John A. Nyman, "Excess Demand, the Percentage of Medicaid Patients, and the Quality of Nursing Home Care," *Journal of Human Resources*, vol. 23 (Winter 1988), pp. 76–92; John A. Nyman, "The Effect of Competition on Nursing Home Expenditures under Prospective Reimbursement," *Health Services Research*, vol. 23 (October 1988), pp. 555–74; John A. Nyman, Samuel Levey, and James E. Rohrer, "RUGS and Equity of Access to Nursing Home Care," *Medical Care*, vol. 25 (May 1987), pp. 363–74; Charlene Harrington and James H. Swan, "The Impact of State Medicaid Nursing Home Policies on Utilization and Expenditures," *Inquiry*, vol. 24 (Summer 1987), pp. 157–71; and William J. Scanlon, "A Theory of the Nursing Home Market," *Inquiry*, vol. 17 (Spring 1980), pp. 25–41.

35. Marylou Tousignant and Patricia Davis, "Nursing Homes in Area, Nationwide Plagued by Reports of Abuse," *Washington Post*, October 13, 1996, pp. B1, B6.

36. The level of detail also reflected Congress's mistrust of the Reagan administration in implementing these rules. In its effort to reduce federal burdens, the Reagan administration had singled out nursing home quality standards for deregulation.

37. State rules are often rigid and bureaucratic as well. According to one official from New York at the May 1996 conference, "We have lots of standards that exceed the federal requirements. They were prescriptive. They required a two-by-four for enforcement. We've had more two-by-fours than you can shake a stick at. And one of the things we're trying to do now is take a look and really try to refocus toward an outcome, and toward continuous improvement in quality without a two-by-four." Nelson S. Rockefeller Institute of Government and the Brookings Center for Public Management, "Devolution and Medicaid: A View from the States" (Washington: unpublished conference transcript, May 23–24, 1996), p. 234.

38. Institute of Medicine, *Improving the Quality of Care in Nursing Homes* (Washington: National Academy Press, 1986); and Joshua M. Wiener, "A Sociological Analysis of Government Regulation: The Case of Nursing Homes" (Cambridge, Mass.: Harvard University, Department of Sociology, 1981).

39. Catherine Hawes, "Assuring Nursing Home Quality: The History and Impact of Federal Standards in OBRA 1987" (New York: Commonwealth Fund, December 1996).

40. One official from New York noted that the state Medicaid program is being sued constantly by people who believe that they are entitled to home-care services or to more home care than they are receiving. "Devolution and Medicaid," p. 199.

41. Burtless, Weaver, and Wiener, "The Future of the Social Safety Net," p. 85.

42. Ibid., p. 105.

43. Pamela Walker and Julie Ann Racino, " 'Being with People': Support and Support Strategies," in Julie Ann Racino and others, eds., *Housing, Support, and Community: Choices and Strategies for Adults with Disabilities*, volume 2 (Baltimore, Md.: Paul H. Brookes Publishing Co., 1993), pp. 81–106.

44. Joshua M. Wiener and Laurel Hixon Illston, "Health Care Reform in the 1990s: Where Does Long-Term Care Fit in?" *Gerontologist*, vol. 34, no. 3 (June 1994), pp. 402–08.

45. Holahan and Liska, "Where Is Medicaid Spending Headed?" p. 6.

46. This section draws heavily from Joshua M. Wiener, "Can Medicaid Long-Term Care Expenditures for the Elderly be Reduced?" *Gerontologist*, vol. 36, no. 6 (December 1996), pp. 800–11.

47. About one-quarter of discharged Medicaid residents were admitted as private-pay residents, exhausted their savings, and then qualified for Medicaid during their course of stay. See Wiener, Sullivan, and Skaggs, "Spending Down to Medicaid," p. iii.

48. Author's calculation based on data in Susan Coronel and Diane Fulton, *Long-Term Care Insurance in 1993, Managed Care and Insurance Operations Report* (Washington: Health Insurance Association of America, March 1995).

49. Ibid.

50. Alice M. Rivlin and Joshua M. Wiener, with Raymond J. Hanley and Denise A. Spence, *Caring for the Disabled Elderly: Who Will Pay?* (Brookings, 1988), pp. 76–77; Robert B. Friedland, *Facing the Costs of Long-Term Care* (Washington: Employee Benefit Research Institute, 1990); Sheila Rafferty Zedlewski and Timothy D. McBride, "The Changing Profile of the Elderly: Effects on Future Long-Term Care Needs and Financing," *Milbank Quarterly*, vol. 70, no. 2 (1992), pp. 247–75; William H. Crown, John Capitman, Walter N. Leutz, "Economic Rationality, the Affordability of Private Long-Term Care Insurance and the Role for Public Policy," *Gerontologist*, vol. 32 (August 1992), pp. 478–85; Wiener, Illston, and Hanley, *Sharing the Burden*.

51. The Omnibus Budget Reconciliation Act of 1993 effectively limits the states that may try this initiative to the ones listed here.

52. Laguna Research Associates, "Partnership for Long-Term Care: National Evaluation Summary Statistics as of December 31, 1995" (San Francisco, May 1996), p. 4.

53. Wiener, Illston, and Hanley, *Sharing the Burden*.

54. Author's estimate based on Coronel and Fulton, *Long-Term Care Insurance in 1993*.

55. Brian Burwell and William H. Crown, "Medicaid Estate Planning: Case Studies of Four States," in Joshua M. Wiener, Steven B. Clauser, and David L. Kennell, eds., *Persons with Disabilities: Issues in Health Care Financing and Service Delivery* (Brookings, 1995), pp. 61–94; Jerry Gray, "Governors Seek to Shed Burdens of Medicaid," *New York Times,* August 4, 1992, p. A8; Julie Kosterlitz, "Middle Class Medicaid," *National Journal*, vol. 23, no. 45 (November 9, 1991), pp. 2728–32.

56. Marilyn Werber Serafini, "Plugging a Medicaid Drain," *National Journal*, vol. 27 (March 18, 1995), p. 687; Stephen A. Moses, "The Magic Bullet: How to Pay for Universal Long-Term Care, A Case Study in Illinois" (Seattle: LTC, Inc., February 1995); Moses, "The Florida Fulcrum: A Cost Savings Strategy to Pay for Long-Term Care" (Kirkland, Wash.: LTC, Inc., April 1994). Speaker Newt Gingrich alleged that transfer of assets by "millionaires" to gain Medicaid eligibility is a "very common problem." See Susan Schmidt and Spencer Rich, "Democrats to Counter GOP Medicare Cuts without New Patient Costs," *Washington Post*, October 2, 1995, p. A7. Cantwell estimated that as much as $5 billion a year—roughly 20 percent of Medicaid nursing home expenditure—could be saved by reducing the incidence of Medicaid estate planning. See James R. Cantwell, "Solutions to the Medicaid Funding Problem" (Dallas: National Center for Policy Analysis, July 1995), p. 10.

57. General Accounting Office, *Medicaid Estate Planning*, GAO/HRD-93-29R, (July 20, 1993).

58. Wiener, Hanley, and Harris found that about two-thirds of the disabled elderly who were admitted to nursing homes from 1982 to 1984 had incomes below 150 percent of the federal poverty line in 1982; about one-third had incomes below the poverty level. Joshua M. Wiener, Raymond J. Hanley, and Katherine M. Harris, "The Economic Status of Elderly Nursing Home Users" (Brookings, 1994).

59. Author's calculations based on Health Care Financing Administration, *Medicare and Medicaid Statistical Supplement, 1996, Health Care Financing Review,* p. 404; and Barbara Bedney and others, "1994 State Data Book on Long-Term Care Program and Market Characteristics" (San Francisco: University of California, October 1995), pp. 1–2.

60. Charles P. Sabatino and Erica Wood, *Medicaid Estate Recovery: A Survey of State Programs and Practices,* Public Policy Institute no. 9615 (Washington: American Association for Retired Persons, September 1996), p. iv.

61. In an analysis of the 1982-84 National Long-Term Care Survey, Wiener, Hanley, and Harris found that 55 percent of disabled elderly persons entering nursing homes owned a home, a percentage that is well below the 75 percent of all elderly who are homeowners, but is still substantial. (See Wiener, Hanley and Harris, "The Economic Status of Elderly Nursing Home Users.") However, the proportion of deceased Medicaid nursing home residents who own houses is probably much smaller, in part because an unknown proportion sell their homes in order to help pay for their nursing home care. Sheiner and Weil found that only 42 percent of all elderly households will leave behind a house when the last member dies. See Louise Sheiner and David N. Weil, "The Housing Wealth of the Aged," Working Paper 4115 (Cambridge, Mass.: National Bureau of Economic Research, July 1992), p. 13.

62. General Accounting Office, *Medicaid: Recoveries from Nursing Home Residents' Estates Could Offset Program Costs,* GAO/HRD-89-56 (March 1989).

63. Most of Oregon's long-term care expenditures are not for nursing homes. Calculated as a percentage of total long-term care expenses, Oregon's estate recovery rate falls to 1.4 percent. Author's calculations based on data from Sabatino and Wood, *Medicaid Estate Recovery,* p. 41; and David Liska, Karen Obermaier Marlo, Anuj Shah, and Alina Salganicoff, *Medicaid Expenditures and Beneficiaries: National and State Profiles and Trends, 1988–1994,* 2d ed. (Washington: Kaiser Commission on the Future of Medicaid, 1996), p. 48.

64. To counter fragmentation within long-term care, several states are considering a reorganization of their programs' administration with an eye toward consolidation of responsibilities. According to several officials at the May 1966 conference, Wisconsin and New York are considering such an initiative. Oregon, New Jersey, and Washington State have already consolidated responsibility in a single agency.

65. Michael Finch and others, "Design of the Second Generation S/HMO Demonstration: An Analysis of Multiple Incentives" (Minneapolis: Institute for Health Services Research, 1992).

66. Charlene Harrington and Robert J. Newcomer, "Social Health Maintenance Organizations' Service Use and Costs, 1985–1989," *Health Care Financing Review,* vol. 12 (Spring 1991), pp. 37–52.

67. Several other initiatives either seek to enroll Medicaid eligibles with disabilities in HMOs for their acute care services or for both their acute and long-term care services. See Joshua M. Wiener and Jason Skaggs, "Current Approaches to Integrating Acute and Long-Term Care Financing and Services," Public Policy Institute #9516, (Washington: American Association of Retired Persons, December 1995).

68. Walter N. Leutz, Merwyn R. Greenlick, and John A. Capitman, "Integrating Acute and Long-Term Care," *Health Affairs*, vol. 13, no. 4 (Fall 1994), pp. 58–74. See also Harrington and others, "Nursing Home Litigation under the Boren Amendment"; Rivlin and others, *Caring for the Disabled Elderly*, p. 18; Walter N. Leutz and others, *Changing Health Care for an Aging Society: Planning for the Social Health Maintenance Organization,* (Lexington, Mass.: Lexington/Heath, Inc., 1985).

69. Marie-Louise Ansak, "The On Lok Model: Consolidating Care and Financing," *Generations,* vol. 14, no. 2 (Spring 1990), pp. 73–74; Rick T. Zawadski and Catherine Eng, "Case Management in Capitated Long-Term Care," *Health Care Financing Review Annual Supplement* (1988), pp. 75–81.

70. Robert L. Kane, Laurel Hixon Illston, and Nancy Miller, "Qualitative Analysis of the Program of All-Inclusive Care for the Elderly (PACE)," *Gerontologist,* vol. 32, no. 6 (December 1996), pp. 771–80; and K. Irvin and others, "Managed Care for the Elderly: A Profile of Current Initiatives" (Portland, Maine: National Academy for State Health Policy, November 1993), p. 22.

71. At the May 1996 conference a Wisconsin official related that two projects are being tried, one for the elderly and the other for younger persons with disabilities. These models incorporate most elements of the PACE model, with the exception that day center attendance will not be required and enrollees will not have to change physicians. Nurse practitioners will attempt to fill the gap created by these two variances in the original model. "Devolution and Medicaid," p. 176.

72. F. Northrup, "Arizona's Integrated Acute and LTC Program," *LTC News & Comment,* vol. 4, no. 11 (July 1994), p. 5; N. McCall, J. Korb, and E. Bauer, "Evaluation of Arizona's Health Care Cost Containment System Demonstration—Third Outcome Report" (San Francisco: Laguna Research Associates, January 1994); N. McCall and others, "Evaluation of Arizona's Health Care Cost Containment System Demonstration—Second Outcome Report" (San Francisco: Laguna Research Associates, April 1993); Irvin, Riley, Booth, and Fuller, "Managed Care for the Elderly," p. 28.

73. On Lok, Inc., "PACE Fact Book: Information about the Program of All-Inclusive Care for the Elderly" (San Francisco, 1995) and "PACE: Who Is Served and What Services Are Used? PACE Progress Report on the Replication of the On Lok Model" (San Francisco, 1993).

74. McCall and others, "Evaluations of Arizona's Health Care Cost Containment System Demonstration—Second Outcome Report."

75. Ibid.

76. William Weissert, "Effectiveness of the Preadmission Screening Instrument and Level of Care Determination," in N. McCall and others, "Evaluation of the Arizona Health Care Cost Containment System Demonstration: Second Implementation and Operation Report" (San Francisco: Laguna Research Associates, April 1992).

77. Joshua M. Wiener and Raymond J. Hanley, "Caring for the Disabled Elderly: There's No Place Like Home," in Stephen M. Shortell and Uwe E. Reinhardt, *Improving*

Health Policy and Management: Nine Critical Research Issues for the 1990s (Ann Arbor, Mich.: Health Administration Press, 1992), pp. 75–110; William G. Weissert, Cynthia Matthews Cready, and James E. Pawelak, "The Past and Future of Home and Community-Based Long-Term Care," *Milbank Quarterly,* vol. 66, no. 2 (1988), pp. 309–88; Rosalie A. Kane and Robert L. Kane, *Long-Term Care: Principles, Programs and Policies* (New York: Springer Publishing Company, Inc., 1987); Peter Kemper, Robert Applebaum, and Margaret Harrigan, "Community Care Demonstrations: What Have We Learned?" *Health Care Financing Review,* vol. 8, no. 4 (Summer 1987), pp. 87–100.

78. Korbin Liu, Jean Hanson, and Teresa Coughlin, "Characteristics and Outcomes of Persons Screened into Connecticut's 2176 Program," in Wiener, Clauser, and Kennell, eds., *Persons with Disabilities.*

79. General Accounting Office, *Medicaid Long-Term Care: Successful State Efforts to Expand Home Services While Limiting Costs,* GAO/HEHS-94-167 (August 1994); and Julie Fralich and others, "Reducing the Cost of Institutional Care: Downsizing, Diversion, Closing and Conversion of Nursing Homes" (Portland, Maine: University of Minnesota National Long-Term Care Resource Center and the National Academy for State Health Policy, February 1995).

80. Rosalie A. Kane and others, "Adult Foster Care for the Elderly in Oregon: A Mainstream Alternative to Nursing Homes?" *American Journal of Public Health,* vol. 81 (September 1991), pp. 1113–20.

81. The effort to increase client autonomy is a common theme among the states. For example, according to a Wisconsin official, "Our goal is to foster independence and quality of life by maximizing an individual's choice of services, providers and care settings, as long as such care and/or support is necessary, meets the adequate level of quality, is cost-effective, and is consistent with the individual's values. . . . The goal of this effort is to look at what is the most cost-effective for each person, and then allowing them a choice of where they would like to go." "Devolution and Medicaid," p. 180.

82. Personal communication with Steven Lutzky of The Lewin Group, Inc., December 28, 1995.

83. Alice J. Stark and others, "Effect on Physical Functioning of Care in Adult Foster Homes and Nursing Homes," *Gerontologist,* vol. 35, no. 5 (October 1995), pp. 648–55.

84. GAO, *Medicaid Long-Term Care;* and General Accounting Office, *Long-Term Care: Current Issues and Future Directions,* GAO/HEHS-95-109 (April 1995).

85. "Devolution and Medicaid," p. 219.

86. Gary A. Smith and Robert M. Gettings, "The Medicaid Home and Community-Based Waiver Program: Recent and Emerging Trends in Serving People with Developmental Disabilities" (Alexandria, Va.: National Association of State Directors of Developmental Disabilities Services, Inc., August 1996), p. 24.

87. K. C. Lakin and others, "Medicaid Institutional (ICF/MR) and Community Based Services for Persons with Mental Retardation and Related Services," report no. 35 (Minneapolis: University of Minnesota, Center on Residential Services and Community Living, 1991).

88. Burtless, Weaver, and Wiener, "The Future of the Social Safety Net."

89. Liska and others, *Medicaid Expenditures and Beneficiaries,* p. 64.

90. Federal spending per elderly resident in 1994 was $1,206 in New York, $796 in

Connecticut, $442 in Alabama, and $491 in Mississippi. Author's calculation based on Liska and others, *Medicaid Expenditures and Beneficiaries*, pp. 41, 64.

91. Harriet L. Komisar, Jeanne M. Lambrew, and Judith Feder, *Chart Book: Long-Term Care for the Elderly* (New York: Commonwealth Fund, December 1996), p. 11.

92. Judith Feder, Jeanne Lambrew, and Michelle Huckaby, *Medicaid and Long-Term Care for the Elderly: Implications of Restructuring* (New York: Commonwealth Fund, December 1996), p. 13.

93. John Holahan and David Liska, "The Impact of the 'Medigrant' Plan on Federal Payments to States" (Washington: Kaiser Commission on the Future of Medicaid, 1995), p.1.

94. Wiener, Illston, and Hanley, *Sharing the Burden*, pp. 138–39; and Health Care Financing Administration (Baltimore, Md.: Office of National Health Statistics, unpublished estimates, 1996).

95. Feder, Lambrew, and Huckaby, *Medicaid and Long-Term Care for the Elderly*.

96. A recent assessment of population groups' relative influence demonstrated that advantage by quoting a state legislator: "If we have $20 million and the choice is between spending it for senior citizens or poor kids, it no contest. The seniors get the money every time." See John D. Deardourff, "Guarantees for the Children," *Washington Post*, June 9, 1996, p. C7, cited in Feder, Lambrew, and Huckaby, *Medicaid and Long-Term Care for the Elderly*, p. 29.

97. In general, home- and community-based services are not as well situated to compete as are nursing homes. Faced with strict budget constraints, states may choose to reduce coverage for home- and community-based services, especially if they are not viewed as cost-effective substitutes for nursing home care. In the political process, home care agencies tend to be politically weak at the state level compared to other provider groups, such as hospitals, nursing homes, and physicians. Moreover, given limited funds, states may decide to allocate resources first to persons with the most severe disabilities without family supports. If they make that allocation decision, then funds will be primarily spent on nursing home care and only secondarily on home care, because the average nursing home resident is far more disabled and has fewer informal supports than the average home care user. If states choose to cut back on home care, then the long-term care delivery system will be even more oriented toward institutional care than it is now.

7

Who Gets What?
Devolution of Eligibility and Benefits in Medicaid

James R. Tallon Jr. and Lawrence D. Brown

Politics: Who Gets What, When, How?

—Harold Lasswell

TRYING TO make sense of Medicaid by working from basic definitions of mission and purpose invites frustration. The program is replete with paradox. It is a federal entitlement that gives states wide discretion on many substantive matters of policy; a poor people's program that covers little more than half of those whose incomes fall below 100 percent of the federal poverty level; a national commitment that intuitively evokes images of poor mothers and children as prime beneficiaries but spends more than 60 percent of its budget on long-term care for the elderly and disabled; a venture in welfare medicine,[1] whose benefit package equals or exceeds that found in many private health insurance plans.

This puzzling programmatic identity reflects Medicaid's unimmaculate conception. In 1965, amid intense political deliberations mainly focused on Medicare—a universal program, linked to Social Security, for those age sixty-five and older and the disabled—late-inning improvisations in the House Ways and Means Committee took up a federal-state model the American Medical Association and congressional conservatives had been promoting for Medicare and used it instead to create Medicaid. Charged with using combined federal and state general revenues to support medical coverage for public assistance recipients, the blind, the disabled, the indigent elderly, plus other groups that states might choose to add to the program (the medically needy), Medicaid has from its start been entangled in tough political issues that Medicare has largely been spared. Who is poor? Who among the poor merit medical benefits? Who beyond the welfare poor should be allowed to qualify? What services should the program's clients get and on what terms? And, not least important, how should the federal and state governments carve up authority for answering these and related questions?

Since Medicaid's inception a measure—and sometimes much more— of political turmoil has hung about it, a condition made chronic by three considerations. The first is philosophical. Medicaid, like the public assistance legislation onto which it was grafted, rests on the range of invidious moral distinctions about desert that Americans like to apply in public policies for the poor. Until the enactment of welfare reform legislation in 1996, those who qualified for welfare (mainly single, poor women who have children and therefore presumably cannot go to work and support the family) also got Medicaid coverage, though states varied widely in setting income thresholds for both programs. The blind, disabled, and indigent aged were deserving—and entitled—more or less by definition. This meticulous social construction of the charmed circle of the entitled naturally invited recurring liberal efforts to win entry for more of those who are "merely" poor and uninsured, as well as conservative challenges to the notion that any citizen deserves income (and perhaps medical) support as a matter of federally conferred right.

Between the mid-1980s and mid-1990s, political tugs-of-war produced shifting policy fortunes. On the one hand, in a series of amendments to Medicaid, Congress broke the link between welfare and welfare medicine by requiring states to offer Medicaid to pregnant women and children who simply met specified age and income criteria, and by permitting states to exceed coverage requirements for these groups while drawing federal matching funds—an invitation that thirty-three states and the District of Columbia had accepted by mid-1994.[2] On the other hand, the welfare reform act of 1996 ended the heretofore automatic connection between Medicaid and welfare eligibility, thereby requiring the (presumably shrinking) public assistance population to navigate its own way through Medicaid eligibility processes.

Required and optional expansions, which brought about 12 million new clients into Medicaid, raised the share of the poor covered by it to about 55 percent and reinforced the program's role as a bulwark of health coverage and care for children, who constitute about half of Medicaid's clients. One of every four American children, and one of every three infants, is covered by the program, which pays for 40 percent of U.S. births and insures fully 83 percent of poor pregnant women and infants and 87 percent of poor preschoolers.[3] This new enrollment arguably enhanced the program's internal equity by defining more needy citizens as deserving, but it also inflamed long-simmering arguments over external equity; that is, the fairness of programmatic distinctions among seemingly similarly situated people. About three-quarters of the uninsured are workers (and their dependents) who often earn low wages, contribute to the general revenues that sustain Medicaid, but enjoy no private or public health coverage whatsoever. The moral claims of universalism dominate the deliberations of most health policy analysts, but the antagonistic moral claims of particularism preoccupy the policy process, as the collapse of the Clinton health reform plan showed.

A second source of unrest in Medicaid is fiscal. On the one hand, federal-state sharing of expenses cushions both funding sources. On the other, it sprinkles the pain among fifty distinct nerve centers that become constituencies for cost control. Between the election of George Bush in 1988 and that of Bill Clinton in 1992, the federal government and most states suffered acute anxiety attacks over high yearly increases in Medicaid spending. In 1988 the federal and state governments spent $51 billion on the program and in 1992, $114 billion—an average annual increase of 21.8 percent. No wonder that in 1993 the National Association of State Budget Officers lamented that the growth of Medicaid spending had become the "single largest budget problem for states."[4]

Some of this fiscal stress derived from medical inflation, recession, and—the states' favorite culprit—federally mandated expansions in Medicaid coverage for poor women and children. A good bit, however, came from the states' creative exploitation of strategies that drew additional federal funds into their Medicaid programs. Many states grew increasingly adept at shifting state-funded maternal and child health and mental programs into Medicaid, transferring costs within and between levels of government, inventing provider taxes and donations with which to fund part of the state's Medicaid match, and attracting ever-larger amounts of federal monies earmarked for institutions facing the burdens of a "disproportionate share" of uncompensated care cases. States, in other words, were "certainly aware that Medicaid was a revenue source as well as an expenditure category"; indeed it was "a novel gold mine."[5] While Medicaid increased by about 22 percent annually between 1988 and 1992, disproportionate share hospital (DSH) payments jumped by 149.9 percent, from a mere $500 million to $17.5 billion. In 1995 DSH monies constituted 12.6 percent of Medicaid spending.[6]

When the figures are adjusted to account for these special programs and payments, the average annual growth in state Medicaid spending falls from 26.6 to 16.7 percent for the period 1990–92.[7] The importance of these strategic sources of budgetary stress appeared in the aftermath of the federal crackdown on them in and after 1991. The average annual growth of Medicaid spending fell to 9.5 percent between 1992 and 1995, and to 3.3 percent (doubtless unsustainably low) in 1996.[8] Medicaid's alleged budget-busting proclivities were nonetheless part of the conventional wisdom of health care policy in the early and mid-1990s, and seemed to validate the proposition that states needed new discretion to get a handle on the program.

Nor, of course, is the program's own spending the sole pertinent economic issue. Money spent on Medicaid obviously cannot go to other programs—like education, nutrition, law enforcement, housing, job training, and income support—that may significantly improve people's health. Some studies suggest that states pay for growth in Medicaid not by raising taxes but rather by cutting public assistance, education, and other social spending—a troubling finding on both efficiency and equity grounds.[9]

Third, as might be expected, the tortured interplay of ethics and economics generates significant political distress. Heavy preordained consumption of state revenues by Medicaid put reform of the program high on state policy agendas in the late 1980s, whether governors and legislators wanted it there or not. Spending so much more so quickly on one set of services for one subset of the poor was politically unsettling, especially because much of the money paid nursing homes to care for the impoverished elderly while the younger poor had readier access to emergency rooms than to preventive and primary care. That some got so much while others (specifically, lower-income uninsured workers) got nothing inspired political efforts to expand coverage while slowing the rise of costs. Innovations ranged from modest public subsidies for employers who bought insurance for workers, to public underwriting of coverage for uninsured children, to Oregon's ambitious plan to trim marginal Medicaid benefits while bringing all Oregonians under the poverty line into the newly prioritized program. Meanwhile, political tempests stretched well beyond the health arena as advocates for education, corrections, and other prominent programs camped in executive and legislative lobbies, demanding to learn why their critically important public priorities must again yield to the Medicaid entitlement.

State leaders coped as best they could, but also carped repeatedly that many of their problems originated in Washington, D.C. The federal government, so the argument ran, set minimum definitions of eligibility and did not hesitate to add new required groups—and costs—when it saw fit. It told states what basic benefits Medicaid must cover. It regulated delivery systems—for instance, Medicaid clients were to have free choice of providers. It limited state discretion and invited litigation over setting payment rates—by requiring, for example, that hospitals and community clinics be paid the reasonable cost of their services. It constrained their creativity in raising funds for the state match by, for instance, objecting when states imposed on providers taxes that were pooled with state dollars to draw down federal monies that were then returned (in part) to providers by means of higher payments. Skeptics countered that these various constraints could not be all that constricting: the states, after all, varied widely in standards of eligibility and services covered. California, for example, covers nearly twice as many Medicaid clients as does New York State while spending half as much.[10] Indeed, 60 percent of Medicaid spending goes for populations and services "offered at state option and not required by federal law or regulation."[11] State policymakers, however, were understandably less impressed by the bigger picture than by the immediate pressures they faced.

Obliged by the force of circumstances to innovate, states repeatedly bumped into federal rules and sought waivers that would allow them to proceed. The arbiter, the federal Health Care Financing Administration (HCFA), tried to protect itself from charges on the left that it was sacrificing the interests of the poor and from the right that it was squandering the federal treasury. As a result, the waiver process sometimes grew protracted, antagonistic, and laden with the red tape that generally accompanies official determination to leave no flank uncovered. Given that the federal government had hamstrung state reform initiatives in other major ways, too—most notably by provisions of the Employee Retirement and Income Security Act (ERISA) of 1974, which preempted state regulation of the contents of employer and union benefit plans and therefore stymied state legislation to cross-subsidize across broad population pools—it seemed clear that the logical solution to Medicaid's problems, affordable universal coverage, must come from Washington. National leaders refused to follow the script, however. When the Clinton reform plan collapsed and no alternative to it commanded much consensus, the sole sensible Plan B for fixing Medicaid appeared to be devolution—give each state a pot of money (perhaps capped, perhaps not) for the program, loosen or eliminate federal strings attached to its use, and let the states redesign public medical insurance coverage—including eligibility standards and benefits—for needy groups as they prefer.

Devolution's Evolution

Devolution flashes and fades in the federalist firmament. There is nothing strange about this. Unlike Medicare, Medicaid embraced devolution as a central tenet and structural principle from the start. A program designed to balance national and state policy goals in caring for the poor naturally invites conflict over how power is divided and deployed by and between the intergovernmental partners. And of course the higher and faster-growing the program's spending, the more intense these conflicts become.

Medicaid was viewed as a policy headache as early as the Nixon administration, whose domestic policy planners worried over where to put it in the principled division of labor between the central and state governments they labored to define.[12] But even if Medicaid survived as a distinct entity in the reconnections among income and medical assistance programs the administration contemplated, its redistributive character made it a poor candidate for the block grants proposed in such policy spheres as employment training and community development.[13]

No such theoretical subtleties troubled the Reagan administration, which hoped both to reduce Medicaid's rate of spending growth and to free state hands in running it. Budget savings had priority over devolution, however. Having flirted unsuccessfully with designs for a grand federal-state swap—in which the federal government would assume responsibilities for the acute care portions of Medicaid and the states would take over long-term care, AFDC, and food stamps—the administration sought and won temporary annual reductions in the rate that set federal matching Medicaid payments.

In the early 1980s Congress began to accept incremental, *de facto* devolution in many nooks and crannies of the program. The Omnibus Budget Reconciliation Act of 1981, for example, let states apply for permission to waive federal rules requiring that Medicaid clients have free choice of provider, which inhibited state plans to experiment with managed care. As the decade proceeded, more states sought more waivers, leaving the devolution glass half-full, half-empty. The federal government was approving endless variations on programmatic themes, but reconciling the objectives pursued—slowing the growth of state Medicaid spending, protecting federal budget neutrality, protecting access and quality for Medicaid clients, and (in some states) extending coverage to some of the uninsured—would have confounded the wisdom of Solomon. As the federal government fiddled, the states burned, and even as waivers offered a measure of liberation from the federal blueprint, Congress mandated that states extend coverage to new clients.

Bill Clinton's arrival in the White House in January 1993 gave the nation its first interval of unified (Democratic) government since the Carter days of 1977-80. Although Clinton styled himself a "new" Democrat, pledged to "end welfare as we know it," the people's choice of Democratic leadership in both the executive branch and Congress seemed to signal stronger national—and therefore presumably federal—support for the poor in general and for their Medicaid entitlement in particular. Two years later, however, the political climate for devolution of Medicaid was the sunniest it had ever been. This about-face derived from several factors. As noted, the late 1980s and early 1990s saw both the expansion of coverage for mothers and children and a flowering of fiscal ingenuity as states combined DSH payments, provider taxes, and other revenue sources to draw new federal dollars. As the political economy of federal-state bargaining grew increasingly fractious and unmanageable, state leaders labored over larger and lesser reforms and learned firsthand about federal constraints. Among those schooled by hard knocks was Bill Clinton himself, who—as governor of Arkansas and chairman of the National Governors' Association (NGA)—resented federal micromanagement and articulated the case against it. With Clinton in the White House, state waiver requests were more readily granted, so the drift toward devolution—state by state, waiver by waiver—accelerated.

The collapse of Clinton's national health reform plan in 1994 ended hopes that the national government would fix the whole system anytime soon and incontestably put reform back in the hands of the states. The congressional elections of November 1994 gave conservative Republicans a majority in both houses of Congress. These electoral returns were widely read as a popular rebuff to big (especially national) government and an unmistakable sign of enthusiasm for both cutting federal spending and handing more social policy decisions to the states. By 1995 far-reaching devolution of Medicaid policy to the states seemed not merely possible but probable.

Devolution: Radical or Restrained

As the introduction to this volume points out, Medicaid devolution can span a continuum of options. What might be called radical devolution would repeal the current Medicaid program (Title 19 of the Social Security Act) and replace it with a block grant. It would end the federally decreed entitlement of those heretofore eligible for Medicaid, repeal all or most federal requirements now binding on the states, give each state a pot of money, and let states decide whom to cover, for what, and how. Restrained devolution, in contrast, would preserve the Medicaid program and entitlement to coverage; repeal many, but not all, federal rules for the states; and allow the states to proceed under what are in effect waivers writ large. Both strategies envision state efforts to rationalize Medicaid; that is, to repair it so as to extract from federal and state monies value that reflects the states', not the federal government's, images of sound public policy. The best way to judge the respective merits of the two versions is to envision the main forms that rationalization would be likely to take if states were magically transported into a political state of nature unmarked by federal rules and then see what, if anything, looks wrong with that picture.

Administrative Improvements

The least ambitious and intrusive approaches to reforming Medicaid modify how the program is managed. Under devolution, three such measures are likely to have special prominence. One seeks savings in redoubled assaults on fraud and abuse. Fear that "morally challenged" clients and greedy providers continually conspire to soak Medicaid evokes indignation and spotlights one of the few features of this complex program that the people and the press think they understand. Unanimous demand for savings from this source combined with uncertainty about the magnitude of the problem saddles Medicaid with a chronic deficit of public confidence. On the other hand, this synthesis of salience and speculation is a boon to public budgetmakers, who can always impute some extra millions of savings from fraud and abuse prevention when outlays need to be brought closer to revenues.

Second, as Frank Thompson and James Fossett suggest in this volume, states may try to fine-tune their managerial technologies and systems. Myriad options include reorganizing the agencies that run Medicaid; acquiring extensive and detailed data on client characteristics, use of services, payment patterns, and clinical outcomes; and upgrading computers and other equipment integral to the very model of a modern management information system (MIS).

Third, states may contend that better administration means more decentralization and devolve key decisions about Medicaid to their counties. The logic that lionizes public closeness to the people, not to mention the apparently growing political distaste for encoding protections for disadvantaged clients who have low status and little clout, supplies principled and pragmatic reasons why the states might pass the federal buck right along to grassroots governments. Because activities combating fraud and abuse now occupy distinct fiscal and administrative niches in Medicaid, devolution might not affect them directly. It is safe to say, however, that well-publicized assaults on malfeasance will continue to be politically prominent in state Medicaid programs, however much or little devolved. Devolution would more immediately change management prerogatives by empowering states to shift program resources toward (or away from) enhancements in managerial infrastructure and to think afresh for themselves about intergovernmental relations within their boundaries.

Redefined Eligibles

Under federal law, the national government specifies the populations that the states must enroll in Medicaid; namely those who meet (state-defined) standards for public assistance plus the blind, disabled, and indigent elderly. States also have the discretion to include additional medically needy clients for whom the federal government shares costs at whatever federal-state matching ratio pertains to the state in question.

By reforming national welfare law in 1996, without accompanying changes in Medicaid, the federal government complicated the states' choices about eligibility for medical assistance. The welfare reform measure ended the entitlement of the poor to public assistance benefits, leaving eligibility decisions to each state. The law also required, however, that states continue to award Medicaid coverage to those who met state standards for inclusion in AFDC as of July 1996. Although the law does not remove Medicaid coverage from those who no longer qualify for public assistance (now called temporary assistance for needy families, or TANF), the end of the automatic link between the latter and the former thrusts on the states a sizable "take-up" problem; namely, how to find non-TANF Medicaid eligibles (who by definition can no longer be tracked in welfare offices) and inform them about Medicaid enrollment. The law adds further complexities by giving states the option to confer Medicaid on legal immigrants who came to the United States before August 1996, while eliminating federal Medicaid funds for five years for legal immigrants who arrived after that date.[14] One likely result is a short-term "decline in Medicaid enrollment and a corresponding increase in the uninsured," whose costs have of course been covered partly by cross-subsidies from Medicaid monies.[15]

Devolution of Medicaid would presumably reopen state decisions on the aforementioned groups and break down federally prescribed coverage categories that are still intact. For example, under the Medicaid substitute before Congress in 1996, the phasing of poor children ages thirteen to eighteen into the program (now mandated by federal law) need not go forward; states could define disability to exclude people with AIDS, substance abusers, and the mentally ill; and Medicaid absorption of Medicare premiums for the indigent elderly would be optional.[16]

Revised Service Packages

Ceaseless innovation in medical technology constantly expands the list of candidates for inclusion in the pantheon of medically necessary procedures. On the other hand, research findings increasingly challenge the efficacy of established procedures for various populations under different conditions, often suggest service substitutions, and highlight services that can be reduced without evident clinical damage. An obvious case in point is the advances in clinical and organizational technologies that have shifted care from inpatient to outpatient settings. Likewise, if some health care, or care in community settings, appears to be as effective as but cheaper than nursing home care, state Medicaid programs may encourage the former by narrowing the criteria for payment for the latter.

Under devolution, states are also likely to refine a time-honored (but sometimes federally constrained) economizing technique; namely cuts in the units of services that Medicaid covers. Allowable days of hospitalization or the number of outpatient visits for mental health services, for example, may be cut—perhaps severely. Or by squeezing global payments to managed-care plans Medicaid budgetmakers may encourage (or compel) these plans to change their benefit packages explicitly (in the contract) or implicitly (in their delivery patterns).

Reduced Payments to Providers

Because states of late have tended to view cost containment as a top priority, they chafe under federal rules that inhibit their plans. Facing few federal constraints on payments to physicians, most states slashed and trimmed rates, watched physician participation decline, and consoled themselves that the institutional safety net—hospital emergency rooms and outpatient departments—was ready, willing, and able to serve Medicaid clients.[17] In a system that treats fee-for-service payments as a norm to be violated only after lengthy efforts to win a waiver, states have worried, however, that too much pressure on payments to hospitals could impair access. Moreover, the Boren amendment, which has obliged states to pay "reasonable" rates to hospitals, limits their fiscal flexibility. Court interpretations holding that managed-care plans lie outside that amendment's reach have added to the list of attractions of Medicaid managed care. With the repeal of the Boren amendment in 1997, states can experiment more freely with payment methods. As they amass data on who uses how much care at what cost, they may try to bargain rates down on the assumption that plans and providers who have entered the Medicaid market in force are unlikely to pull out and cede precious market share to competitors.

Reorganized Use of Services

Devolution will very likely accelerate the object of so many waiver exercises: enrollment of Medicaid clients in managed-care plans. Absent federal hoops intended to protect the disadvantaged, states will presumably implement mandatory enrollment of all or most Medicaid clients in managed care in short order. As traditional fee-for-service Medicaid seemed increasingly to offer diminishing access and quality at rising cost, the prospect that managed care could supply reasonable access to good care (including preventive and primary-care services) at more slowly rising costs grew more attractive. Changing the service mix by means of managed care, moreover, is the natural institutional vehicle for such related strategies as revised service packages and reduced payments to providers. In the states' eyes, managed care has come to constitute the answer to the problem of value for money in Medicaid: it is widely expected to deliver more bang for fewer bucks. Under devolution, states that have jumped on the managed-care bandwagon will push it farther and faster; those that have held back will probably hasten aboard.

Risks of Rationalization

The five strategies sketched here would probably form the heart of state Medicaid agendas if radical devolution were adopted, and they might produce a leaner, if somewhat meaner, program. None of them is a dramatic invention; all have been tried (though sometimes gingerly) in one or another state setting and all merely correct long-noticed problems with fee-for-service Medicaid—indeed, with fee-for-service medicine generally. None of these steps, however, is entirely free of risk, and the cumulative effect of their interactions invites justified anxiety about both the parts and their sum.

Savings annually imputed to attacks on fraud and abuse can create a public impression that Medicaid is a hopeless den of iniquity, and thereby encourage indiscriminate cutbacks and crackdowns on clients. Public relations and budget maneuvers aside, the administrative costs of detecting and deterring malfeasance may (depending on time, settings, and circumstances) exceed the costs of abuses.

In a devolved program, states will doubtless pay ardent lip service to the importance of reorganized agencies, better data, and the rest, but whether they will back rhetoric with action is questionable. As in fighting fraud and abuse, it takes money to make money, and whereas the budgetary costs of managerial improvements are plainly portrayed in the public record, the benefits realized cannot be easily isolated from other influences on the program or clearly attributed to the enhanced capacity and sagacity of the public sector. Budget savings from, say, a new MIS are not likely to make the six o'clock news, and other managerial innovations—for example, better identification and faster enrollment of eligibles—may raise costs. Staff downsizing and administrative "outsourcing" to cut bureaucratic ranks and costs could deplete the supply of state managerial skills even as the demand for them rises sharply under devolution. Better data and managerial systems are crucial to effective and fair discharge of state duties under devolution, but the constituency for them is not large or vocal. Likewise, shifting Medicaid decisions from the state level to counties will remove pressure from the states only to ignite controversy at a policymaking level that may be administratively and otherwise underdeveloped.

Removing federal rules that oblige states to cover specified groups in Medicaid could have at least three troubling consequences: States might drop coverage for those poor deemed least deserving—immigrants (legal and other) and repeat drug offenders, for instance—whose health needs and kindred vulnerabilities are substantial. Vanished federal regulation would, moreover, pit the "deserving" poor against powerful constituencies in such arenas as education and corrections, which have long deplored Medicaid's favored entitlement status and will eagerly display their political prowess on a newly leveled playing field. Finally, devolution would oblige remaining groups of Medicaid eligibles to compete with one another for the sums that are left once the program has been adjusted to conform with indigenous cultural and political preferences.

Redefinitions of service packages that favor primary-care providers and outpatient treatments over emergency room visits and hospital admissions make good theoretical sense, but in practice less is known about what is appropriate in concrete cases than is sometimes supposed. (Witness the federal commitment to—and slow and contentious evolution of—the development of medical practice guidelines for a handful of clinical conditions and the less-than-stunning returns on federally supported research on medical outcomes.) Analysts and advocates will not know whether Medicaid officials and health plans in a devolved regime define their package appropriately unless states (and plans) invest money and staff time in evaluating clients' access, satisfaction, and clinical outcomes. Such monitoring could fall by the wayside for several reasons: the federal government no longer requires such reporting and the states do not care enough about the answers to ask good questions; health plans demand relief from burdensome governmental red tape; state administrators do not recognize their information needs or cannot credibly sell the case for upgraded systems to political superiors. If states turn to managed-care plans in hopes of getting program responsibilities off public backs and into the private sector where they supposedly belong, they may not care to play backseat driver.

Substituting less costly for more costly services may promote efficiency but will not enhance quality too unless the social and personal circumstances of Medicaid clients fit the script. For instance, caring for the chronically disabled at home instead of in nursing homes presupposes that the clients in question have a home, that it is more or less safe and stable, and that family members or other caregivers are on hand to give care. These assumptions do not hold for some Medicaid clients, so advancing quality as well as efficiency requires careful planning and dialogue between state officials and health plans. Nor is it easy to judge *a priori* or in general whether constrictions in covered units of service enforce reasonable economies or serious hardship on such populations as the mentally ill and substance abusers. More may not be better, but less may not be enough. Will states take the trouble to gather and study sufficient information to make the distinctions within these complex populations that good care requires? If they do, will they marshal the political will to devise monitoring, regulatory, and incentive systems adequate to induce plans and providers to follow the evidence and arguments where they lead?

If the federal government simultaneously cuts the growth of Medicaid funds and removes restrictions on how states manage them, most states will be tempted to cut payments to providers. States negotiating mainly with managed-care plans may conclude that earlier payment levels, set generously high in order to entice plans into the then-suspect Medicaid market, should come down, and that few big participating plans will withdraw from that market and surrender thousands of members. The accuracy of such conjectures depends on a range of factors, including a plan's mix of commercial and public enrollees and the tolerance of plan management for protracted private bargaining and public conflict with state officials. In some states, a vibrant market handsomely populated with plans could dwindle in local settings into a handful of dominant players who estimate that state purchasers will not call their financial bluff lest Medicaid clients lose their medical home. What such bargaining games may do to entry and exit, continuity of enrollment and care, and the clinical value plan proponents believe they are able to offer for the money they get is anyone's guess. They could, however, wreak havoc on undercapitalized, provider-sponsored health plans that have traditionally served Medicaid clients, have little commercial penetration, depend on state Medicaid rates for survival, cannot credibly bluff and bargain, but are an important bulwark of choice for many Medicaid populations. Federal rules, though burdensome, impose some stability on health care markets, the dynamics of which may toss about vulnerable citizens who lack market power and savvy.

In well-run managed-care plans, reorganization of use patterns can secure access and quality while slowing the growth of costs. But as the ups and downs to date of Medicaid managed care in many states suggest, there is nothing automatic about the right number or the right kinds of plans. Moreover, states have so far adopted managed care mainly for AFDC-eligible Medicaid clients, notably poor mothers and children, who account for about 70 percent of the program's clients but only about 30 percent of its spending. If states want major savings from managed care they must negotiate coverage for the indigent elderly, the disabled, and other groups. Few managed-care plans have much experience yet with the complex (and hard-to-manage) interweaving of medical and behavioral conditions these groups present. The worlds of managed and long-term care have hardly begun to meet, and the prospects for harmony between them are largely speculative.

Furthermore, these "chronic" populations are better positioned politically than are mothers and children to voice their demands. The ripple effect in state political arenas no longer fenced in by federal directives could be troublesome. Incorporating these new clients into managed care may conflict with states' growing desire to ratchet payments to plans down to the levels that experience, data, and growing analytical sophistication suggest are reasonable reflections of the true cost of managing care in Medicaid. More heterogeneous clients complicate cost estimation, risk adjustment, negotiation, and rate setting. And mothers and children could find themselves losing a race to the bottom of the political priority list of Medicaid populations.

Safety net hospitals and clients that now serve sizable populations of Medicaid patients and the uninsured (subsidizing care of the latter, in part, with funds for the former) may also look askance at devolution. Earmarked federal DSH payments that now give these vulnerable institutions a measure of reliable relief would presumably disappear into larger pots. As states bargain hard with managed-care plans in the Medicaid market, the fiscal fate of these so-called essential community providers will depend on a combination of the plans' willingness to help keep them in business and the individual states' determination to require or pressure plans to do so.

Some may see in the portfolio of rationalizing strategies that states would most likely deploy in a devolved program the normal range of potential benefits and costs that public policy innovations generally present. If nothing is very new about the stakes of devolution, why not craft a block grant, turn states loose, and record what transpires in the federal system's famous laboratories of democracy?

This argument is not absurd and may end up carrying the day. But the critical counterpoints are equally, and maybe more, compelling. First, although individual items on the list of reform strategies might not hurt Medicaid clients, all-out implementation of the whole package might not be so benign. A quasi-block grant entrusting states with "complete flexibility in defining amount, duration, and scope of services . . . without any guarantee of how many services from what providers at what cost to beneficiaries," Karen Davis warns, is "a hollow promise of coverage."[18]

Second, state policymakers will be able to understand and modify adverse consequences of reform only if they invest significantly in MIS and evaluation systems that track the program, and then summon the political energy to act on this information. These low-visibility projects on behalf of a low-status population may slide far down state policy agendas.

Third, if states fail to monitor and repair the program, radical devolution will add insult to injury by removing the checks and balances of congressional rules and federal administrative oversight. Moreover, if the NGA has its way, devolution will also curtail opportunities for judicial relief. Disputes about covered services, says the NGA, "should be resolved as a contractual matter" between client and plan and should use alternate dispute resolution before going into state courts. Moreover, the governors would allow "no private right of action for providers or health plans regarding payment rates."[19] All these disquieting possibilities will surely not converge for the worst in all, nor necessarily in many states, but the risks are high enough to warrant second thoughts about how much farther Medicaid eligibility and benefit policies should devolve.

Dissolving or Devolving

The enthusiasm for Medicaid devolution draws strength from several converging forces: growing skepticism about the wisdom of federal policy rules, increased confidence in the capacities of the states, declining legitimacy of the poor (and of social programs that assist them), state resentments over federal mandates, and mounting federal irritation over state "scams" to attract extra federal funds. The old devolutionary battle cry—more stable budgets, fewer constraining strings—may at long last become the foundation of political compromise.

Arguably the mid-1990s enthusiasm for devolution of Medicaid simply writes the final act to a thirty-year drama that proves once again that poor people's programs are inherently poor programs, unable to find and keep a core constituency strong enough to preserve them from erosion, and incapable of replacing stigma with the legitimacy of universal programs that embrace the middle class. The answer of course is universal coverage under federal legislation that guarantees fair access and coverage to all citizens by right. The free-fall of the Clinton plan is a chilling comment on the prospects for such reform today. But if neither radical devolution nor national health insurance looks like a promising solution to Medicaid's problems, what about an alternative that is less dramatic than these two options yet more ambitious than restrained devolution: namely, dissolving Medicaid into innovative strategies that (arguably) preserve its goals while averting its strains? Three models merit quick inspection.

State Coverage Subsidized by Income

One strategy is to dissolve the stark categorical definitions that make Medicaid eligibility a dichotomous variable. An appealing model is the Basic Health Plan, enacted by Washington State in 1987 and expanded subsequently. In the BHP, uninsured individuals and families (mostly working) get coverage from designated managed-care plans whose premiums are paid mainly by state-appropriated funds and, in part, by premiums from enrollees. Subsidies and premiums vary along a sliding income-based scale. The absence of an employer mandate averts the formidable opposition of the business community, though employers can buy BHP coverage for their workers if the latter qualify for the program. Public subsidies are generous, averaging around 87 percent of premiums in 1997.[20]

To date the BHP has stayed administratively distinct from Medicaid, with which uninsured workers often prefer not to be associated; BHP applicants deemed eligible for Medicaid are referred to that program. In principle, however, the BHP could absorb Medicaid, whose clients would take their place at the heavily (perhaps wholly) subsidized end of the scale, with monies coming from federal funds and state general (or other) revenues.

Ending the sharp line between publicly defined haves on Medicaid and working uninsured have-nots who are eligible for the program would seem to enhance fairness and salve social resentment. The strategy has its problems, however. A big one is cost. The BHP now covers about 130,000 subsidized members (plus about 21,000 who pay their own premiums) at a cost of $214 million for the 1995-97 state budget biennium. The state has about 600,000 uninsured residents, so by extrapolation the annual price of universal coverage would be nearly $1 billion. How far the federal government would cover the costs of Medicaid in a new, integrated program depends on how federal funding formulas were set and how Washington State fared under them.

The budgetary stakes of expanded, not to mention universal, coverage would doubtless induce states to try to evaluate benefits against criteria of cost-effectiveness or other measures of value for money. They could follow the example of Oregon by redrawing benefits in the public plan, thus generating enough imputed savings to build political support for expanded enrollment. Still, a major increase in public funds and coverage would not be simple politically. Conservatives would undoubtedly deplore both the government takeover of parts of the health care system and the terrifying single-payer system supposedly hiding behind the necessary tax increases.

Moreover, such a plan might induce employers to drop or curtail their own contributions to the coverage of lower-income workers who qualify for a subsidy. If this crowding out of private insurance caused much curtailment of workers' benefits, the costs of the public program would rise with little or no net increase in coverage. Adverse selection by uninsured individuals (those who most expect to use services would be most inclined to pay premiums to get the subsidy) could drive the plan's costs higher still.

Even if a state willingly bit these budgetary bullets for the sake of universal coverage, doing so might not be good public policy. The poor and near-poor need many things besides health insurance—better schools, housing, law enforcement, job training, and nutrition to name a few. Some of these social services may promote health more effectively than do some types of medical care. And although the public-private patchwork that constitutes the safety net should not be an excuse for inaction on universal coverage, the health arena at least extends this modicum of protection, which has no counterpart in some other salient policy spheres.

A Public Health Model

If public purchase of health insurance for a subset of the poor in a largely private health coverage market is inherently unstable, perhaps policymakers should abandon the insurance model altogether. The rationale for this approach—that it would empower the poor to secure mainstream care in a single national tier—has not worn well and will evaporate if Congress repudiates the entitlement of eligibles to Medicaid coverage. Why not then discharge public health duties with a public health delivery model? States (or counties, or both) could pay community health centers and public hospitals directly to care for those who are now eligible for Medicaid.

Despite the appeals of eliminating the insurance middleman, such a model would not be easy to implement. For years states and counties have been trying to hold the line on budgets of public health institutions on the assumption that excess capacity in the private and voluntary sectors makes government delivery of care superfluous. This conviction has been seconded by much public health thinking, which contends that the public health field should concentrate on measuring needs, planning a more rational connection of needs to resources, and evaluating the health status of local populations, not on direct delivery of personal health services. Many communities therefore lack the capacity to take over Medicaid, and few states would welcome the invitation to plan, fund, and build a bigger, better public health system as a corollary of devolution. One suspects that the combined and "synergistic" appeal of devolution and managed care is that they take state and local policymakers off the hook for Medicaid, and that the superior accountability of the public health model is anything but a selling point.

Another New Federalism

One can also picture a rationalized, streamlined division of labor between the federal and state governments, one that centralizes and devolves duties according to some cogent theory of intergovernmental problem-solving and views federal-state relations as an exercise in cooperation, not a zero-sum power game. That federal systems can perform such feats is plain from a glance across the border to Canada. There, the central government devolves extensive authority and money to the ten provinces, which do most of the work of managing the national health insurance system. The providers are not smothered in red tape; on the contrary, national law succinctly sets forth a few general principles that the provinces must obey, and beyond that they are largely free to tailor their programs (and funding sources) as they please.[21]

It is an intriguing mental exercise (but, alas, perhaps no more than that) to picture the short list of principles the U.S. federal government might adopt for the administration of a devolved Medicaid program. The key problem is disentangling the effects of coherent federalism from those of universal coverage and a single-payer system. In Canada, health benefits must be universal, comprehensive, and portable across provincial lines. The United States views creation of a uniform benefit package for Medicaid, binding on all states and available to all Medicaid clients across the land, as inconsistent with devolution, which is understood to mean tolerance for extensive interstate variations in benefits. Canada's national law requires that health insurance be publicly administered by the provinces; that is, it cannot simply be devolved or contracted to competing for-profit health plans. This is easy to say in a single-payer system; in the United States, the content of minimum national standards imposed on the states is a hot controversy. Measures that embody a nationally protected universalism cannot readily be exported to rationalize a program predicated on state decisions about eligibility and benefits for medical care for a subset of the poor. Canada deliberately removes from the provincial ball game matters that the United States—which values state freedom, flexibility, and diversity as civic virtues in themselves—insists on keeping in constant intergovernmental play. If the United States could get clear about universal coverage and government's role in securing it, it would not now be debating the devolution of Medicaid. Ironically, it is precisely this lack of national clarity that offers the best arguments for restrained devolution.

Conclusion

Perhaps the best route toward an answer to the policy question "devolution for what?" is to explore a question of political history: devolution *from* what? Radical devolution challenges the increasingly inexplicit logic of a grants-in-aid system that has traditionally balanced uniformity and diversity in programs for which the federal and state governments share authority. At Medicaid's inception, that logic seemed clearly to fit the political facts. In a nation that finds national health insurance too much to swallow, stakeholders could agree at least on this: that assuring adequate (perhaps indeed mainstream) medical care to those poor who presumably could not fend for themselves was both a legitimate national goal and a defensible federal role; that the goal lent itself to diverse state interpretation and expressions; that too much variation degenerated into objectionable inequities; that a delicate balance between national uniformity and subnational variation made sound policy sense; and that joint federal-state funding and management of Medicaid embodied the checks and balances that make such programs work in the distinctive American context.

By the thirtieth anniversary of Medicaid, the fiscal bargaining intrinsic to grants-in-aid had overshadowed the program's original intent, which had grown increasingly obscure anyway as the rightward drift of political opinion prompted the view that the sole defensible national goal in social policy was to reduce the dependence of state and local governments on federal will and whim and of individuals on public support. For proponents of thoroughgoing devolution, state autonomy is a powerful national objective in itself. Uniformity in a federal system is no virtue, diversity no vice.

Advocates of restrained devolution, in contrast, defend the legitimacy of federal-state balancing while acknowledging that the balance—of policy, power, and purse—is and should be dynamic and evolutionary. Medicaid was, after all, born devolved and, national exertions and intrusions notwithstanding, still leaves the states vast discretion over decisions on eligibility, benefits, and more. The real question then is whether Medicaid is now so broken that it merits fixing by the wholesale excommunication of national interest and the removal of national checks on the expenditure of $100 billion or so of federal dollars on behalf of nearly 40 million vulnerable citizens.

Karen Davis's assertion that "all Americans should be concerned with assuring that a baby gets a healthy start in life—not just the residents of the state in which that child is born" frames the question vividly.[22] Behind that exhortation lies a world view on which Medicaid is a compelling, if sometimes convoluted, commentary. It holds (in effect) that the national interest is not an empty locution, that it can be more than the sum of the subnational parts, that securing a minimum level of well-being (not to mention a fair start in life's swift competitive race) is a national priority, and that public action to ease avoidable suffering is a cardinal indicator of a good society. Such sentiments, never at the top of the American cultural dance card, today seem quaint and picturesque, but they lie somewhere embedded in the social fabric and arguably deserve to be unearthed. These social principles are compatible with devolution but not with abandonment of the balancing act that animates a grant system devised precisely to accommodate a measure of purposive national leadership to the centrifugal values of American federalism.

On this view, Medicaid *should* combine federal mandates with federally supported state options. The feds can lead, the states can choose, and if federal direction grows too intrusive, the states can collectively protest and seek political redress. If states want to pursue Medicaid managed care, let them do so without tightly constraining federal rules and laborious waiver procedures—but not without reasonable standards and safeguards that oblige states to monitor access and quality of care and minimally connect federal means to national ends. Likewise, states should enjoy creativity and choice in funding their Medicaid matching shares and assisting uninsured citizens and hard-pressed provider institutions. But when such strategies go haywire—as they did in the period 1988-92—the federal government may properly restore balance. One observer's stifling, centralized stasis is another's normal political give-and-take as policymakers argue over the application of scarce resources to deep-seated problems.

Today the governors have a long agenda for reform of federal-state relations in Medicaid.[23] Given the big picture—slowing of enrollment growth and spending and increased willingness in Washington, D.C., to give states a freer hand in such weighty matters as managed-care initiatives and payments to providers—one may hope that these demands can be accommodated by restrained steps toward devolution within the basics of an intergovernmental policy system that has probably coped about as well as can be expected with American ambivalence about the role of national power in protecting the poor.

Notes

Valuable comments by Tanya Ehrmann, Cindy Watts Madden, Diane Rowland, and Michael Sparer much improved this chapter.

1. Robert Stevens and Rosemary Stevens, *Welfare Medicine in America: A Case Study of Medicaid* (Free Press, 1974). See also Michael S. Sparer, *Medicaid and the Limits of State Health Reform* (Temple University Press, 1996).

2. Alpha Center, "The Medicaid Expansions for Pregnant Women and Children: A Special Report" (Washington, undated document), p. 3.

3. Karen Davis, "Medicaid: The Nation's Health Care Safety Net for the Poor," testimony at Hearing on Welfare and Medicaid Reform before the Senate Committee on Finance, 104 Cong. 2 sess. (Government Printing Office, 1996), p. 2; Diane Rowland, "Medicaid's Role," testimony at Hearing before the Subcommittee on Health and Environment of the House Committee on Commerce, 105 Cong. 1 sess. (GPO, 1997), pp. 3, 6.

4. Teresa A. Coughlin and others, "State Responses to the Medicaid Spending Crisis: 1988 to 1992," *Journal of Health Politics, Policy and Law*, vol. 19 (Winter 1994), pp. 843, 838.

5. Ibid., pp. 861, 845.

6. Rowland, "Medicaid's Role," p. 4.

7. Coughlin and others, "State Responses," p. 857.

8. General Accounting Office, "Medicaid: Recent Spending Experience and the Administration's Proposed Program Reform," statement of William J. Scanlon before the Subcommittee on Health and Environment of the House Committee on Commerce, GAO-T-HEHS-97-94 (March 11, 1997), p. 1.

9. C. Eugene Steuerle and Gordon Mermin, "Devolution as Seen from the Budget," *Assessing New Federalism: Issues and Options for States*, series A, no. A-2 (Washington: Urban Institute, January 1997), p. 3. For a skeptical view on crowding out see James W. Fossett and James H. Wyckoff, "Has Medicaid Growth Crowded Out State Educational Spending?" *Journal of Health Politics, Policy and Law*, vol. 21 (Fall 1996), pp. 409–32.

10. Sparer, *Medicaid and the Limits of State Health Reform*, p. 66.

11. Rowland, "Medicaid's Role," p. 10.

12. Richard P. Nathan, *The Plot That Failed: Nixon and the Administrative Presidency* (Wiley, 1975), chap. 2.

13. Lawrence D. Brown, "The Politics of Devolution in Nixon's New Federalism," in Lawrence D. Brown and others, *The Changing Politics of Federal Grants* (Brookings, 1984), pp. 54–107.

14. Leighton Ku and Teresa A. Coughlin, "How the New Welfare Reform Law Affects Medicaid," *Assessing New Federalism: Issues and Options for States*, series A, no. A-5 (Washington: Urban Institute, 1997).

15. Sylvia Fubini, "Medicaid under Welfare Reform," *Health Care Trends Report*, vol. 11 (February 1997), p. 2.

16. Davis, "Medicaid," p. 6.

17. Sparer, *Medicaid and the Limits of State Health Reform*, pp. 39–41.

18. Davis, "Medicaid," p. 7.

19. National Governors' Association, "NGA Policy: EC-8, Medicaid," Section 8.3.1. (The statement is a revision in Winter 1997 of language adopted two years earlier.)

20. Data on the BHP kindly supplied by Keenan Konopaski of the Washington State Health Care Authority. For background on the BHP, see Carolyn W. Madden and others, "Washington State's Health Plan: Choices and Challenges," *Journal of Public Health Policy*, vol. 13 (Spring 1992), pp. 81–96.

21. On the evolution and workings of the Canadian system, see Malcolm G. Taylor, *Insuring National Health Care: The Canadian Experience* (University of North Carolina Press, 1990).

22. Davis, "Medicaid," p. 9. See also Forrest P. Chisman, "A National Approach to Health Care Reform," in Chisman and others, eds., *National Health Care Reform: What Should the State Role Be?* (Washington: National Academy of Social Insurance, 1994), pp. 25–39.

23. National Governors' Association, "NGA Policy."

8

Federalism and the Medicaid Challenge

Frank J. Thompson

THE DEBATE over Medicaid devolution is a small episode in a federalism drama that has been playing since the birth of the United States. Writing more than 200 years ago, James Madison in the *Federalist Papers* captured the core of this drama when he observed that "the proposed Constitution is . . . neither a national nor a federal Constitution, but a composition of both." Although working to strengthen the national government, Madison understood that the new political system would in many ways preserve the "faculty" of federal and state governments "to resist and frustrate the measures of each other."[1]

From the outset, the division of labor between the national and state governments was murky. To be sure, the Tenth Amendment to the Constitution, ratified in December 1791, attempted some clarification by insisting that, "The powers not delegated to the United States by the Constitution, nor prohibited by it to the States, are reserved to the States respectively, or to the people." Moreover, many early students of American government adhered to a view known as "dual federalism"[2]—a perspective that saw the roles of the federal and state governments as relatively distinct and sharply drawn. For instance, writing at the dawn of the twentieth century, the distinguished scholar James Bryce observed:

The characteristic feature and special interest of the American union is that it shows us two governments covering the same ground, yet distinct and separate in their action. It is like a great factory wherein two sets of machinery are at work, their revolving wheels apparently intermixed, their bands crossing one another, yet each doing its own work without touching or hampering the other.[3]

The coming of the New Deal and the contemporary welfare state, however, increasingly made the theory of dual federalism obsolete. As the federal government expanded its role in domestic policy, the imagery of federalism as a "marble cake" with "no neat horizontal stratification" of functions prevailed.[4] Driven by the proliferation of federal grant programs, domestic policies came to be seen as involving federal-state and often local partnerships. The federalism drama increasingly revolved around the quality of these partnerships—especially on whether one level of government had too much power in the relationship. Issues of the appropriate balance of power between the federal government and the states were not, of course, simply matters for abstract discourse about the design of political institutions. As the debate over Medicaid devolution illustrates, stakeholders sense that decisions about the division of labor in a federal system ultimately affect who gets what from government.

By the mid-1990s no systematic assessment of American federalism could safely slight Medicaid; arguably, the program had become the single most important intergovernmental initiative on the American policy stage. From 1980 to 1996, for example, Medicaid grew from 22 percent of all federal aid to the states to 40 percent.[5] Hence modifications in Medicaid loom large not only from the perspective of health policy, but also from the vantage point of American federalism.

In addressing the Medicaid partnership between the federal and state governments in providing health care to the needy, the chapters in this volume benefit greatly from the insights provided by a conference of Medicaid officials and other experts held in May 1996. This conference plus subsequent research strongly suggests that neither the states nor the federal government can appropriately be portrayed as the strong senior partner in the Medicaid program as of the mid-1990s. In certain aspects of the intergovernmental dance, the federal government leads; in other areas, the states do. Clearly, states possess vast discretion to tailor Medicaid to their tastes. Like many partnerships, tensions beset the relationship between the federal and state governments over Medicaid. The partners, for instance, each look for ways to shift costs to the other; each would like the other to be more cooperative and deferential. In some cases the relationship looks less like a dance than a shoving match, but on balance federal and state officials work in a relatively harmonious fashion.

Proponents of devolution seek to alter this partnership by enlarging state power and influence over Medicaid. Given the potential significance of devolution for the delicate balance among cost, quality, and access in the health care arena, this chapter zeroes in on the overarching question of whether states are up to the challenge. Could states readily shoulder substantially increased responsibility for Medicaid, such as that envisioned by the Medigrant legislation or other proposals for major devolution?

In broaching this topic, the chapter first assesses the governing capacity of the states—the degree to which they possess the wherewithal in terms of institutions and other resources to assume significantly greater responsibility for Medicaid. Although many states have made progress in bolstering their governing capacity, serious issues persist concerning the ability of states to formulate and implement policy effectively. Second, the fiscal capacity of the states to cope with major devolution receives attention. What fiscal resources do states have and how readily can they be tapped for public programs such as Medicaid? Third, this chapter focuses on the related issue of state commitment to the Medicaid program—the degree to which state officials place a priority on providing health care to the needy. In the face of major devolution, will officials intensify their commitment or let it erode via the race to the bottom or a related dynamic? Based on this assessment of state capacity and commitment, a final section recommends a more incremental, calibrated approach to Medicaid devolution that pays particular attention to implementation (especially with respect to eligibility for children) and assigns a critical scorekeeping role to the national government.

The Governing Capacity of the States

Major devolution of Medicaid becomes more viable to the degree that states have substantial governing capacity—the ability to formulate coherent, creative, plausible policy *and* carry it out efficiently, effectively, and accountably. In this regard the states have by most accounts made considerable progress over the past thirty years. Until the 1960s most state governments had reputations for being political and administrative backwaters. Their legislatures and bureaucracies lacked professional staffs; their governors did not have authority over many line agencies; relatively low pay and patronage characterized personnel administration; election processes assured that urban areas lacked proportionate representation in state legislatures; and many southern states denied minorities the right to vote and engage in meaningful political participation. By the mid-1990s this dismal view of state governments had given way to optimism that states had made great strides in bolstering their ability to sustain well-performing, democratic governance.[6] Any advantage the federal government had once enjoyed over the states now seemed to have vanished.

A Slippery Concept

In acknowledging state progress, however, two critical points should be kept in mind. First, political scientists have made only modest headway in defining and measuring such capacity satisfactorily, because it is a very slippery concept. R. Kent Weaver and Bert A. Rockman have gone further than most in advancing understanding when they suggest that governing capacity increases to the degree that states have the ability to:
—Set and maintain priorities among many conflicting demands;
—Target resources where they are most effective;
—Coordinate conflicting objectives into a coherent whole;
—Impose losses on powerful groups;
—Innovate when old policies have failed;
—Represent diffuse, unorganized interests as well as concentrated, well-organized ones;
—Manage political cleavages so that society does not degenerate into violent or other costly conflict;
—Sustain enough policy stability that policies have time to work; and
—Ensure the effective implementation of government policies that have been decided on.[7]
These criteria speak to fundamental questions of the degree to which state governments are democratic and efficacious in formulating and implementing theoretically sound policy. But exactly how these factors interact to yield greater governing capacity and the relative importance of each remain far from clear. Part of the problem in this regard springs from difficulties in measuring the presence of these conditions. Even more fundamentally,

different normative views about the nature of democracy and efficacy make conceptual resolution concerning governing capacity a Sisyphean task.

Second, and relatedly, the link between various institutional arrangements and governing capacity is far from settled. In fact, challenges to the conventional wisdom about how to do "good government" have multiplied and intensified. Consider, for instance, the question of whether legislative professionalism should be construed as an indicator of greater governing capacity. Reformers have tended to portray better paid legislatures with abundant supporting staffs as a plus for the formulation of coherent policy and the preservation of democratic accountability. Following this line of reasoning, states with more professionalized legislative institutions would, other things being equal, be better equipped to handle Medicaid devolution.

More recent discussions of health policy reform at the state level, however, have tended to turn the case for legislative professionalism on its head. In this revisionist view, such professionalism fuels gridlock, especially in an era when most states have divided governments (that is, the same party does not control the governorship and both houses of the legislature). These revisionists detect a silver lining in factors that tend to undercut the expertise of state legislatures in forging health policy: relatively high turnover rates (which may well be fueled by the spread of term limits), the absence of committee systems that reward seniority, limited professional staffs, and an environment with far fewer think tanks than is the case in the nation's capital. From a revisionist perspective, their "amateurism" may make legislators more open to creative reform. These policymakers may avoid the analysis paralysis that can be brought on by having countless analytic units dissect a given proposal—the prevailing pattern when the national government considers policies. They may also avoid the crippling memories of failed health reform efforts that are so common in the nation's capital.[8]

Whether in fact less professionalism in legislatures would galvanize more innovative approaches to providing health care for the needy under Medicaid devolution is, of course, highly debatable. To a considerable degree, the question boils down to whether executive-driven political systems, on balance, produce better policy. Less legislative professionalism means that the governor and top officials in the executive branch gain comparative advantage in terms of expertise and time. With the executive gaining clout, Medicaid policy might come to be formulated in a less fragmented and fractious environment. Any claims for the virtues of legislative amateurism in the context of Medicaid devolution, however, should be juxtaposed with other findings. Various studies suggest that more professionalized legislatures (especially those with higher salary levels) are more likely to be Democratic and more inclined to expand government programs. Controlling for a range of potentially important factors, legislative professionalism is associated with higher state expenditures.[9] If this dynamic applied to Medicaid, amateurism could mean leaner times.

Questions of state governing capacity not only intersect with complex issues related to institutional configurations but also pertain to state cultures. Although devilishly difficult to prove, one cannot escape impressions that some states have civic cultures more conducive to "good government" than others. One of the more promising lines of inquiry here focuses on the impact of social capital on government performance. Social capital refers to networks, norms, and trust that enable citizens to act together more effectively to pursue shared objectives. Certain forms of this capital expedite the pursuit of civic ends. Recent research has found that states vary greatly in their scores on a social capital index based on four indicators: social trust, associational memberships, voting turnout, and the incidence of nonprofit groups. Measured in this way, social capital helps explain school performance in the states even after controls are imposed for other possible explanatory factors.[10] Whether and how much variations in social capital among states would affect their efficacy in dealing with increased responsibility for Medicaid remains an open question. But at a minimum these findings lend credence to the view that students of devolution should pay heed not only to the Alabama syndrome[11] (how bad things can happen when states get too much discretion), but also to the Minnesota syndrome (why some states almost always seem to respond in innovative and effective ways).

Issues of political institutions and culture ultimately intersect with the question of whether Medicaid devolution would shift power to more democratic political systems. Again, conceptual and measurement issues, as well as great variation among the states, make it hard to assess claims that state governments are closer to and represent their citizens better than their national counterpart. To be sure, existing studies do suggest that state policy choices reflect to a remarkable degree the general political ideology of their populations as measured by the proportion of citizens in each state who identify themselves as political liberals, moderates, or conservatives.[12] In this volume Donald Boyd has found citizen ideology to be a statistically significant predictor of Medicaid policy.[13]

But findings such as these take us only a limited distance toward settling the question of the relative degree to which the states and the national government approach democratic ideals. Skeptics about the states note that citizens often seem to have less knowledge of state issues and tend to participate less in state elections.[14] Furthermore, nagging questions persist about the extent to which state policy processes reflect a broad spectrum of societal interests—not just those of the affluent but also of the poor. As will be discussed later, business firms and the affluent can more readily use the threat of exit in state politics to buttress their power position than they can at the national level.[15] Moreover, policymakers in many states may well lack the tools that their federal counterparts have to conduct oversight and hold administrative agencies accountable. Ironically, critical administrative transactions of the federal government are often more transparent than those at the state level due to numerous analytic units (for example, the General Accounting Office) that focus on the details of implementation. For these and other reasons, questions about devolution and democracy are as slippery as other issues of governing capacity in the states.

Administrative Capacity

The ability of states to formulate coherent, plausible, and broadly responsive Medicaid policy is a key ingredient of governing capacity. But as the chapters in this book emphasize, the ability of states to implement these policies efficiently, effectively, and accountably may well be an even more critical component of such capacity. Administrative capability tends to increase to the degree that agents responsible for delivering the Medicaid program possess several qualities. These include:

—Resources such as authority, money, personnel, information or expertise, status, physical facilities, and equipment;

—Skilled leadership and management sensitive to the technical requirements of health care provision and the strategies required to assemble and sustain the diverse networks needed to make the program work; and

—Administrative institutions with cultures and standard operating procedures conducive to accomplishing Medicaid objectives.

State governments have, over the last thirty years, seen an increase in their general administrative capacity as well as their specific ability to deliver Medicaid. Their work forces have, for instance, become more professional. But in many areas, troubling questions persist. In fact, the 1990s have fueled a conviction among many advocates of "reinvention" that the progressive reforms of the past have come full circle to emerge as obstacles to more efficient and effective implementation. For instance, the National

Commission on the State and Local Public Service concluded that states often "hamstring their chief executives by diffusing their power. They operate with antiquated and obsolete personnel, procurement, and budget systems. They fail to invest in the most critical resource they have: their rank and file personnel."[16] By standards of "best corporate practice," training budgets in virtually all state governments are woefully inadequate.[17] Nor can one assume that state administrators enjoy a more trustful, nurturing environment than their federal counterparts—one that would presumably provide more fertile soil for innovation and learning from mistakes. When surveys ask citizens about their confidence in different levels of the federal system, state governments appear to enjoy a marginal advantage, if any, over the national government.[18]

In the late 1990s the pervasive ideology of downsizing, and its attendant bureaucracy bashing, particularly threaten administrative capacity. Ironically, many state and local governments have turned to downsizing at precisely the time when the fervor for this approach in the private sector has met growing skepticism. As many downsized companies have seen profits and growth shrink, management experts have increasingly questioned the wisdom of a strategy based on "shrinking to greatness."[19]

Although they can point to an impressive set of achievements, state Medicaid agencies cannot insulate themselves from the general forces that threaten implementation capacity. One study of these agencies notes the presence of significant administrative problems flowing from such forces as staff cutbacks, civil service restrictions, rapid turnover in top leadership positions, structural fragmentation, and a crisis atmosphere.[20]

And, of course, the chapters in this book highlight a potpourri of management challenges that may intensify under devolution and sorely tax the administrative capacity of the states. Among these challenges, none are more pressing than those associated with contracting for health care services. The successful implementation of Medicaid has always depended on the capacity of not only state bureaucracies but also a wide range of other public and private agents—physicians, hospitals, nursing homes, managed-care companies, local governments, and more. As Michael Sparer demonstrates in chapter 5, the future of Medicaid in no small way depends on whether states and others act to preserve the safety net institutions that have done so much to provide services to Medicaid enrollees and other low-income citizens. His chapter cautions against doctrines of competitive procurement that charge government solely with employing the most efficient agent over the short term to deliver services. It suggests that state governments should also pay attention to preserving a mix of suppliers for the future—especially those with a tradition of reaching out to disadvantaged populations.

As the chapters in this book emphasize, Medicaid contracting has undergone transition as devolution has elevated the importance of managed care. In some respects, this development has simplified matters for state governments. In the past, for instance, states essentially had contracts with a vast array of health care providers (that is, individual physicians, nursing homes, hospitals) that stipulated that these providers would be paid according to a particular formula every time they delivered service to a Medicaid enrollee. State Medicaid officials were largely preoccupied with claims processing and bill paying. More recently, Medicaid waivers have given states more opportunity to shift to a model where HMOs and other managed-care firms assume responsibility for providing Medicaid beneficiaries with health care for a capitated payment. State governments have thereby moved toward an indirect relationship with many health care providers whose fortunes increasingly depend on their ability to sign subcontracts with large managed-care firms rather than state governments.

On the surface, this development may seem to make life easier for state officials, allowing them to hand off problems that used to be in their domain to managed-care contractors. But the authors in this volume persuasively argue otherwise. They suggest that the rise of managed care may mean just the opposite—the need for increased state administrative capacity to oversee contractors.[21] James Fossett, James Tallon, and Lawrence Brown note in their chapters that the movement by Medicaid officials to contract with large managed-care companies does not, as many originally thought, mean that the staffs of state governments can easily be streamlined. To the contrary, the effective management of managed care puts pressures on state agencies to hire additional personnel. Failure to do so seriously threatens the access of Medicaid enrollees to health care of adequate quality. Whether state agencies will be able to build and sustain adequate staffs to deal with managed care in an era dominated by the dogma of downsizing remains an open question.

In this vein the greater reliance on managed care also puts to the test the capacity of states to secure the information they need to hold contractors to high standards of efficiency and effectiveness. The fundamental logic of a fee-for-service system, where Medicaid pays an array of vendors for providing specific services, naturally yields key program data on the encounters of Medicaid enrollees with providers. In contrast, lump-sum payments to capitated managed-care plans do not automatically call for a careful recording of the services provided to enrollees. Managed-care firms have less financial incentive to keep track of the cost of every transaction between patients and providers. In fact, it may be more efficient for them not to do so.

Many see the development of electronic information systems that routinely produce encounter data as a solution to this problem. Ideally, these systems facilitate utilization review and an assessment of the quality of care that providers deliver to Medicaid enrollees and others. But designing and operating these systems pose many problems. The federal government and the states have not reached a consensus on the answers to certain fundamental questions. For instance, what exactly is an encounter between a patient and provider? What information about it should be routinely coded? Assuming that agreement can be reached on the answers to these questions, officials face the fact that encounter systems require an investment in administrative capacity. As one analysis of such systems notes, "Developing useful encounter data is a time-consuming, labor-intensive effort." In this regard, "the lack of internal staff capacity is one major impediment to development of an operational encounter data system." The analysis concludes that many financially strapped states do not have the requisite staff and resources to develop such systems and that the Health Care Financing Administration (HCFA) program to assist states has been "late to arrive, is limited in scope, and will not be sufficient."[22]

Greater devolution will also test the administrative capacity of the states in ways that go beyond the special challenges of contracting for managed care. For instance, Medicaid's eligibility intake processes will be subject to new trials and possibly tribulations. Great numbers of children and qualified Medicare beneficiaries who are legally entitled to benefits currently fail to receive them. For reasons to be discussed later in this chapter, the gap between the number of potentially eligible beneficiaries and those who actually sign up may well grow sharply unless states build an administrative infrastructure that does more to publicize Medicaid benefits and develop client-friendly intake offices that are readily accessible to potential recipients. In dealing with this challenge, Medicaid managers confront the possibility of working at cross-purposes with policymakers in their states who may lack the commitment to provide such capacity because enrolling more beneficiaries will drive up program costs.

The evidence related to managed care, eligibility determinations, and other factors suggests that most states will have to shore up and enhance their Medicaid administrative capacity if they are to realize greater efficiency and effectiveness in the wake of devolution. Many states may be up to the challenge. However, the perennial propensity of policymakers to slight implementation issues and underinvest in administration could well undercut the ability of state Medicaid officials to achieve positive results.

Federally Imposed Incapacity: ERISA and Medicaid

State capacity to formulate and implement sound health care policy depends on much more than the factors indigenous to the state. The general policies of the federal government also enlarge or shrink that capacity. In this regard, the national government has seriously limited the number of arrows in the quivers of state governments through the Employee Retirement Income Security Act (ERISA).

Although ERISA permits states to regulate health insurance, it also shields self-funded business plans from many forms of state intervention. These self-funded plans make up an increasing proportion of the health care market, covering an estimated 17 percent of all citizens in 1993. Firms with fewer than one hundred employees have recently shown particular interest in moving to self-funding.[23] ERISA prevents states from taking pressure off Medicaid by passing a law that requires all employers to provide some specified health benefit package to their workers. It also prevents states from imposing a premium tax on all contributions to health plans in order to fund a universal health insurance system or subsidize care for the poor. ERISA allows self-funded firms to dodge state requirements concerning community rating, uniform data reporting and claims procedures, any-willing-provider laws, and more. The law has made it more difficult for eligibility workers to obtain the information needed to determine whether applicants for Medicaid already have access to health benefits under a self-funded plan.[24] Efforts to revise ERISA in order to free states from these shackles or to grant certain states waivers from these restrictions have run into a political brick wall. Strong opposition to ERISA reform by business lobbies has undercut whatever modest propensity Congress might otherwise have to empower the states in this sphere.[25]

One should emphasize, however, that although ERISA erodes state governing capacity in the health care arena, it still leaves policymakers with an array of Medicaid options. As one legal analysis notes, "ERISA does not prohibit a tax law with only tangential impacts on an employee health plan. Therefore, it is fairly clear that a state can tax employers or use an income tax to finance a less-than-universal program."[26] Hence states could legally use expanded discretion under devolution to impose taxes that would substantially expand the number of poor and uninsured covered by Medicaid. Nor does it appear likely that ERISA prevents states from using provider or excise taxes to fund expanded Medicaid coverage. ERISA may well be the nightmare for state-driven health reform that some claim,[27] but it should not be construed as the principal barrier to expanded coverage under Medicaid. As will be discussed later, an array of other factors does much more to inhibit states' aggressiveness than ERISA does.

Fiscal Capacity: Variation and Handcuffs

The response of the states to Medicaid devolution also depends on their fiscal capacity—their wealth and their formal right to tax and appropriate their assets for public purposes. As the chapter by Boyd shows, state wealth predicts the generosity of state Medicaid programs to a remarkable degree. State fiscal capacity continues to vary greatly. Although the period from 1940 through 1970 saw variation in state per capita income steadily decline, the last twenty-five years have brought no significant movement toward greater equality among states. As of 1996 personal income per capita [in current dollars] ranged from $17,471 in Mississippi to $33,189 in Connecticut. States also differ appreciably in the proportion of their citizens who live in poverty. As of 1995 the state with the highest poverty rate (New Mexico at 25 percent) exceeded the lowest state (New Hampshire at 5 percent) by a factor of five.[28] Of course state fiscal fortunes fluctuate over time. States face the conundrum that an increasing proportion of their citizens need Medicaid during economic downturns when their fiscal capacity to provide coverage diminishes.

As Boyd points out, the existing Medicaid formula for distributing funds among states is somewhat redistributive but does not level the playing field. If poorer states were to make their Medicaid programs as broad and deep as those of richer states, they would need to exert greater tax effort. None of the major devolution proposals espoused in 1995 and 1996 would have significantly increased the redistribution of funds from richer to poorer states. Moreover, several of these proposals would have undercut states' ability to counter the effects of economic recessions. As an open-ended entitlement, the current Medicaid program assures states that they can count on a certain federal match no matter how much they spend. If they budget more for Medicaid during business downturns, the federal government will also provide more money. Medigrant and the devolution proposals of the National Governors' Association (NGA) in 1996 would have undercut this countercyclical dynamic.

Variations in state wealth provide only a partial picture of state fiscal capacity. The degree to which state constitutions and statutes authorize policymakers to tax these assets also looms large in importance. In this regard, the repeated triumphs of the anti-tax movement over the past twenty-five years has placed fiscal handcuffs on a growing number of states. In the process, this movement has also raised nagging concerns about state governing capacity—especially the degree to which states can respond to the preferences of a majority of their citizens.

The National Conference of State Legislatures reports that as of 1996, twenty-seven states had adopted tax and expenditure limits. These provisions assume myriad forms, but most of them remove state fiscal policy still further from the realm of majoritarian politics to an arena where extraordinary majorities must be mobilized for a state to increase its tax effort or appropriations at all or beyond a certain increment.[29] For instance, such diverse states as Arizona, California, Louisiana, South Dakota, and Washington require a two-thirds majority in both houses of their legislatures to raise taxes. Many states also limit the amount of money that they can generate in revenues or spend in a given year. For example, in any fiscal year state revenue in Michigan may not exceed 9.49 percent of total personal income for the prior year. To transcend this ceiling the governor must specify an emergency and each chamber of the legislature must approve the exemption by a two-thirds vote. As a result of strictures such as these, state efforts to increase their financial support for Medicaid in response to any federal cuts wrought by devolution would depend heavily on economic growth that helps them sustain benefits at current tax rates, or on decisions to strip funds from other state programs such as higher education.

The proliferation of state revenue and expenditure constraints means that states may be less likely than in the past to compensate for declining federal support. In their seminal study of state responses to devolution during the Reagan administration, Richard Nathan and associates found considerable effort by most of the states in their sample to deflect or otherwise compensate for the cuts in funding brought on by block grants. They noted, however, that California proved to be a major exception and suggested that the "minimal response" of that state in no small measure reflected the enactment of major fiscal limitations through referendums.[30] Since the time of that study, other states have followed in California's footsteps—a circumstance that seems likely to vitiate their ability to respond creatively to certain forms of devolution.

Viewed broadly, developments related to state fiscal and governing capacity caution against state boosterism in the debate over Medicaid devolution. Capacity has increased on some fronts and receded on others. Variation among states continues to be great. Certain types of devolution might well ignite creative innovation in the states, but other forms would push states beyond their abilities.

State Commitment to Medicaid

Even if states possess the capacity to provide health care services of high quality to the needy through the Medicaid program or a devolved substitute, policymakers and administrators may lack the commitment to do so. The interaction between state capacity and commitment will shape the degree to which the Medicaid lifeline is preserved, enhanced, shortened, or shredded. The concept of state commitment to Medicaid poses complex issues of conceptualization and measurement. In general terms, however, it gauges the efforts state governments exert to provide access to quality health care to the needy under Medicaid.[31] In this regard, Medicaid devolution could lead to: (1) less commitment where, for example, empowered states cut back on the resources they expend on the program from their own sources; (2) sustained commitment where state officials continue their current level of effort to provide coverage and quality assurance under Medicaid; and (3) enhanced commitment where, for instance, state governments spend more of their own monies to compensate for reduced federal support.

In considering likely reactions to devolution, some scenarios primarily emphasize the response of state policymakers to the behavior of other states. In this regard, much of the debate about state commitment has revolved around the question of whether devolution would fuel a race to the bottom.

A Race to the Bottom?

Some analysts see interstate economic competition as the driving force in shaping overall levels of commitment to redistributive social programs such as Medicaid. Rather than focus on the values of state policymakers and the forces of voice in the state political system (that is, interest groups) they stress the potency of exit and entry as pivotal political resources in state politics. In a time marked by the increased geographic mobility of labor and capital, business leaders and the affluent gain power in state politics by threatening to leave if tax support for redistributive programs, such as Medicaid, becomes too onerous. The specter of entry also underpins this model. It holds that states can in fact become welfare magnets if their benefit levels become too generous, thereby creating considerable fiscal stress and unleashing pressures to make benefit levels less alluring.

The race-to-the-bottom theory assumes that state policymakers pay particular attention to benefit levels in states contiguous to their own. In the interest of economic development, each state prefers to offer somewhat lower benefits than its neighbors; if one state cuts benefits, a chain reaction may well occur with neighboring states also reducing them. The model predicts that if Medicaid devolution takes the form of reduced federal funding and the relaxation of mandates concerning service packages, eligibility, and fiscal maintenance of effort, Medicaid benefits will spiral downward as states try to avoid exit by the affluent and entry by the needy.

The validity of the race-to-the-bottom theory depends in part on whether the affluent, business firms, and the poor react to welfare policy in the predicted manner. The key factor is whether state policymakers believe that the model applies. The public rhetoric of politicians who have proposed cuts in Medicaid often emphasizes that interstate economic competition leaves them with little choice other than to cut benefits. In New York State, for instance, both Governor George Pataki and the senate majority leader, Joseph Bruno, have repeatedly proclaimed that New York's economy will prosper and the outward migration of its citizens diminish only if taxes are cut and support for such government programs as Medicaid is reduced. Other policymakers proclaim the potency of welfare magnets. Noting the generous health care benefits offered by his home state of Minnesota, for example, one legislator observed: "We see an influx in Minnesota because of the benefits. To give you a sense, in my home county, about 25 percent of the people that signed up last year for medical assistance came from out of state. In one of the other counties, it was almost 40 percent. . . . The welfare magnet kind of thing is a phenomenon we see in fact happening."[32]

Although the race to the bottom has been a central metaphor in the debate about Medicaid devolution, the model has yet to be adequately tested. A systematic search uncovered only one empirical study explicitly focused on the subject—a state-by-state analysis of Medicaid benefits each year for the period from 1976 through 1989 by Peterson, Rom, and Scheve.

This study measured benefits as the annual average expenditure per Medicaid recipient adjusted for a state consumer price index. Among other things, the authors hypothesized that state policymakers would tend to reduce expenditures per recipient if their benefits were higher than those of neighboring states and in response to increasing numbers of poor persons in the state. Overall they found support for their view that interstate economic competition negatively affected Medicaid benefit levels and concluded: "The evidence is consistent with a theory of state policy change that emphasizes the sensitivity of states to the benefit levels of their neighbors and to changes in their poverty populations."[33] But as the authors of this study themselves acknowledge, their analysis is only a first step in efforts to test the race-to-the-bottom hypothesis in the case of Medicaid.

Although policymakers should not dismiss the possibility that major devolution of Medicaid would trigger a race to the bottom, the limits to the metaphor as a vehicle for understanding state commitment should also be understood. Some of these limits emanate from prickly conceptual and methodological problems concerning how to test the model. Consider, for instance, matters related to measuring the dependent variable, Medicaid benefits. A thorough test of the race to the bottom would require shining the spotlight on a broad spectrum of these benefits. For instance, Boyd's chapter suggests the need to focus on not only a state's Medicaid expenditures per enrollee, but also Medicaid enrollees as a percentage of the poor. Other pertinent indicators include state policies on eligibility and the scope of service to be covered by Medicaid. In fact, optimal assessment of the race to the bottom would factor in issues of quality. Given that the quality of care is less easy to track and measure than access to and the cost of health care, state officials will be sorely tempted to sweep quality issues under the rug if devolution ushers in significant federal funding cuts. As Fossett notes in this volume, reductions in federal support would increasingly drive managed-care firms to emphasize cost cutting above all else, and to scrimp on the investments required to assure quality in managed-care plans.

Aside from the problem of determining the appropriate dependent variables to test the race-to-the-bottom hypothesis, other perplexing questions persist. What is the bottom in this model—almost certainly not zero, so then what? Will states race or instead drift downward? Will states respond to neighboring states, or will they focus on more distant ones? To what degree will the variation in state commitment to Medicaid grow as more affluent states with relatively small poverty populations continue to provide relatively generous benefits? These and other questions beg for answers. For present purposes, it deserves emphasis that even if states in the aggregate demonstrate a decline in commitment to Medicaid, the pattern of state behavior may not fully mirror the dynamic predicted by the race-to-the-bottom model.

The race to the bottom has not been the only metaphor used to suggest likely state responses to devolution. Others, who see state policies as strongly driven by the behavior of other states, have pointed to the utility of the convoy metaphor. The reasoning runs as follows: during wartime, no single ship (read state) in a naval convoy can afford to be too far out ahead or behind other vessels in a given policy area. In this vein, states could vary in their Medicaid programs but not by too much.[34] Unlike the race to the bottom, this metaphor does not predict that states would have incentive to do less but, rather and more simply, not to be too different from each other. Like the race to the bottom, the convoy metaphor contains a germ of insight. But it also begs certain critical questions. It does not, for instance, predict the extent to which different forms of devolution would cause the convoy to spread out, with the distance between the leading states and those bringing up the rear becoming larger. Nor does it adequately acknowledge that devolution built on a diminution in federal funding might well cause the convoy to reduce its speed (that is, on average, lead to an erosion in eligibility, the scope of service packages, or quality).

Internal Forces in State Politics

Ultimately, of course, fathoming the magnitude and nature of state commitment to Medicaid will require going beyond the motivational impact of interstate competition to the internal dimensions of state politics—ideology, political leadership, interest group activity, and much more.[35] These factors vary greatly across the states.

Consider political ideology, for example. As Boyd's analysis in chapter 3 reflects, one important measure of a state's ideology turns out to be the degree to which its citizens consider themselves to be politically liberal, moderate, or conservative. Recent research suggests that this measure strongly correlates with the social policies adopted by states. Although self-identified conservatives outnumber liberals in all states, their preponderance is much greater in some than others. Among the five most populous states in the country, Texas ranked as most conservative (23 percentage points more conservatives than liberals) followed in order by Florida, Pennsylvania, California, and New York (with only 3 percentage points more conservatives than liberals).[36] Major devolution to the states would open the door for state ideologies to have an even greater effect. Variation in state commitment to Medicaid would probably increase.

Just as broad ideological forces shape commitment to Medicaid, so too do the values and skills of particular political leaders in the executive, legislative, and, at times, judicial branches of government. Governors and legislators in such states as Tennessee and Minnesota have, for instance, served as catalysts for innovations that strive to achieve a better balance among access, quality, and cost in the Medicaid program. In shaping the program, state policymakers respond to multiple factors, including the policy legacy of their state as reflected in previous decisions of political leaders concerning Medicaid and the institutional configurations that have evolved over time from these choices. At an early point in Medicaid's history, for example, the governor and legislature in New York State determined that the state and local governments should split the costs of the nonfederal share of Medicaid almost equally. Thus when state policymakers in New York choose to expand Medicaid, they do so with the knowledge that they will not have to find the funds to pay fully for the initiative; local governments will pay a significant portion. This financing arrangement has made it easier for legislators to favor generous Medicaid policies and has contributed to New York's position as a state that spends much more than most others per enrollee.

Interest group pressures will also mold the outcomes of Medicaid devolution. To the degree that meaningful discretion over Medicaid shifts to the states, new groups may form to support the program and existing groups may intensify their efforts. The pushes and pulls of interest group activity will shape the overall level of spending on the program. In this regard, Medicaid may fare better than other redistributive initiatives that provide cash assistance to the needy, because certain groups of health care providers have a stake in preserving the program.

Interest group activity will not only affect overall commitment to providing health care to the needy, but also shape which Medicaid stakeholders win and lose in the wake of devolution. Pressures to preserve certain features of Medicaid will be more intense than others. Institutional providers, for instance, will toil diligently to sustain their payment levels. Moreover, as the chapters by Fossett and Joshua Wiener suggest, the elderly and disabled may well be in a better position to hold their own in the struggle for resources than poor mothers and children. Fossett emphasizes the political dynamics created by geography. Poor mothers and children tend to be concentrated in urban areas and dependent for political advocacy on the safety net institutions described by Sparer in chapter 5. The elderly and disabled, in contrast, can typically count on vigorous support from nursing home operators and advocacy groups distributed across legislative districts in the entire state. Wiener sees the political punch of the elderly and disabled as flowing from their higher status as "deserving poor" and from the fact that long-term care institutions, which depend on Medicaid for a substantial proportion of their revenues, are well organized politically, contribute significant sums to the campaigns of state legislators, and know the leverage points in state Medicaid bureaucracies.

Of course, the permeability of governments to interest group pressures varies greatly from state to state. For instance, a comparative study of Medicaid programs in California and New York found that groups in the latter—especially institutional providers and labor unions—had many access points to the policy process and exercised much more influence over the decisions of top Medicaid officials. In contrast, Medicaid officials in California enjoyed greater insulation from these pressures.[37]

Interest group activities, state ideologies, the particular values and skills of top political leaders, and other factors indigenous to a state's political fabric will do much to leaven the effects of interstate economic competition in shaping state Medicaid policies. They will test the limits of the race-to-the-bottom model.

Whatever the exact dynamics that shape state commitment to Medicaid, one likelihood deserves emphasis: devolution that substantially curtailed federal funding to the states, such as the Republican Medigrant proposal, would in all probability lead to an attenuation of the Medicaid lifeline.[38] Most states would find it difficult to elevate their commitment to a level that would fully compensate for significant reductions in federal aid. Whether through formal policy changes or the opaque and silent politics of implementation, they would instead tend to reduce eligibility for Medicaid, narrow the range of services available to enrollees, erode the quality of care delivered, or all three. Only if state policymakers proved willing to shift funds to Medicaid from other policy sectors, such as education; achieved extraordinary gains in program efficiency; enjoyed the revenue windfall of extremely robust growth in their state economies; or (against formidable political odds) enhanced their tax effort would this weakening of the Medicaid lifeline be avoided.

Medicaid Devolution in Perspective

Taken as a whole, the chapters in this volume present an image of state capacity and commitment that translate into a flashing red light about devolution—stop, and proceed with caution. The late 1990s offer a political opportunity to remain at the traffic light a bit longer. The pressures to do something big about Medicaid have abated at least for the time being, and a more measured response to program reform seems possible. To be sure, the widely shared desire to forge a balanced budget will subject entitlement programs to intense scrutiny. But Medicaid has stopped devouring state and federal budgets at a growing clip. In early 1997 the Congressional Budget Office projected that federal Medicaid spending would rise by an average of 7.8 percent a year from 1997 to 2002, rather than the 9.7 percent it had estimated in mid-1996. The savings in federal outlays this recalculation generated surpassed what the Republican Medicaid proposals in 1995 and 1996 would have yielded.[39] Fueled in part by this development and also by the reelection of President Clinton, the country has shifted at least temporarily away from the politics of big Medicaid devolution—a sort of fire, ready, aim approach—to a more technical politics of calibration.

In a context that provides more time for reflection about the proper balance between the federal government and the states in providing health care to the needy, a wide range of options deserves attention. Space does not permit a comprehensive review of them here. Instead, three general points relevant to the Medicaid debate are discussed. First, the politics of calibration concerning federal-state responsibility for Medicaid has many sanguine features. Although lacking in drama, it can nonetheless yield significant movement to devolve more authority to the states. Second, gains in narrowing the gap between Medicaid promise and performance will only materialize if policymakers do what does not come naturally to them: focus on improving implementation. Nothing illustrates this point better than the incomplete efforts of Medicaid to provide benefits to children who are legally entitled to them. Third, devolution will pose the greatest risk if the federal government loses its capacity to keep score in the health care arena. Preservation of this capacity provides the foundation for a genuinely evaluative, as opposed to a dogmatic, approach to devolution.

Calibration Rather Than the Big Plunge

For years Medicaid has been stuck in the middle, getting little respect from either conservatives or liberals. The former brought their natural distaste of costly entitlement programs to their assessment of Medicaid. The latter saw the program as a Band-Aid on a wound that required surgery; they saw it as a feeble substitute for the real solution—that is, national health insurance for all Americans. In the context of the late 1990s, however, Medicaid appears in a softer, more favorable light. It has provided and could continue to provide a health care lifeline to millions of citizens during a time when the private sector is retreating from its role in providing health insurance. Moreover, the current Medicaid program embodies a model of cooperative federalism. In this model, neither the states nor the federal government plays senior partner. Instead, each wields substantial power over the program in a manner relatively devoid of intense conflict and impasse.[40]

Viewed from this vantage point, a calibrated approach to issues of Medicaid devolution becomes more appealing. This approach closely resembles the restrained devolution discussed in this volume by Tallon and Brown. But calibration does not automatically assume that devolution would imply cuts in funding, and it holds out the prospect that at least marginal centralization in some areas may be desirable.

Above all, a calibrated approach shines the spotlight on discrete questions about different aspects of the Medicaid program. Should states have more flexibility to determine eligibility for the program? Should they have more discretion to define the service package and the approach to quality assurance? Should they have greater freedom to choose providers and set payment rates for them? Should they have more discretion to determine the level and sources of state financing? Should states have more opportunity to shape their administrative systems and the data they report to the federal government? Careful assessment of each of these questions may well lead to a conclusion that devolution, in some instances, will improve the balance among access, quality, and cost in the provision of health care for the needy. But in other cases it may lead to the opposite conclusion—toward preference for the status quo or greater centralization of authority in the federal government.

The resolutions emanating from an NGA meeting in early 1997 reflect the politics of calibration. Rather than trumpeting their ability to take over Medicaid under a block grant, the governors announced that they "adamantly oppose[d] a cap on Federal Medicaid spending in any form." Rather than seeking sweeping discretion, the governors endorsed more modest steps toward devolution, including (1) giving states more authority to require the Medicaid-eligible to enroll in managed-care plans without first obtaining a federal waiver, and (2) repeal of the Boren provisions on provider payment.[41] The Balanced Budget Act of 1997 included both of these provisions and represented a triumph for the NGA.

Devising means to make the waiver process less cumbersome for states committed to managed care may well be a step in the right direction. State officials understandably resent the need to answer "ten questions phrased 650 different ways" when they approach HCFA for a waiver. Even when they got an audience with the White House concerning a waiver, state officials sensed that HCFA could block a favorable response. As a Medicaid director from one state put it, "HCFA knows, frankly, like any good bureaucrat knows, just the poisoned question to ask which ties you in knots because you can't explain it in two and a half minutes."[42]

It is also difficult to view the protracted and convoluted legal struggles over provider payment spawned by the Boren amendment without some sympathy for the states' desire to be freed from this provision. Perhaps outright repeal of Boren goes too far, but it makes considerable sense to develop and legitimate state institutions that can make decisions about provider payment that are substantially insulated from appeals to the court system.

Access for Children: Incomplete Implementation

The full benefits of the politics of calibration will not be achieved unless policymakers pay more attention to administration. The details of implementation strike most as dreary and dull, but they are critically important. Without adequate attention to implementation capacity and commitment, Medicaid policy risks becoming the triumph of dazzle over delivery—a symbolic exercise long on promise but short on performance.

In noting the tendency of policymakers to neglect and underestimate issues of administration, the point is not to portray the Medicaid program as a tale of implementation woe. To the contrary, the program has been remarkably successful in certain respects. Federal and state administrators, as well as many private sector agents, have often demonstrated ingenuity and acumen in providing insurance and service to Medicaid enrollees. They have established administrative systems that, on balance, work well. But this circumstance should not provide an excuse for policymakers to ignore the gap between policy promise and performance that greater sensitivity to implementation issues could help close. In no aspect of Medicaid management does the relevance of this point loom larger than in the provision of health insurance to needy children.

Eligibility: The Gap between Policy and Performance. In early 1997 Democratic senators Thomas Daschle and Edward M. Kennedy announced as one of their top legislative priorities measures to provide health insurance to an estimated 10 million children who lacked such coverage. The senators opted for different policy tools to accomplish that end. Daschle indicated that he favored an approach based on tax credits, while Kennedy proposed the use of vouchers.[43] In March 1997 Republican senator Orrin Hatch announced his support for Senator Kennedy's initiative, suggesting that his endorsement was proof that the Republican Party "does not hate [poor] children."[44] This growing bipartisan interest ultimately led to the passage of a new child health block grant in August 1997. The legislation committed the federal government to provide states with more than $20 billion in federal funds over a five-year period in order to reduce the number of low-income uninsured children. To be eligible for the new federal monies, states were not to reduce their current Medicaid eligibility levels for children. States had the choice of using the new matching funds to expand Medicaid or to develop other child health insurance programs. Debate persisted over the best vehicle for extending health care to the nation's uninsured children.[45]

Whatever the merits of the new law, one conspicuous feature of the debate leading to its passage stands out: partisans directed scant attention to eligibility mandates embedded in current Medicaid law and the implementation issues they pose. Failure to consider the Medicaid experience in this regard eroded the quality of the debate and increases the risk that the resulting policy will be long on promise and short on delivery. If implemented, existing Medicaid mandates would go a considerable distance toward providing health insurance coverage to children. As of early 1997 federal law required Medicaid coverage for all children under age six if their family income was below 133 percent of the federal poverty line. Children from ages six through thirteen were eligible if their family income fell below 100 percent of poverty. By 2002 Medicaid requires that all poor children under age nineteen be eligible for Medicaid.

The problem is, of course, that legislating mandates is one thing and getting them implemented is another. Estimates of the number of uninsured children entitled to Medicaid coverage but who fail to enroll were approximated at between 2.7 million and 2.9 million in 1994.[46] Nearly half of all uninsured children under age eleven were eligible for Medicaid in that year. Children entitled by law to Medicaid but not to cash assistance under AFDC or SSI were especially likely to fall through the cracks. In 1994 Medicaid administrators managed to enroll only 38 percent of eligible children under age eleven who did not receive cash assistance under these programs. This performance gap cannot be attributed to the failure of poor, conservative states to comply with federal mandates. If one examines estimates of uninsured children under age eleven who did not receive AFDC or SSI but were income-eligible for Medicaid between 1992 and 1995, liberal and wealthier northern states did not fare appreciably better than their southern counterparts. For example, from 23 to 37 percent of income-eligible, uninsured children not on AFDC or SSI from New York did not enroll in Medicaid; in Pennsylvania the range was from 24 to 41 percent. Two populous southern states had similar rates—from 24 to 37 percent in Florida and from 29 to 41 percent in Texas.[47]

The difficulties in getting eligible children enrolled for Medicaid springs from many sources. To a degree it reflects the stigma some people attach to applying for "welfare medicine." But the failure to enroll also emanates from the administrative strategies states use to review eligibility and disseminate information about Medicaid. Applicants for Medicaid must typically jump several hurdles. They often have to present documentation of their citizenship, residency, income (that is, copies of tax returns, verification of child support), assets (that is, deeds, fair market and book value of all owned vehicles, statements of current bank accounts), and expenses (that is, copies of canceled checks or receipts from child care providers). Failure by the applicant to furnish the required paperwork or meet other procedural requirements frequently leads to denial. For example, an analysis of Medicaid applications by non-cash-assisted individuals in three states—Georgia, Illinois, and Massachusetts—found that the overall denial rate ranged from roughly 35 to 50 percent of applicants. Over 60 percent of those rejected in Illinois and Massachusetts met that fate for procedural reasons; that is, applicants did not give welfare officials enough paper documentation or failed to show up for the eligibility interview. To some degree this may reflect belated awareness by applicants that they are not poor enough to be eligible. But it no doubt also stems from the procedural gauntlet they must run.[48] Since many needy individuals know that hospital emergency rooms are legally required to treat them without regard to their ability to pay, the hassle of applying for Medicaid may not seem worth the effort.

Nor do the agents responsible for implementing Medicaid typically adopt proactive strategies for enrolling those entitled to program benefits. Concerns about making eligibility errors of generosity and driving up overall program costs have inhibited the development and implementation of aggressive outreach programs. It is primarily when uninsured individuals need acute inpatient care in hospitals that enrollment efforts intensify. Many hospitals have established units to assist people in signing up for Medicaid. Considerable numbers of them have contracted with private firms to enroll Medicaid patients. Working as a kind of bounty hunter where they receive payment only for success in getting hospital patients enrolled in Medicaid, these firms identify people who are eligible for the program, assist in overturning previously denied Medicaid applications, and generally help individuals initiate and complete the application process.[49] The larger bills and higher payment rates that prompt hospitals to fight obstacles to Medicaid eligibility tend to be absent for providers offering more routine preventive and other ambulatory care.

Three factors threaten to widen the gap between the number of children legally entitled to Medicaid and those who actually sign up for the program: first, under current law the number of children entitled to Medicaid will continue to grow through 2002, when all poor children under age nineteen without insurance will be eligible. The enrollment task will therefore become more formidable.

Second, the welfare reform act of 1996 will reduce the number of individuals automatically deemed eligible for Medicaid by virtue of their enrollment in AFDC and SSI. The new law severs the link between the new cash assistance program for the needy (temporary assistance for needy families, or TANF) and Medicaid eligibility. It mandates that low-income families receive Medicaid if they meet the state's old AFDC income and related standards for enrollment, regardless of whether they qualify for cash benefits under TANF. Whereas in the past social service agencies had used a single application form to judge an applicant's eligibility for cash assistance and Medicaid, the new law allows states to use separate application forms for TANF and Medicaid. As a consequence, an even greater proportion of those children legally entitled to Medicaid benefits will fail to enroll unless states become more aggressive about outreach and make their eligibility processes more user friendly. The 1996 policy changes aimed at making it more difficult for children to qualify for SSI benefits may well pose similar challenges. Many of the children at risk of being ineligible for SSI benefits will nonetheless continue to qualify for Medicaid. But the change means that their families will have to go the additional mile of applying for Medicaid.[50]

Third, the emphasis in at least some states on reducing caseload in part by transforming the culture of eligibility offices may increase the number of Medicaid-eligible children who do not enroll. Focusing on applications for cash assistance, Lawrence Mead has observed that "The goal of reducing the caseload is now paramount, with economic gains for the recipients secondary."[51] The welfare reform act of 1996 embodies this perspective. While acknowledging the importance of a number of performance measures, it emphasizes "reducing the overall welfare caseload and, when a practicable method for calculating this information becomes available, diverting individuals from formally applying to the State program and receiving assistance."[52] In this regard, several states with welfare waivers have emphasized the diversion of formal applications. In Wisconsin, for example, intake workers used to process applications for assistance automatically to determine eligibility for AFDC benefits. Under the new approach, officials in that state encourage staffs to work with clients and discuss whether applying for benefits is desirable at all.[53] The emphasis on diversion applies most directly to cash assistance programs, but one cannot gainsay the potential spillover into eligibility determination processes for Medicaid.

Some state officials will no doubt view the delinking of Medicaid and TANF as a plus—an opportunity to remove the welfare stigma from Medicaid enrollees. They may well develop highly innovative strategies to facilitate enrollment. But for state policymakers who place a premium on cutting costs, phlegmatic outreach, an emphasis on diversion, and the maintenance of procedurally cumbersome eligibility processes may, in a sense, enable them to have their political cake and eat it too. Formal eligibility policies may appear generous while administrative processes dampen actual enrollments.

To the degree that federal policymakers pass mandates that the states will not or cannot implement, the symbolic aspects of Medicaid policy become more pivotal. This possibility adds a twist to the predictions of Fossett and Wiener in this volume. They expect that in the face of devolution the elderly and disabled may well be in a better political position to protect their benefits than poor women and children. It deserves note, however, that this dynamic may play out more fully in the implementation arena than in the legislative chambers of state capitols. Some states may respond to devolutionary pressures by keeping formal requirements covering children on the books but skimping on administrative capacity so severely that the gap between entitlement and enrollment widens.

The degree to which states succeed or fail in their enrollment practices possesses implications for the health of children. Recent research points to important gains from Medicaid's eligibility expansions in terms of improved use of preventive care and reduced mortality among infants and children; the expansions are estimated to have lowered infant mortality by 8.5 percent and child mortality by 5.1 percent. According to the study, this translated into a cost per life saved of roughly $1 million to $1.6 million, a lower figure than many other programs aimed at preventing death.[54] And these data neither take into account the benefits to children in the form of reduced morbidity nor apprehend the health gains that might well have been achieved had more children made it through the gates to Medicaid eligibility.

Other Problems with Eligibility. The Medicaid enrollment gap with respect to children is not, of course, an isolated example of the disparity between what federal law requires and what states actually do.[55] For example, as indicated earlier, many states have not implemented the requirement that Medicaid pay for Medicare premiums, deductibles, and copayments for all elderly individuals at or below 100 percent of poverty—the qualified Medicare beneficiaries (QMBs). The issue here may well be less one of state capacity than of commitment. States such as Maine, Massachusetts, Vermont, and Washington have signed up nearly all of those entitled to be QMBs. In contrast, an estimated 84 percent of those eligible for QMB coverage in California had not enrolled in the program as of 1993.[56]

Medicaid mandates designed to inhibit crowding out also point to the propensity of federal policymakers to pay inadequate attention to the implementation demands of enrollment. Crowding out refers to the process whereby private employers shirk the obligation to provide insurance to their workers because they know that their employees can secure Medicaid coverage.[57] Concerned about this issue, Congress approved provisions in 1990 that required state Medicaid programs to buy into private employer coverage when it was available to a Medicaid applicant. Federal law stipulated that states were to pay the employees' share of the costs for covering themselves and their families when the cost of these buy-ins would be less than the anticipated expenditure of enrollment in the regular Medicaid program. In addition, the federal government required the states to cover services generally available under the Medicaid program but not provided to needy workers by their private sector plans.

Although many working Medicaid enrollees should be covered by this provision, the staggering complexities of administering it have undercut its implementation. Medicaid applicants do not always disclose the availability of coverage from their employer. They do not know the specifics of these plans and their employers often drag their feet in providing this information. Questions persist as to whether ERISA exempts self-insured firms from any state requirement to submit insurance information about their employees to Medicaid officials. Even if administrators can fathom the private coverage that a Medicaid applicant has, they cannot always readily calculate the degree to which it would be cheaper to pay the private insurance costs of the employee, or to sign him or her up for the regular Medicaid program.[58] These and other factors make it hard for even the most committed states to comply with federal mandates concerning private employer coverage. And doing so clearly requires an investment in administrative capacity, a step many states seem reluctant to take in an era of downsizing.

Fix Implementation or Approve New Programs? In order to bolster state capacity to enroll a higher proportion of legally entitled children in Medicaid, the federal government could appropriately assume a leadership role in providing incentives and technical assistance. For example, federal officials could set the pace in developing and disseminating a new software system to link Medicaid with TANF eligibility processes.[59] The development and promulgation of information systems based on this software would be neither cheap nor a panacea, but such an initiative could well yield positive enrollment results. So, too, could state willingness to allow certain medical providers to enroll children "presumptively" in Medicaid. Under this approach, Medicaid would pay for certain health services while the child awaited the final eligibility determination. The Balanced Budget Act of 1997 gives states the option of establishing presumptive eligibility systems.

Ultimately, the most potent step to closing the gap between enrollment promise and performance would be to focus less on process and more on results—to assign the federal government a significant role in providing financial bonuses to states that signed up a higher proportion of needy citizens entitled to Medicaid (or penalties for those that did not). This would give states incentive to launch aggressive outreach programs and to streamline their eligibility processes. But political opposition to such a policy from key groups representing the states make it unlikely that such an approach could muster congressional approval. In early 1997, for instance, the NGA asserted that any federal strategies to reach out to families of children eligible for Medicaid but not receiving benefits should "be developed in conjunction with the states." In doing so, the governors stressed: "because the group of children currently eligible for Medicaid but not enrolled has proved difficult to accurately quantify and has been resistant to previous outreach efforts, the Governors would oppose tying receipt of Medicaid funds to achieving increased enrollment targets."[60]

Even if adopted, a payment-for-performance system targeted at Medicaid enrollments would not be simple to implement. As the governors suggest, devising and legitimating a sampling system that pinpoints the exact proportion of uninsured children eligible for Medicaid in a state would present HCFA administrators with significant methodological problems. Moreover, underperforming states threatened with loss of funding would resort to time-honored tactics in the American intergovernmental system; they would attempt to rally political allies in Congress, the executive branch, and the judiciary in an effort to derail the imposition of penalties. Despite these limitations, giving HCFA the authority to reward states with more positive enrollment records would at least improve the bargaining position of the federal government in dealing with the states on the enrollment of children entitled to Medicaid.

Although the more vigorous implementation of Medicaid mandates would go a long way toward ameliorating the nation's problem of uninsured children, its political appeal relative to other approaches is limited. The tendency of state governments to underinvest in administrative capacity, the limits to their commitment to aggressive implementation, and the ideological and other barriers to vigorous federal intervention undercuts the viability of the approach. So does the tendency of lawmakers to prefer the glamour of creating new policies to the unheralded drudgery of fixing the administrative machinery of current programs. In this regard, a complex redundant approach—one based on creating new programs such as the child health block grant of 1997—may well be the only feasible way to provide needy children with more health insurance at least over the next few years. Rather than enhance the Medicaid lifeline, policymakers may, in essence, throw several other lifelines out, none all that long or strong, but with the potential to do some good. Throwing a basket of programs at the problem may improve the health prospects of children in the aggregate. But it will also add to the fragmentation and transaction costs of an administrative system that is already complex and confusing for even the most diligent citizen. The proliferation of government programs in the United States in part reflects a national reluctance to pay careful attention to, repair the implementation of, and build on existing initiatives.

A Central Scorecard

Beyond issues of calibration and eligibility intake, the devolution debate over Medicaid will benefit from keeping a basic point in mind: whatever the degree of devolution preferred with respect to Medicaid eligibility, services, provider payment, and financing, the capacity to evaluate and learn from program experience depends on the federal government serving as the central scorekeeper. According to Robert Behn, one of the three big questions of public management is: "How can public managers measure the achievements of their agencies in ways that help to increase these achievements?"[61] The twist added by devolution to this big question is, of course, "whose performance measures, those of the states or the federal government?" Although the selection of these measures should be the subject of negotiation between the national government and the states; once decided, learning will be enhanced if federal officials take the lead in assuring the systematic collection of comparable data from the states. Individual states could, of course, also collect data of particular use to themselves. But the national government would establish the basic parsimonious requirements.[62]

As indicated earlier in this volume, some proponents of devolution chafe under federal information requirements and want states to have much greater latitude to determine the specific Medicaid information they collect and routinely report to the national government. While HCFA should guard against imposing needless information costs on the states, a strong case exists that the federal government should be assertive about its role as scorekeeper. States cannot be perfect laboratories of democracy in a way that satisfies the highest standards of social science research. But unless federal officials impose a reasonable degree of uniformity in determining what Medicaid data states report and how, prospects for fruitful comparisons that contribute to policy learning will be minimal. In the absence of such requirements, the temptation for states to game the numbers in order to portray their programs in a favorable light will grow. Without comparable information on an array of indicators, the tendency to pay too much attention to one measure (for example, reductions in caseload) may lead to substantial program distortions.

Two general types of data will be important for the federal government to assemble and disseminate: those related specifically to Medicaid and those dealing more broadly with the health care system and its outcomes. With respect to the former, the current Medicaid Management Information System (MMIS) provides useful data on the numbers enrolled in Medicaid by various categories (for example, children, the disabled, the elderly) and the general services they receive. This system feeds off Medicaid's fee-for-service approach whereby health care providers submit bills to Medicaid for services they deliver to specific enrollees. Since significant numbers of Medicaid recipients (especially the disabled and the elderly) will continue to receive care on a fee-for-service basis, the federal government should continue working with the states to preserve and enhance the validity and reliability of the data that this approach yields.

But, as noted earlier in this chapter, the emergence of capitated managed care necessitates that information systems move beyond this. In this regard, the federal government in partnership with state Medicaid officials and the private sector should encourage the development of electronic data systems that record patient encounters in managed-care settings. It also makes sense for the federal government to persist in its efforts to require state Medicaid programs to comply with a standardized health plan employer data and information set (known as HEDIS 2.5).[63] This data system calls for Medicaid's managed-care contractors to report information on specific indicators concerning the membership of these plans, utilization, quality, access, finances, and general management. The measures embedded in HEDIS 2.5 are far from perfect. Building the administrative capacity within managed-care firms and state governments to provide the data demanded by HEDIS and related systems will, as Fossett points out in this volume, be a formidable task. But without a measure of federal success in establishing this information beachhead for Medicaid, the long-term prospects for promoting policy learning and program accountability will plummet.

To ensure proper assessment of devolutionary initiatives under Medicaid, the federal government should also continue as the lead player in gathering and disseminating information related to the health care system and the health of the populace. The federal government enjoys a considerable advantage over the states in the capacity to perform this function well. Its statistical agencies achieve high standards for professional competence. For example, much of the understanding of the degree to which citizens with different incomes have health insurance comes from the Bureau of the Census. The National Center for Health Statistics gathers important data about such critical matters as access to the health care system, morbidity, and mortality. Preserving and enhancing the capacity of these statistical agencies should be a central priority of the federal government. The temptation, very much in evidence in recent sessions of Congress, to slash the budgets of these agencies and narrow the range of data they collect would poorly serve those who seek to understand the implications of devolution in the health care arena.

The preservation of federal statistical agencies and uniform Medicaid reporting requirements for the states could become the foundation for the construction of a health care report card for each state. The report cards would allow a state's policymakers to gauge whether they are gaining or losing ground in the struggle to advance health. Medicaid will be only one part of the system affecting access and health outcomes, but it will be a big part. If changes to Medicaid by state officials coincide with a decline in a state's grades on its health care report card (such as the number of uninsured within the state), it can signal the need to reappraise and possibly recalibrate Medicaid policy.

The Long View

The endorsement of a calibrated, implementation-focused approach to Medicaid with the federal government as central scorekeeper will, of course, hardly satisfy certain stakeholders. It will not, for example, please those who favor devolution principally as a means to reduce government's role in the economy and society. From this perspective, Medicaid devolution featuring a significant cut in federal financial support for the states mixed with the preservation, or even tightening, of ERISA constraints fills the bill. Proponents of this view, in essence, espouse what Robert Rich and William White have called opportunistic federalism. Under this approach, "tension between downsizing and decentralization is resolved in favor of downsizing, through selectively applying devolution to those situations in which it is likely to reduce government intervention, while reserving the right to preempt the states when federal control seems more favorable to the market."[64] Proponents of this approach anticipate great general benefits (for example, robust economic growth) for society as government plays a smaller role. But those who advance this option should at least acknowledge that for many needy citizens (probably a growing number), their prescription would be debilitating and in some instances lethal.

A calibrated approach to Medicaid will also fail to satisfy those who believe that it is a travesty that a country as wealthy as the United States does not, as virtually all other industrialized democracies do, provide health insurance to all of its citizens. They can appropriately charge that a calibrated approach will do little to ease the hard questions of rationing that will increasingly confront the Medicaid program even at current funding levels. Several forces seem destined to fuel these pressures. First, the retreat of the private sector from providing health insurance to low-skilled workers seems unlikely to abate in the foreseeable future. Second, the demand for Medicaid subsidies will increase as the number of elderly citizens grows both in absolute terms and as a proportion of the population. Third, advances in medical technology continue to elevate the quality of care possible but also tend to push up health care prices. Hence Medicaid officials will increasingly confront painful choices concerning how much to spend on the "best" treatments for enrollees. Their rationing decisions will not just involve "Hail-Mary" interventions such as bone marrow transplants for those in the terminal stages of cancer.[65] It will also center on expensive treatments that have a very high probability of improving health. For instance, several newly developed drugs appear to be quite effective in suppressing HIV, the virus that causes AIDS. But these drugs frequently cost as much as $10,000 to $15,000 per year per infected enrollee, a circumstance that prompts states to limit the numbers who receive a subsidy for this medicine.[66]

Dispiriting as these developments may seem, the political realities of the late 1990s make comprehensive reform unobtainable. As Tallon and Brown suggest in this volume, the best hope over the short term may well be to keep Medicaid from doing more poorly by the poor. Although Medicaid is a highly flawed lifeline, it has greatly reduced death, disease, disability, discomfort, and dissatisfaction for millions of Americans. Moreover, Medicaid could eventually serve as a building block for major reform. Sobered by the debacle of the Clinton health plan, advocates of comprehensive reform have come to see the states as key players in making reform politically tenable. Rather than attempt the politically perilous task of crafting a massive, detailed blueprint like the Clinton comprehensive health plan, reformers could propose a parsimonious plan that left key details to the states. Under this scenario, the national government would set certain basic requirements for the receipt of a significant federal subsidy, including a mandate that states make health insurance accessible to all of their citizens. In a spirit of genuine devolution, Congress would repeal those ERISA provisions that vitiate state governing capacity in the health care arena. In a manner similar to Medicaid, the national government would also accept great variation in state approaches on a broad range of policy and administrative issues.[67]

Whatever direction the United States pursues—a constant recalibration of the federal and state roles in the existing Medicaid program, major devolution with reduced federal funding, or movement toward a state-based approach to national health insurance—the twin challenges of state commitment and capacity will persist. Contemplation of state involvement should not be the fount of boosterism or pessimism. This volume has certainly called into question optimistic assumptions about the governing and fiscal capacity of the states, as well as their willpower to meet fully the challenges of providing health care to the needy. But the experience with Medicaid also cautions against becoming a Cassandra even with respect to the short suit of American government—implementation. Virtually all states have established administrative systems that perform certain Medicaid functions reasonably well; some states have been remarkably creative. To be sure, getting the implementation glass from one-half to three-quarters full will, as the chapters in this book suggest, be difficult. It will require policymakers and the citizenry to move beyond clichés and stereotypes about public programs and the scapegoating of public administrators. Hard as it will be to sensitize the political system to issues of state capacity and commitment in the health care arena, the stakes are too high not to try.

Notes

1. James Madison, Alexander Hamilton, and John Jay, *The Federalist Papers,* ed. Isaac Kromnick (London: Penguin Books, 1987), no. 39 (p. 259) and no. 46 (p. 298).

2. See Richard P. Nathan, "Federalism—The Great 'Composition,'" in Anthony King, ed., *The New American Political System,* 2d ed. (Washington: AEI Press, 1990), p. 246.

3. James Bryce, *The American Commonwealth,* vol. 1 (Macmillan, 1910), p. 324.

4. Morton Grodzins, "The Federal System," in *Goals for Americans: The Report of the President's Commission on National Goals* (Prentice-Hall, 1960), p. 265.

5. Frank J. Thompson, ed., *Revitalizing State and Local Public Service: Strengthening Performance, Accountability, and Citizen Confidence* (San Francisco: Jossey-Bass, 1993), p. 16; *Analytical Perspectives: Budget of the United States Government, Fiscal Year 1998* (Government Printing Office, 1997), pp. 193, 201.

6. See, for instance, Ann O'M. Bowman and Richard C. Kearney, *The Resurgence of the States* (Prentice-Hall, 1986); U.S. Advisory Commission on Intergovernmental

Relations, *The Question of State Government Capability* (Washington, A-98, 1985); and John D. Donahue, *Disunited States* (Basic Books, 1997), pp. 9–13.

7. R. Kent Weaver and Bert A. Rockman, eds., *Do Institutions Matter? Government Capabilities in the United States and Abroad* (Brookings, 1993), p. 6; for another effort to measure government performance, see Robert D. Putnam, *Making Democracy Work: Civic Traditions in Modern Italy* (Princeton University Press, 1993).

8. For a particularly forceful statement of this view, see Howard M. Leichter, "State Governments and Their Capacity for Health Care Reform," in Robert F. Rich and William D. White, eds., *Health Policy, Federalism, and the American States* (Washington: Urban Institute Press, 1996), pp. 151–79.

9. See Morris P. Fiorina, "Divided Government in the American States: A Byproduct of Legislative Professionalism?" *American Political Science Review*, vol. 88 (June 1994), pp. 304–16; Morris P. Fiorina, "Professionalism, Realignment and Representation," *American Political Science Review*, vol. 91 (March 1997), pp. 156–62; and Paul E. Peterson, *The Price of Federalism* (Brookings, 1995), pp. 101–06.

10. Jay Braatz and Robert D. Putnam, "Families, Communities, and Education in America: Exploring the Evidence" (Cambridge, Mass., unpublished paper, July 1996); see also Tom W. Rice and Alexander F. Sumberg, "Civic Culture and Government Performance in the American States," *Publius*, vol. 27 (Winter 1997), pp. 99–114.

11. Leichter, "State Governments," p. 156.

12. Robert S. Erikson, Gerald C. Wright, and John P. McIver, *Statehouse Democracy: Public Opinion and Policy in the American States* (New York: Cambridge University Press, 1993).

13. Other students of Medicaid have reached a similar conclusion. See, for instance, Charles J. Barrilleaux and Mark E. Miller, "The Political Economy of State Medicaid Policy," *American Political Science Review*, vol. 82 (December 1988), pp. 1089–1107; and Colleen M. Grogan, "Political-Economic Factors Influencing State Medicaid Policy," *Political Research Quarterly*, vol. 47 (September 1994), pp. 589–622.

14. See, for instance, Michael S. Sparer, *Medicaid and the Limits of State Health Reform* (Temple University Press, 1996).

15. Of course, in a genuinely global economy, firms can also use the threat that they will ship jobs overseas as a bargaining chip with the federal government. But the greater ease with which firms can move from one state to another makes state governments more vulnerable to this threat. One review of existing studies suggests that firms have become increasingly sensitive to state tax policies in deciding where to locate; see Donahue, *Disuninted States*, pp. 171–82.

16. National Commission on the State and Local Public Service, *Hard Truths/ Tough Choices: An Agenda for State and Local Reform* (Albany, NY: Nelson A. Rockefeller Institute of Government, 1993), p. 4.

17. See Thompson, *Revitalizing State and Local Public Service*, pp. 320–23.

18. Ibid., pp. 10–11. A nationwide survey completed in December 1995 found that 25 percent of the citizenry trusted the federal government to do the right thing "just about always" or "most of the time," while 35 percent expressed this view of their state government. The *Washington Post*/Kaiser Family Foundation/Harvard University Survey Project, "Why Don't Americans Trust the Government" (Kaiser Family Foundation Web Page [http://www.kff.org:80/kff/library.html?document_key=131&data_type_key=160] June 1997).

19. Bernard Wysocki Jr., "Some Companies Cut Costs Too Far, Suffer 'Corporate Anorexia,'" *Wall Street Journal,* July 5, 1995, p. A1. See also Donald F. Kettl and John J. DiIulio Jr., *Cutting Government* (Brookings, 1995); and Alex Markels and Matt Murray, "Call it Dumbsizing: Why Some Companies Regret Cost-Cutting," *Wall Street Journal,* May 14, 1996, p. A1. The downsizing of administrative agencies in response to government actions to eliminate certain programs (often called load shedding) is not the main concern in this context. The more serious problems for implementation capacity arise when policymakers continue or increase the number of programs but continue to cut the agency personnel to carry them out.

20. Michael Sparer and Lawrence D. Brown, "Between a Rock and a Hard Place: How Public Managers Manage Medicaid," in Frank J. Thompson, ed., *Revitalizing State and Local Public Service,* pp. 279–306.

21. For a general discussion of this point, see Donald F. Kettl, *Sharing Power: Public Governance and Private Markets* (Brookings, 1993).

22. Embry M. Howell, "Medicaid Managed Care Encounter Data: What, Why, and Where Next?" *Health Care Financing Review,* vol. 17 (Summer 1996), pp. 94–95.

23. General Accounting Office, *Employer-Based Health Plans: Issues, Trends, and Challenges Posed by ERISA,* GAO/HEHS-95-167 (July 1995), pp. 3, 11.

24. Richard Curtis, Mark Merlis, and Ann Page, "Finding Practical Solutions to 'Crowding Out,'" *Health Affairs,* vol. 16 (January/February 1997), pp. 201–03.

25. See, for instance, Marilyn W. Serafini, "Up against ERISA," *National Journal,* vol. 27 (February 11, 1995), pp. 349–52.

26. Jesselyn Alicia Brown, "ERISA and State Health Care Reform: Roadblock or Scapegoat?" *Yale Law & Policy Review,* vol. 13 (1995), p. 361.

27. Leichter, "State Governments," p. 154.

28. Richard F. Winters, "The Politics of Taxing and Spending," in Virginia Gray and Herbert Jacob, eds., *Politics in the American States: A Comparative Analysis,* 6th ed. (Washington: CQ Press, 1996), pp. 319–60; Bureau of the Census, *Statistical Abstract of the United States, 1997* (Government Printing Office, 1997), pp. 457, 477.

29. Communication from the National Conference of State Legislatures (June 19, 1996).

30. Richard P. Nathan and others, *Reagan and the States* (Princeton University Press, 1987), p. 19.

31. Constructing a valid and reliable index of state commitment to Medicaid presents formidable methodological problems. At a minimum, the index should incorporate such variables as a state's expenditures for Medicaid from its own revenue sources, an indicator of the ease with which greater numbers of people can become eligible for the program, a measure of the scope of services covered, and a proxy for state efforts on behalf of quality assurance.

32. Nelson A. Rockefeller Institute of Government and Brookings, Center for Public Management, *Devolution and Medicaid: A View from the States* (Washington: unpublished transcript, May 23–24, 1996), pp. 84–85.

33. Paul E. Peterson, Mark C. Rom, and Kenneth F. Scheve Jr., "State Welfare Policy: A Race to the Bottom?" Paper prepared for the National Association for Welfare Research and Statistics Annual Research Conference, Jackson, Wyoming, September 1995, p. 15.

34. See John Shannon, "Federalism's 'Invisible Regulator'—Interjurisdictional

Competition," in Daphne A. Kenyon and John Kincaid, eds., *Competition among States and Local Governments: Efficiency and Equity in American Federalism* (Washington: Urban Institute Press, 1991), pp. 117–26. See also Daphne A. Kenyon, "Health Care Reform and Competition among the States," in Rich and White, eds., *Health Policy, Federalism and the American States*, pp. 253–74.

35. In their analysis of the race to the bottom, Peterson and others control for such internal state factors as Democratic Party strength and state tax capacity. See Peterson and others, "State Welfare Policy."

36. Erikson and others, *Statehouse Democracy*, p. 12. To derive this estimate, the authors pooled data from each state for the period 1976-88. In 1996, 17 percent of respondents to the *New York Times*/CBS poll classified themselves as liberals, 32 percent as conservatives, and 43 percent as moderates. Over the last twenty-one years, the conservative advantage over liberals has ranged from eight points in 1976 to seventeen points in 1995. In all of the years except three (1976, 1977, 1991), the conservative margin over liberals has been at least ten points. Data furnished by Michael R. Kagay of the *New York Times* in personal correspondence (April 24, 1997).

37. Sparer, *Medicaid and the Limits of State Health Reform.*

38. See, for instance, John Holahan and others, *Cutting Medicaid Spending in Response to Budget Caps* (Washington: Urban Institute Press, 1995); and Howard Chernick and Andrew Reschovsky, *State Responses to Block Grants: Will the Social Safety Net Survive?* (Washington: Economic Policy Institute, 1996).

39. Robert Pear, "Medicaid Costs Are Seen Rising at Slower Rate," *New York Times*, January 17, 1997, p. A1.

40. Rich and White, eds., *Health Policy, Federalism, and the American States*, pp. 298–99.

41. National Governors' Association (Washington: unpublished report on the resolutions of the Winter 1997 meeting), pp. 17, 21–22.

42. Rockefeller Institute and the Brookings Center for Public Management, *Devolution and Medicaid*, pp. 33, 63.

43. Pear, "Medicaid Forecast," p. A1.

44. Robert Pear, "Hatch Joins Kennedy to Back a Health Program," *New York Times*, March 14, 1997, p. A24.

45. See Jane Koppelman, "Crafting a Children's Health Insurance Plan: Design and Implementation Issues," *National Health Policy Forum Issue Brief No. 701* (Washington: George Washington University, 1997); Andy Schneider, "Reducing the Number of Uninsured Children: Building on Medicaid Coverage is a Better Approach Than Creating A New Block Grant to the States" (Washington: Center on Budget and Policy Priorities, 1997); Alan Weil, "The New Children's Health Insurance: Should States Expand Medicaid?" (Washington: Urban Institute, 1997).

46. The higher estimate comes from the General Accounting Office, *Health Insurance for Children: Private Insurance Coverage Continues to Deteriorate*, GAO/HEHS-96-129 (June 1996), p. 3; the lower estimate is from Laura Summer, Sharon Parrott, and Cindy Mann, "Millions of Uninsured and Underinsured Children are Eligible for Medicaid" (Washington: Center on Budget and Policy Priorities, 1997), p. 2.

47. Summer and others, "Millions of Uninsured and Underinsured Children," p. 3.

48. General Accounting Office, *Health Care Reform: Potential Difficulties in Determining Eligibility for Low-Income People*, GAO/HEHS-94-176 (July 1994).

49. Ibid.

50. Jane Koppelman, "Impact of the New Welfare Law on Medicaid," *National Health Policy Forum Issue Brief No. 697* (Washington: George Washington University, 1997).

51. Lawrence M. Mead, "Welfare Policy: The Administrative Frontier," *Journal of Policy Analysis and Management*, vol. 15 (Fall 1996), p. 590.

52. *Personal Responsibility and Work Opportunity Reconciliation Act of 1996*, Public Law 104-193, 104 Cong. 2 sess. (August 22, 1996), 110 Stat. 2105.

53. General Accounting Office, *Welfare Waivers Implementation: States Work to Change Welfare Culture, Community Involvement, and Service Delivery*, GAO/HEHS-96-105 (July 1996), p. 24.

54. David M. Cutler and Jonathan Gruber, "Medicaid and Private Insurance: Evidence and Implications," *Health Affairs*, vol. 16 (January/February 1997), p. 199.

55. For an overview, see Frank J. Thompson, "The Evolving Challenge of Health Policy Implementation," in Theodor J. Litman and Leonard S. Robins, eds., *Health Politics and Policy*, 3d ed. (Delmar, N.Y.: Delmar Publishers, 1997), pp. 155–75.

56. Amanda H. McCloskey, Danielle Holahan, Normandy Brangan, and Evelyn Yee, *Reforming the Health Care System: State Profiles 1996* (Washington: American Association of Retired Persons, 1996), p. 248. See also Susan L. Ettner, "Medicaid Participation among the Eligible Elderly," *Journal of Policy Analysis and Management*, vol. 16 (Spring 1997), pp. 237–55.

57. Although analysts tend to agree that some crowding out has occurred, they also concur that the phenomenon cannot adequately explain the growing proportion of workers who lack health insurance. For instance, John Holahan concludes: "For the most part, during the late 1980s and 1990s, Medicaid extended coverage to persons who otherwise would be uninsured." John Holahan, "Crowding Out: How Big a Problem?" *Health Affairs*, vol. 16 [January/February 1997], p. 204. Various studies suggest that from 10 to 20 percent of the decrease in employment-based insurance can be linked to Medicaid expansions. General Accounting Office, *Employment-Based Health Insurance: Costs Increase and Family Coverage Decreases*, GAO/HEHS-97-35 (February 1997), p. 23.

58. Curtis and others, "Finding Practical Solutions to 'Crowding Out.'"

59. Koppelman, "Impact of the New Welfare Law," p. 8.

60. National Governors' Association, unpublished report, pp. 21–22.

61. Robert D. Behn, "The Big Questions of Public Management," *Public Administration Review*, vol. 55 (July/August 1995), p. 315.

62. More generally, Paul Starr calls for government policy to impose common data dictionaries and standards for electronic interchange to improve the availability and quality of information in the health sector. "Smart Technology, Stunted Policy: Developing Health Information Networks," *Health Affairs*, vol. 16 (May/June 1997), pp. 91–105.

63. *Medicaid HEDIS* (Washington: National Committee for Quality Assurance, 1995).

64. Rich and White, eds., *Health Policy, Federalism and the American States*, p. 298.

65. Rockefeller Institute and the Brookings Center for Public Management, *Devolution and Medicaid*, p. 472.

66. Robert Pear, "Expense Means Many Can't Get Drugs for AIDS," *New York Times*, February 16, 1997, p. A1. In the spring of 1997 the Clinton administration began to explore ways to use Medicaid waiver authority to expand access to these drugs among low-income individuals with HIV. See Robert Pear, "Medicaid May Be Extended to Early Treatment of AIDS," *New York Times*, June 1, 1997, p. A20.

67. See Theodore Marmor, Jerry Mashaw, and Jonathan Oberlander, "National Health Reform: Where Do We Go From Here?" in Rich and White, eds., *Health Policy, Federalism, and the American States*, pp. 277–91.

Contributors

Donald J. Boyd
Center for the Study of the States
The Nelson A. Rockefeller Institute
  of Government

Lawrence D. Brown
School of Public Health
Columbia University

John J. DiIulio Jr.
The Brookings Institution and
  Princeton University

James W. Fossett
Department of Public Administration
  and Policy
Nelson A. Rockefeller College of
  Public Affairs and Policy
University at Albany, State University
  of New York

Richard P. Nathan
The Nelson A. Rockefeller Institute
  of Government

Michael S. Sparer
Division of Health Policy and
  Management
Columbia University School of
  Public Health

James R. Tallon Jr.
United Hospital Fund

Frank J. Thompson
Graduate School of Public Affairs
Nelson A. Rockefeller College of
  Public Affairs and Policy
University at Albany, State University
  of New York

Joshua M. Wiener
The Urban Institute

Conference Participants
May 23–24, 1996

Joyce Allen
State of Wisconsin

Peggy Bartels
State of Wisconsin

Pris Boroniec
State of Wisconsin

Representative Francis Bradley
State of Minnesota

Ken Cameron
State of Washington

Richard Cody
State of New York

Doug Cook
State of Florida

Gary Crayton
State of Florida

Jeff Harris
National Governors' Association

Michael Hanson
State of Florida

W. David Helms
Alpha Center

Jane Horvath
National Academy for State Health Policy

Peter Klemperer
*New York City Health and Hospital
   Corporation*

Kala Ladenheim
Intergovernmental Health Policy Project

Michael Murphy
State of Alabama

Karen Peed
State of Minnesota

Rush Russell
Robert Wood Johnson Foundation

Karen Schimke
State of New York

John Walker
State of Michigan

Alan Weil
State of Colorado

Index